THROMBOSIS AND CARDIOVASCULAR DISEASES

Recent Volumes in this Series

Volume 159
OXYGEN TRANSPORT TO TISSUE–IV
Edited by Haim I. Bicher and Duane F. Bruley

Volume 160
PORPHYRIN PHOTOSENSITIZATION
Edited by David Kessel and Thomas J. Dougherty

Volume 161
MYOCARDIAL INJURY
Edited by John J. Spitzer

Volume 162
HOST DEFENSES TO INTRACELLULAR PATHOGENS
Edited by Toby K. Eisenstein, Paul Actor, and Herman Friedman

Volume 163
FOLYL AND ANTIFOLYL POLYGLUTAMATES
Edited by I. David Goldman, Joseph R. Bertino, and Bruce A. Chabner

Volume 164
THROMBOSIS AND CARDIOVASCULAR DISEASES
Edited by Antonio Strano

Volume 165
PURINE METABOLISM IN MAN–IV
Edited by Chris H. M. M. De Bruyn, H. Anne Simmonds, and Mathias M. Müller

Volume 166
BIOLOGICAL RESPONSE MODIFIERS IN HUMAN ONCOLOGY AND IMMUNOLOGY
Edited by Thomas Klein, Steven Specter, Herman Friedman, and Andor Szentivanyi

Volume 167
PROTEASES: Potential Role in Health and Disease
Edited by Walter H. Hörl and August Heidland

A Continuation Order Plan is available for this series. A continuation order will bring delivery of each new volume immediately upon publication. Volumes are billed only upon actual shipment. For further information please contact the publisher.

THROMBOSIS AND CARDIOVASCULAR DISEASES

Edited by

Antonio Strano

Institute of Clinical Medicine and Medical Therapy
University of Palermo
Palermo, Italy

PLENUM PRESS • NEW YORK AND LONDON

Library of Congress Cataloging in Publication Data

Main entry under title:

Thrombosis and cardiovascular diseases

(Advances in experimental medicine and biology; v. 164)
Proceedings of the second European Symposium held Dec. 5-8, 1980 in Palermo, Italy.
Includes bibliographical references and index.
1. Thrombosis—Congresses. 2. Thrombosis—Complications and sequelae—Congresses. I. Strano, Antonio. II. Series. [DNLM: 1. Blood coagulation disorders—Complications—Congresses. 2. Blood platelet disorders—Complications—congresses. 3. Vascular diseases—Etiology—Congresses. 4. Fibrinolysis—Congresses. W1 AD559 v. 164 / WG 500 A244 1980]
RC694.3.T4584 1984 616.1'35 82-24579

DOI 10.1007/978-1-4684-8616-2

Proceedings of the Second European Symposium
held December 5-8, 1980, in Palermo, Italy

A Division of Plenum Publishing Corporation
233 Spring Street, New York, N.Y. 10013

PREFACE

Four years ago when the first European Symposium on the relationship between alterations of blood clotting mechanisms and atherosclerosis was organized, we asked ourselves which would be the best way to obtain both scientific and practical contributions.

We have been interested in cardiovascular diseases for several years now and have therefore focused our attention on the "container" (i.e. the blood vessel) rather than on the "contents" (i.e. the various components of blood) as considered only from a haemodynamic point of view.

In recent years correlations were found between alterations of vascular wall and alteration of coagulative, fibrinolytic, and platelet factors as well as of haemorheological phenomena in the thrombogenic evolution of atherosclerotic lesions.

A close cooperation between cardiologists and workers interested in atherosclerosis and thrombosis is therefore necessary. We think that the most appropriate approach to the various problems concerning correlations between thrombogenic and atherosclerotic lesions is co-operation between experts in these different fields of research.

We thus decided to organize the 2nd Symposium taking into account the great progress achieved in this field during the past few years, and hope that discussions on diagnostic and therapeutical perspectives will yield useful elements both for the cardiologist and for the cardiologist and for the general practitioner.

The invalidating consequences of thrombotic pathology may thus be treated and cardiovascular diseases - still ranging first in morbidity and mortality statistics of economically developed countries - may be prevented; for this reason the European Society of Cardiology has created a work group on Thrombosis and Platelets that will meet for the first time during this Symposium in Palermo.

Antonio Strano
Symposium Chairman

CONTENTS

THROMBOSIS IN CORONARY HEART DISEASE:
AN ASSESSMENT OF THE PRESENT STATE

Working Group of the European Society of Cardiology

COAGULATION AND VASCULAR DISEASES

VASCULAR COMPLICATIONS OF DIABETES MELLITUS

PLATELET FUNCTION AND VASCULAR DISEASES

PART 1

THROMBOSIS IN CORONARY HEART DISEASE: AN ASSESSMENT OF THE PRESENT STATE

HAEMOSTATIC FUNCTION AND ISCHAEMIC HEART DISEASE

T.W. Meade

MRC Epidemiology and Medical Care Unit
Northwick Park Hospital
Harrow, HA1 3UJ, England

The Northwick Park Heart Study (NPHS) (Meade and North, 1977; Meade et al., 1980) is a prospective study of haemostatic function in the pathogenesis of ischaemic heart disease (IHD). It is based on the traditional application of epidemiology - that is, the comparison of groups to draw general inferences about causation and pathogenesis.

There are two main reasons for prospective rather than case-control or cross-sectional studies of IHD when the results of blood tests (as opposed to personal or medical histories) are involved. One is that a myocardial infarct may have long-term effects on many biochemical or haematological characteristics (Meade, 1981). In these circumstances, data collected after the event make it impossible to distinguish cause and consequence. The second is that a high proportion of all first major IHD episodes manifest themselves as sudden death. Cross-sectional studies cannot contribute to the study of this major component of the syndrome.

The early prospective results of NPHS, based on 1510 men aged 40-64 at recruitment, show that those who later died of cardiovascular disease had significantly higher entry values of factor VII_C^* and VIII_C^*, fibrinogen and cholesterol than those who survived. The figure gives the numbers of deaths in the low, middle and high thirds of the distributions of the four variables. The range of factor VII_C values, for example, has been subdivided so that there are equal

---

*The subscript $_C$ is used here to denote factor VII or VIII measured by a biological or clotting assay. No subscript is used when a clotting factor is referred to in general terms and without specifying a method of measurement.

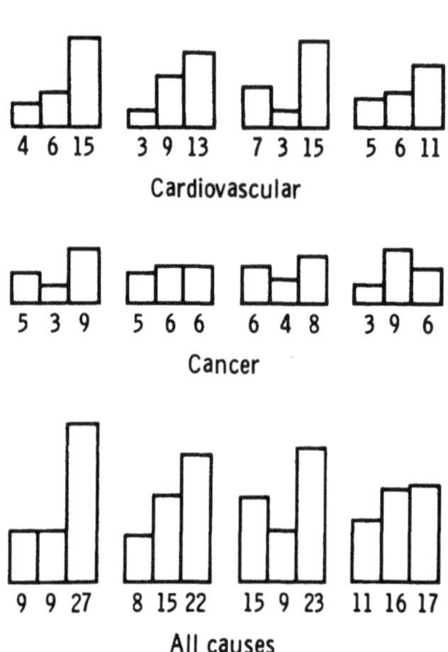

Figure. Numbers of deaths by low (L), middle (M) and high (H) thirds of distributions of the variables specified. NPHS men.

numbers of men - about 500 - in each third. If there were no association between factor VII_C and cardiovascular death there would be equal numbers of deaths in each third. In fact there is a steady rise. About 60% of the cardiovascular deaths occurred in the high third of the factor VII_C distribution. There are similar patterns for factor VIII_C and cholesterol. Though highly significant, the trend for fibrinogen is not entirely consistent - there is some reason for believing this is the result of small numbers. There was a marked tendency for those who died of cardiovascular disease to have had high levels of two, or all three, of the clotting factors in question (Meade et al., 1980). There is no firm evidence of any association between clotting factor levels at recruitment and death from cancer. In other words, the associations seem to be specific for cardiovascular disease.

The increasingly important question is what interpretation to put on the prospective findings. They are compatible with the idea of a hypercoagulable state which contributes to the causation of IHD. It is worth bearing in mind that the coagulation system, in producing thrombin, may influence platelet behaviour as well as fibrin formation. But the high clotting factor levels associated with later cardiovascular death might simply be a secondary response to vessel wall damage or atheroma. Factor VIII_C and fibrinogen are acute phase proteins which may rise in response to many stimuli of a non-specific nature. They may presumably do the same in response to chronic stimuli. Factor VII_C, on the other hand, falls in response to acute stimuli (Brozović, 1977; Meade, 1981) and possibly chronic ones as well. So it seems unlikely, from the outset, that the association between factor VII_C and cardiovascular death (see Figure) is to be explained in terms of the response of factor VII_C to atheroma.

One approach to the biological significance of the NPHS prospective data is to see whether the general epidemiology of the three clotting factors in question is consistent with the hypothesis that they are of causal significance in IHD. Table I suggests that it is so. (The Table summarizes the direction but not the magnitude of the effects. For example, the effect of alcohol on factor VII_C, while significant, is small. The effect of the ethnic group on factor VIII_C is very large.) Increasing age, white ethnic group, blood group other than O, cigarette smoking, obesity, oral contraceptive use and diabetes all apparently lead to an increase in one or more of the three clotting factors. Moderate alcohol intake and a vegetarian diet, both associated with some protection against IHD (Kozarevic et al., 1980; Phillips et al., 1978), appreciably lower fibrinogen and factor VII_C respectively. It can be argued that these are no more than comparisons of situations characterized by different degrees of vessel wall disease and that they do not, therefore, really provide evidence on the causal significance of the high clotting factor levels in the prospective results. However, if the high levels of all three factors were simply due to vessel wall disease the general epidemiology of the three individual clotting factors should be very similar. In fact, it is clear that the characteristics of each on its own are rather different. Table II illustrates this point. Smoking appears to raise fibrinogen, has no effect on factor VII_C and lowers factor VIII_C. The factor VIII effect (also described (Schwartz et al., 1980) in baboons) is particularly interesting. Smokers probably have more atheroma than non-smokers. If the high factor VIII_C levels associated with cardiovascular death (Figure) were merely a response to atheroma, then smokers should have higher, not lower, factor VIII_C levels than non-smokers. It should be noted that the smoking/factor VIII_C effect is not incompatible with a causal role for factor VIII_C in IHD. Other features determine the factor VIII_C level, in particular ABO blood group. Those of groups other than O have higher factor VIII_C levels (Meade et al., 1978) and an increased risk of IHD (Medalie et al., 1971) by comparison with those of group O.

There are thus several respects in which the general epidemiology of the clotting factors under discussion does not really support

Table I. General epidemiological characteristics of factors VII_C and VIII_C and of fibrinogen.

		VII_C	VIII_C	Fibrinogen
Age	Young → Old	+	+	+
Ethnic group	White → or → Black	+	–	0
Blood group	0 → or → (A+B+AB)	0	+	0
Cigarette smoking	None → Heavy	0	–	+
Alcohol consumption	None → Heavy	+	0	–
Obesity	Non-obese → Obese	+	(?+)	+
Oral contraceptives	Non-users → Users	+	0	+
Vegetarianism	Vegetarian → Non-vegetarian	–	0	0
Diabetes	Non-diabetic → Diabetic	+	0	+

Signs show direction of change according to the progression indicated by the arrow, e.g. + for effect of age indicates a rise with advancing age.

+ signifies rise
– " fall
0 " no effect

Original NPHS and related publications on which the Table is based are given in the list of references.

Table II. Effects of smoking on factors VII_C and VIII_C and fibrinogen in NPHS men.

	Smokers	Non-smokers	P
Factor VII_C, %	106.7	107.0	NS
Factor VIII_C, %	79.9	83.0	< 0.02
Fibrinogen, g./l.	3.03	2.81	< 0.001

NS: Not significant.
Results adjusted to age 40.

the idea that the high levels associated with cardiovascular death are simply a reflection of vessel wall disease.

The epidemiological points can be considered alongside theoretical and experimental evidence, particularly on factor VII.

Unlike the other clotting factors, factor VII circulates in an active or semi-active form. This is certainly true of bovine factor VII (Esnouf, 1977) and probably of human as well. It is crucial in initiating the very rapid coagulation characteristic of activation through the extrinsic pathway. This pathway is poorly covered by antithrombin activity (Broze and Majerus, 1980). Quite a small excess of factor VII could have increasingly marked effects at later stages in the coagulation system (Esnouf and Macfarlane, 1968). Indeed, the extent to which factor VII levels can vary without a high chance of a major thrombosis is likely, at least on theoretical grounds, to be quite small. A relatively recent development is recognition that factor VII may activate factor X *via* factor IX (Zur and Nemerson, 1980). This gives added interest to the possible role of factor VIII, which regulates the activation of factor IX. The implication is that high levels of both factors VII and VIII would be particularly likely to pre-dispose to thrombosis - a hypothesis for which NPHS now provides quite strong support.

The inclusion of activated factors in concentrates used in haemophilia B have led to diffuse intravascular coagulation (Hirsh, 1977). This is a rather extreme situation, but it confirms what is to be expected theoretically. Factor VII deficient beagles seem to be protected to a large extent against the thrombogenic influence of *E. coli* toxin (Garner and Evensen, 1974). And we should not forget the light that may be shed on pathogenetic mechanisms by the experience of the anticoagulant trials, reinforced as these now are by the results of the Dutch Sixty Plus trial (Sixty Plus Reinfarction Study Research Group, 1980). Taken as a whole, these trials add to the evidence that the coagulation system is involved in the pathogenesis of IHD. Finally, substantial reductions in factors VII_C, VIII_C and X_C and an increase in fibrinolytic activity followed the dietary treatment of hyperlipidaemia (Elkeles et al., 1980). Thus, dietary modifications aimed at lessening the risk of IHD may exert their effects through the haemostatic system as well as through changes in lipid metabolism.

The questions about causality raised by NPHS cannot be fully answered by epidemiological techniques alone. But the evidence so far, complemented by clinical and laboratory findings, is compatible with the idea that a "hypercoagulable state" is one determinant of clinically manifest IHD.

REFERENCES

Broze, G.J. & Majeurs, P.W. (1980) Purification and properties of human coagulation factor VII. Journal of Biological Chemistry 255:1242-7.

Brozović, M. (1977) Physiological mechanisms in coagulation and fibrinolysis. Br. Med. Bull. 33:231-8.

Elkeles, R.S., Chakrabarti, R., Vickers, M., Stirling, Y. and Meade, T.W. (1980) Effect of treatment of hyperlipidaemia on haemostatic variables. Br. Med. J. 281:973-4.

Esnouf, M.P. & Macfarlane, R.G. (1968) Enzymology and the blood clotting mechanism. In: Advances in Enzymology and related areas of molecular biology. Ed. Nord, F.F. Interscience Publishers, New York.

Esnouf, M.P. (1977) Biochemistry of blood coagulation. Br. Med. Bull. 33:213-8.

Fuller, J.H., Keen, H., Jarret, R.J., Omer, T., Meade, T.W., Chakrabarti, R., North, W.R.S. & Stirling, Y. (1979) Haemostatic variables associated with diabetes and its complications. Br. Med. J. 2:964-6.

Garner, R. & Evensen, S.A. (1974) Endotoxin-induced intravascular coagulation and shock in dogs: the role of factor VII. Br. J. Haematol. 27:655-68.

Haines, A.P., Chakrabarti, R., Fischer, D., Meade, T.W., North, W.R.S. & Stirling, Y. (1980) Haemostatic variables in vegetarians and non-vegetarians. Thromb. Res. 19:139-48.

Hirsh, J. (1977) Hypercoagulability. Seminars in Haematology 14:409-25.

Kozararević, D.J., McGee, D., Vojvodic, N., Racic, Z., Dawber, T., Gordon, T., & Zukel, W. (1980) Frequency of alcohol consumption and morbidity and mortality. Lancet 1:613-6.

Meade, T.W. (1981) The epidemiology of atheroma and thrombosis. In: Haemostasis and Thrombosis, ed. Bloom, A.L. & Thomas, D.P. Published by Churchill Livingstone, Edinburgh. In press.

Meade, T.W., Brozović, M., Chakrabarti, R., Howarth, D.J., North, W.R.S., & Stirling, Y. (1976) An epidemiological study of the haemostatic and other effects of oral contraceptives. Br. J.

Haematol. 34:353-64.
Meade, T.W., Chakrabarti, R., Haines, A.P., Howarth, D.J., North, W.R.S., & Stirling, Y. (1977) Haemostatic, lipid, and blood-pressure profiles of women on oral contraceptives containing 50 µg. or 30 µg. oestrogen. Lancet 2:948-51.
Meade, T.W. & North, W.R.S. (1977) Population-based distributions of haemostatic variables. Br. Med. Bull. 33:283-88.
Meade, T.W., Brozović, M., Chakrabarti, R., Haines, A.P., North, W.R.S. & Stirling, Y. (1978) Ethnic group comparisons of variables associated with ischaemic heart disease. Br. Heart J. 40:789-95.
Meade, T.W., Chakrabarti, R., Haines, A.P., North, W.R.S. & Stirling, Y. (1979) Characteristics affecting fibrinolytic activity and plasma fibrinogen concentrations. Br. Med. J. 1:153-6.
Meade, T.W., North, W.R.S., Chakrabarti, R., Stirling, Y., Haines, A.P. & Thompson, S.G. (1980) Haemostatic function and cardiovascular death: early results of a prospective study. Lancet. 1:1050-54.
Medalie, J.H., Levene, C., Papier, C., Goldbourt, U., Dreyfuss, F. & Oron, D. (1971) Blood groups, myocardial infarction and angina pectoris among 10,000 adult males. New Engl. J. of Med. 285:1348-53.
Phillips, R.L., Lemon, F.R., Beeson, W.L. & Kuzma, J.W. (1978) Coronary heart disease mortality among Seventh Day Adventists with suffering dietary habits; a preliminary report. Am. J. Clin. Nutr. 31:(supplement) S191-4.
Schwartz, C.J., McGill, H. & Rogers, W.R. (1980) Smoking and cardiovascular diseases. In: Banbury Report 3: A Safe Cigarette? Cold Spring Harbour Laboratory, 81-91.
Sixty Plus Reinfarction Study Research Group. (1980) A double-blind trial to assess long-term oral anticoagulant therapy in elderly patients after myocardial infarction. Lancet 2: 989-94.
Zur, M. & Nemerson, Y. (1980) Kinetics of factor IX activation via the extrinsic pathway. Journal of Biological Chemistry 255:5703-5.

PATHOPHYSIOLOGY OF ARTERIAL THROMBOSIS

E.F. Lüscher

Theodor Kocher Institute
University of Berne
Freie Strasse, 1
Berne, Switzerland

It is today an established fact that myocardial infarction in most cases is due to the obstruction by thrombi of the coronary vessels (5, 15, 2 as well as 3 for further references). Thus Bulkley and Hutchins (5) find, in 88% of all post-mortem examinations, in patients with aterosclerotic coronary artery disease, evidence for the existence of thrombi. Thus, arterial thrombosis is a major contributing factor to myocardial infarction and its pathophysiology therefore deserves every attention. Arterial thrombi as a rule start from a vascular lesion, most often from ruptured atheromas and have been shown to progress from a primary deposite of blood platelets. Thus, arterial thrombosis in many respects appears as the pathological deviation from a physiological process, i.e. the formation of a hemostatic plug. It appears appropriate to deal first with the mechanisms which are involved in the production of a platelet aggregate, which by its self, or by virtue of its procoagulant properties and subsequent fibrin formation, is capable of occluding a blood vessel.

A. Blood platelets

1. The circulating platelet has a discoid shape; on electron microscopical examination, a wealth of subcellular structures becomes discernible, among them 2 prominent types of storage organelles, the dense bodies (DB) and the α granules (for review cf. 14). Although devoid of a nucleus and hence barely capable of protein synthesis, platelets nonetheless possess a well developed energy metabolism, which forms the basis of their manifold activities. Considerable progress has been made in recent year in the characterization of essential membrane costituents, which may act as receptors or substrates in platelet activation, as well as in their interaction with

other cells and tissues and among themselves (for review cf.17).

2. Platelet adhesion. Platelets adhere almost instantaneously to sites of vascular injury, whereby a high molecular weight plasma glycoprotein, von Willebrand factor (vWF, which forms part of the factor VIII complex) is required. vWF combines with a receptor on the platelet surface, glycoprotein Ib (GPIb), thus forming a link to subendothelial structures (2).

3. Activated platelets. A remarkable variety of agents is capable of transforming the resting platelet into activated forms. Depending on the nature and the concentration of the inducer, at least 4 easily discernible steps can be distinguished.
These are:

- "Rapid shape change", i.e. the transformation, within 20 sec of the discoid platelet to a "spiny sphere", i.e. a spherical structure with long, filiform protrustions (10).
- Aggregation (which depends on the presence of external Ca^{2+} ions).
- The release reaction, consisting of the specific and rapid release of materials from storage organelles. In human platelets the dense bodies release essentially ADP, ATP, serotonin, small amounts of adrenaline and Ca^{2+} ions, whereas substances of higher molecular weight originate from the α granules. Among them are β-thromboglobulin (βTG), two heparin-binding materials (platelet factor 4 and a low affinity heparin-binding factor, which is structurally related to βTG), fibrinogen, thrombospondin, and mitogenic factor(s) (16).
- The active contraction of the primarily loose aggregate, corresponding in vivo to the consolidation of the hemostatic plug and responsible for making intravascular thrombi capable of withstanding the eroding forces of the blood stream.

4. The mechanism of platelet activation

a. Activating agents. An astonishing variety of agents is capable of bringing about platelet activation. Among them are:

- Several proteolytic enzymes, in particular thrombin.
- High molecular weight substances, all of them characterized by a repetitive structure: Collagen, polymerizing (but not polymerized) fibrin, antigen-antibody complexes involving IgG and aggregated IgG.
- Lower molecular weight agents such as ADP, serotonin, vasopressin and adrenaline. It should be noted that some of them are in turn released from fully activated platelets, thus giving rise to a positive feedback mechanism. It is noteworthy, though, that e.g. ADP will induce aggregation followed by release only in suspension media with a low Ca^{2+} concentration. Thus, it appears as if under these circumstances it is not ADP per se, but rather the cell-cell contact which acts as an inducer of the release reaction. At physiological Ca^{2+}-concentrations, ADP is unable to trigger release, although aggregates are formed. ADP-induced aggregation depends

on the presence of external fibrinogen, which is bound to a receptor which becomes available only upon stimulation of the platelets (11).

- Prostaglandins, thromboxanes and platelet activating factor (PAF) are products of the lipid metabolism. Thromboxane A_2 (TXA_2) is a most powerful, though short-lived stimulator of aggregation and release. Whereas PGE_2 also activates platelets, other products of the PG series, such as PGD_2 and E_1 are inhibitors of platelet activities. PAF in minute amounts induces activation of rabbit platelets. Human platelets are also capable of synthesizing this material, which is also produced by stimulated leukocytes; however they are considerably less sensitive to it (7).

b. Sequence of intracellular events leading to platelet activation.

Most of the listed inducers of platelet activation are unable to enter the cell. It must be assumed, therefore, that they interact with structures localized on the platelet surface, which either are substrates (for proteases, in particular thrombin) or receptors (cf.17). In every case, the sequence of events which follows primary stimulation, is identical, suggesting a common pathway of reactions which are set in motion by a membrane-localized mechanism. Evidence has been accumulating that it is the intracellular mobilization of Ca^{2+} ions which is decisive. Thus, shape change, is linked to the release, from a membrane-bound form, of Ca^{2+}ions (4), and ionophores which allow the passage of Ca^{2+} through membranes, are perfect inducers of platelet activity (12). Thus, there is good reason for the assumption that the signal created by the plasma membrane in response to stimulation says: "Release Ca^{2+}ions". This intracellular release (which should not be confused with Ca^{2+} release to the outside from DB) probably occurs in several steps, which depend upon the intensity of the stimulus: First from a membrane-bound form, then from the "dense tubular system" (DTS), the platelet equivalent of the sarcoplasmic reticulum of muscle, and perhaps, although with a certain delay, also from mitochondria. Lastly, the plasma membrane of stimulated platelets becomes permeable for Ca^{2+}ions (13).

The rise in cytoplasmatic Ca^{2+} from 10^{-7}M (resting state) to 10^{6}-10^{5}M (activated state) is accompanied by a series of important manifestations:

- Activation of the contractile system. Platelets contain large amounts of actomyosin, which is first assembled from its non-polymerized components, and then induced to contract. It is assumed that the rapid shape change is a first consequence of the contraction of a membrane-linked layer of actomyosin. Further activation leads to gross contractile phenomena, such as the contraction of aggregates and, in the presence of fibrin, of clot retraction.
- Prostaglandin synthesis. The substrate for PG- and TX-synthesis is arachidonic acid, which is incorporated into phospholipids. It is made available by the action of phospholipases, in particular phospholipase A_2, an enzyme which for activity depends on Ca^{2+}ions.
- Other, hitherto ill defined processes, perhaps indirectly linked

to the availability of cytoplasmic Ca^{2+} are most likely involved in the release reaction, which infact is the result of a fusion of the organelle - with the plasma - membrane. At present the process of Ca^{2+} mobilization from the DTS is also poorly understood; perhaps PG-endoperoxides which infact are produced right on the DTS, play an important role (8). It should be noted, though, that the total blocking of PG-synthesis by inhibition of the key enzyme, cyclooxygenase (e.g. by aspirin) still allows the activation of platelets, provided a powerful enough stimulus, such as that provided by thrombin or collagen (but not by ADP, serotonin or adrenaline) is given. Therefore, a PG-indipendent, alternative pathway of platelet activation must be postulated.

5. Blood platelets and the blood clotting system. At the onset of thrombus formation, the primary stimulators of platelets adhering to a site of endothelial damage are collagen, thrombin, and perhaps immune complexes, all of them belonging to the class of powerful inducers of platelet alterations. Serious vascular lesions go along with the availability of tissue thromboplastin, which locally initiates thrombin formation. For the propagation of the aggregation-release cycle, thrombin is of particular importance, since it may be formed right on the platelet surface via the intrinsic pathway of coagulation. In fact, activated platelets acquire on their surface procoagulant properties: they make available via a structural rearrangement of the phospholipids within the membrane, so-called platelet factor 3, an essential component of intrinsic thrombin formation. According to some authors, activated platelets also participate in the activation of factor XI (18). The final consolidation of a thrombus is achieved via fibrin formation, which for the reasons given above, will generally start from the procoagulant platelet aggregate.

B. Scheme of thrombus formation

The formation of an arterial thrombus starting from platelets deposited at the site of a vascular lesion must be looked at as resulting from the interplay of cellular and humoral factors. In Fig.1 a simplified scheme of these events is presented. It is obvious that with collagen of subendothelial origin, a cascade of events just involving platelets can be started, which, via released materials and TXA_2 theoretically can lead to the establishment of a consolidated platelet thrombus. Most likely, however, the participation of the clotting system is essential and thrombin as an amplifier and powerful activator on its own, plays a decisive role. This is born out best by the fact that an efficient hemostatic plug will still form in subjects whose platelets (e.g. after aspirin ingestion) are unable to produce TX, the only "intrinsic" agent capable of inducing not only aggregation (such as ADP), but also the release reaction.

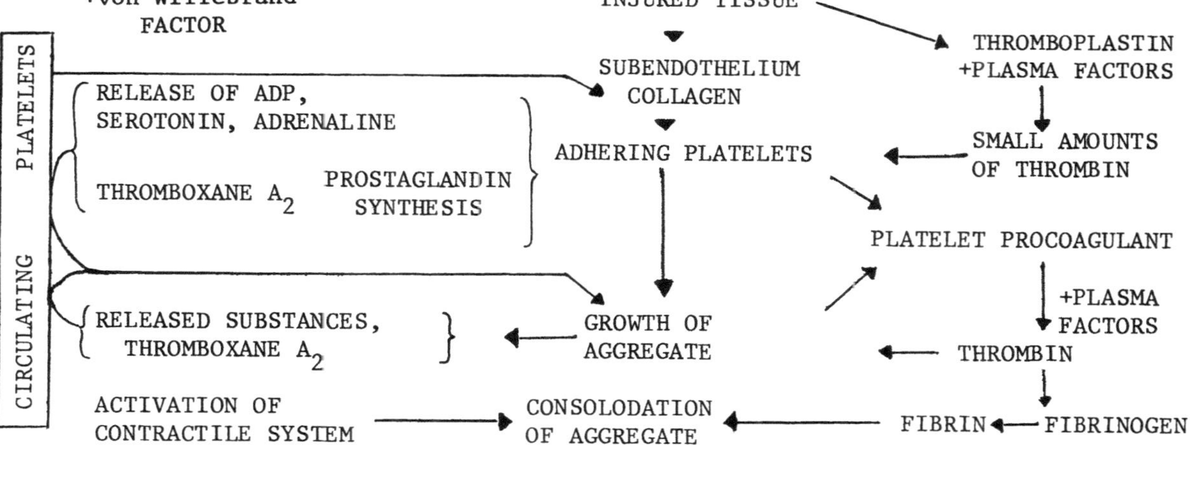

Fig. 1. Schematic representation of formation of a consolidated platelet thrombus.

C. Inhibitors of platelet activity

A series of substances is capable of interfering with platelet activation. The physiological inhibitor par excellence is prostacyclin (PGI_2), a short-lived prostaglandin produced by cells of the vascular wall. PGI_2 exerts its effect by activating adenylate cyclase, the cAMP-synthesizing enzyme. A high level of cAMP exerts a stimulating effect on the elimination of intracellular Ca^{2+}ions (9) and in this respect is comparable to other efficient inhibitors such as PGE_1 and adenosine. In view of the importance of TXA_2 in platelet activation, measures taken to interfere with PG synthesis lead to an impairment of platelet function. This approach has found widespread application in a variety of "antiaggregating agents", most of them non-steroidal anti-inflammatory agents (e.g. aspirin, indomethacin etc) are based on this mode of action.

D. What are the prerequisites for arterial thrombus formation?

According to theory, and in analogy to the hemostatic process, a large enough endothelial lesion should invariably lead to a consolidated platelet thrombus, which by slowing down circulation would favor fibrin formation thus leading to vascular occlusion. Animal experiments, however, show that even the total removal of the endothelium of the aorta only leads to transient platelet thrombus formation; within a relatively short time these thrombi are carried away and what remains is more or less a "monolayer" of degranulated platelets which offers no obstacle to the blood stream whatsoever (1). The question arises, what the prerequisites for formation of a stable, obstructing aggregate are.

First, local factors may be quite decisive. Coronary thrombosis in most instances starts out from a ruptured atheromatous lesion and this alone may be linked to unfavorable flow conditions due to a thickened arterial wall and to the availability of a continuing supply of tissue activator, particular from a bleeding atheroma. Second, conditions in the circulation may exist, which favor a more rapid and vigorous responce of the platelet, once they are deposited at the site of endothelial injury. Obviously, it is the time required for the establishment of a consolidated aggregate, capable of withstanding the eroding forces of arterial circulation, which is decisive for the fate of the primary platelet deposit. It appears rather unlikely that the processes within the cell, i.e. PG-synthesis, the release reaction, and contractile, i.e. morphological manifestations, can be accelerated. However, the extent of stimulation - whether all or only part of the adhering platelets are triggered into activity - may vary. This in turn most likely depends on the extent and the speed with which inducers are produced, whereby the prime interest undoubtedly is focussed on thrombin formation. Thus, a "preactivated" clotting system may indeed be able to provide in a short time amounts of thrombin which are large enough to involve all platelets within an aggregate in the activation process. It has indeed been shown that the in vivo activation of the contact system of blood coagulation favors the formation of occluding thrombi in the denuded rabbit aorta (7). It is obvious that this "prothrombotic state" of the clotting system may be due to a wide variety of causes, both on the side of activators as well as of the inhibitors. Finally, the reactivity of the specific defence mechanisms, particularly of prostacyclin availability must also be considered. It may be envisaged that conditions exist, where local PGI_2 production is inadequate and lastly, the possibility that platelets do not adequately react to the inhibitor must also be considered.

E. Conclusion

Arterial thrombosis is the result of the interaction of an amazing variety of mechanisms and factors. Platelet reactivity plays a key role; however, equally important are the contributions of the vascular wall and of the humoral and tissue constituents of the blood clotting system. The formation of obstructing thrombi is the result of an imbalance in a most complex system of activators and inhibitors, further influenced by rheological factors. In this context, the fact that TXA_2, as well as serotonin and ADP, all of them released from platelet aggregates, are powerfull vasoconstrictors, deserves special attention. Also in this respect, they are counteracted by the vasodilator prostacyclin. It is obvious that more knowledge on the decisive elements in this puzzling array of factors and mechanisms is badly needed.

REFERENCES

1. H.R. Baumgartner, The subendothelial surface and thrombosis. In: Pathogenesis and clinical trials. Trans. IV Int. Congr. on Thrombosis and Haemostasis. E. Deutsch, K.M. Brinkhous, K. Lechner, S. Hinnom, Ed., Shattauer, Stuttgart, N.Y. (1974).
2. P.A. Bolhuis, K.S. Sakariassen, J.J. Sixma, Adhesion of blood platelets to human arterial subendothelium: Role of factor VIII - von Willebrand factor. Haemostasis 8:312-323 (1979).
3. G.V.R. Born, Die Rolle der Blutplättchen in der Pathogenese des Herzinfarktes. In: "Neue Aspekte der medikamentösen Behandlung des Herzinfarktes". F. Gross, ed., Huber, Bern Stuttg., Wien, S. 119-123 (1979).
4. G.C. Le Breton, R.J. Dinerstein, L.J. Roth, H. Feinberg, Direct evidence for intracellular divalent cation redistribution associated with platelet shape change. Biochem. Biophys. Res. Comm. 71:362-370 (1976).
5. B.H. Bulkley, J.M. Hutchins, Coronary thrombosis: The major cause of acute myocardial infarction in atherosclerotic coronary artery disease. Circulation 56/II, III-64 (1977).
6. J.W. Burch, P.W. Majerus, The role of prostaglandins in pla-

telet function. Sem. Hemat. 16:196-207 (1979).
7. M. Chignard, J.P. le Couedic, M. Tence, B.B. Vargaftig, J. Benveniste , The role of platelet-activating factor in platelet aggregation. Nature, Lond. 279:799-800 (1979).
8. J.M. Gerrard, A.M. Butler, G. Graff, S.F. Stoddard, J.G. White, Prostaglandin endoperoxides promote calcium release from a platelet membrane preparation. Prostaglandins Med. 1:373-385 (1978).
9. R. Käser-Glanzmann, M. Jakábová, N.J. George, E.F. Lüscher, Stimulation of calcium uptake in platelet membrane vesicles by adenosine 3', 5' cyclic monophosphate and protein kinase. Biochim. Biophys. Acta 466:429-440 (1977).
10. P. Latimer, G.V.R. Born, F. Michal, Application of light-scattering theory to the optical effects associated with the morphology of blood platelets. Arch. Biochem. Biophys. 180: 151-159 (L977).
11. G.A. Marguerie, T.S. Edgington, E.F. Plow, Interaction of fibrinogen with its platelet receptor as part of a multistep reaction in ADP-induced platelet aggregation. J. Biol. Chem. 255:154-161 (1980).
12. P. Massini, E.F. Lüscher, Some effects of ionophores for divalent cations on blood platelets - comparison with the effects of thrombin. Biochim. Biophys. Acta 372:109-121 (1974).
13. P. Massini, E.F. Lüscher, On the significance of the influx of calcium ions into stimulated human blood platelets. Biochim. Biophys. Acta 436:652-663 (1976).
14. E. Morgenstern, Ultracytochemistry of human blood platelets. Progr. Histochem. Cytochem. 12, 4 (1980).
15. R. Okada, T. Konoh, A morphological study on relationship between coronary thrombosis and myocardial infarction. Blood and Vessel 9:510-515 (1978).
16. D.S. Pepper, Macromolecules released from platelet storage organelles. Thrombos. Haemostas. 42:1667-1672 (1979).
17. D.R. Phillips, An evaluation of membrane glyciproteins in platelet adhesion and aggregation. Progr in Thrombosis and Haemostasis 5:81-108 (1980).
18. P.N. Walsh, Platelet coagulant activities: Evidence for multiple, different function of platelets in intrinsic coagulation. Ser. Haemat. 6:579-592 (1973).

CLOTTING SYSTEM IN PRETHROMBOTIC STATE

M.R. Boisseau and H. Bricaud

Hôpital Cardiologique de Bordeaux
Avenue de Magellan
33 604 Bordeaux-Pessac, France

A short time ago, hypercoagulability in circulating blood was appreciated as an increased activation of coagulation related to more elevated factors than in controls. Thus Whole Blood Thromboelastography illustrated this state like heparin consumption in vivo and in vitro also did. Meanwhile it quickly appeared that these tests were poorly correlated to thrombogenesis and were much more related to a compensated intravascular disseminated coagulation.

Two main discoveries have produced changes in ideas. First the identification of fibrinopeptide A in blood, direct proof of a thrombin activity recently appeared (1). Second, the notion of consumption of coagulation factors inhibitors, starting from the observation of Egeberg (2). These two ideas have led to another conception of hypercoagulability and also to a different management of the clotting tests in view of the prediction of thrombosis.

In this review we are going to study the actual concepts, the used tests, the analysis leading to consider laboratory results in the comprehensive condition of the patients or of the chosen population. Finally practical hypotheses are also set up.

CONCEPTS IN HYPERCOAGULABILITY

(1) Hypercoagulability as unbalanced haemostasis

The possibility we have in patients to observe concomitantly a thrombin activity and a decrease of antithrombin III (AT III) favours the hypothesis of a strong correlation. This association appears as a good definition of the hypercoagulability. Particularly the defect of inhibitors is dangerous, stimulating thrombin activity.

(2) Hypercoagulability as a continuous activation and inhibition of coagulation factors

In this concept noted by different authors (3, 4), activation does not exist from time to time, neither from one vascular position to another, but exhibits a continuous evolution throughout the vessel wall. In fact this phenomenon concerns essentially the arterial wall and arteriosclerosis. In venous thrombosis the activation is more probably related to environmental factors and therefore activation should be unexpected (4). The continous activation concerns also blood platelets and fibrinolysis. It obviously appears necessary to lower this state all the time and therefore to have a continuously acting inhibitory system.

They are both of them in fact (Table 1) some move from the vessel wall, inhibiting platelets and sharing fibrinolysis. The others are plasmatic including the antiprotease system. Several molecules are here concerned: α 1 antitrypsin (α1 AT.), α 2 macroglobulin (α2 M) and the most effective, antithrombin III (AT III). This latter product actually represents a quite specific inhibitor of the coagulation, very active on thrombin but also on activated factor X.

(3) Thrombosis and haemostasis

The balanced haemostasis system must also be considered as a thrombo-haemorrhagic balance (5). Indeed activation of coagulation and platelets lead to deposits of fibrin throughout the vessel wall. This fibrin only appears in small quantities, if inhibitor systems work actively, either the extrinsic system (AT III) or the intrinsic one (feed-back inactivation and clearance of factors). Fibrin is also destroyed by the wall induced fibrinolysis. But also defects in factors lead to haemorrhages, the balance moving in the opposite side. The same phenomena concern also platelets.

Finally these new concepts lead us to study hypercoagulability in the following four ways:

<u>Study of the coagulation factors</u>. But it is not obvious that their high level in blood is by itself sufficient, except for hereditary states. Furthermore their level in thrombosis is variable and difficulties exist also in the standardization of laboratory methods. Only and epidemiological study can profit from their variations (6).

<u>Study of thrombin related products</u>. In the case of unbalanced state, thrombin is able to let new factors appear in the blood, after degradation of the substrates. Presence of fibrinopeptide A (Fp A) in plasma is the best example and further, quite simple laboratory techniques are available.

<u>Study of defect in inhibitors</u>. The hereditary defect in AT III and acquired decerased levels appear as an interesting discovery in

Table 1. Inhibitory system in Haemostasis

Factor	Origin	Nature
Platelets	Wall	PGI_2 PGI_3 ADP-ase
Fibrin	Wall	Activator of Plasminogen
Thrombin	Plasma	AT III α1 AT α2 M

hypercoagulability. More and more prospective studies, either in populations (6, 7, 8) or in patients (9) show a correlation between the defect of AT III and thrombosis. It also appears that the notion of defect in AT III is useful for a given patient and important in heparin treatment. In other respects different inhibitions also exist, which are to be considered and certainly new inhibitors have to be discovered.

The turnover rate of the coagulation factors. Theorically isotopic study of factors half-life is important, especially for fibrinogen. But in practice, techniques are difficult to use, concerning standardization and the necessary time needed. In return the technique of V.V. Kakkar, using 125 iode labelled fibrinogen, is able to discern superficial fibrin deposits, and is of great interest. This technique favours the concept of unbalanced factors resulting in fibrin formation. Also this method is able to control the prophylactic management and the effect of drugs. in the prevention of thrombosis (10).

THE USED CLOTTING TESTS IN HYPERCOAGULABILITY

Numerous works have been done about the level of factors and decrease in AT III. Actually the detection of thrombin related products concomitantly to the detection of decrease in AT III appears to be more useful.

(a) Increase of clotting factors in hypercoagulability

Increased fibrinogen is a risk factor in thrombosis, as it has been shown in epidemiological studies or in series of patients, especially in deep venous thrombosis (DVT). But interpretation of this test is related to a general situation which has to be taken into account. Furthermore the standardization of methods is difficult. Works about women taking oestrogens are numerous and exhibit an increase in factors II, VII, X and VIII, as well as a decrease in AT III (11). In venous thrombosis and pulmonary embolism an increase has been found in factors V, VII and VIII as well as a decrease in AT III (12). It must be noted however that in the course of venous occlusion hypercoagulability is very close to the phenomenon of intravascular coagulation and that variations appear. Thus Denson (13) showed the interest of increase of factors VIII RA and VIII C, and further of the unbalanced ratio between them. In arterial thrombosis these phenomena are less frequent as any variations in clotting factors, perhaps because they are cleared rapidly out of the blood stream (5). The following have also been reported: an increase of factor VII in serum (14), the risk of quick increase in factors II, XII, IX, X after withdrawal of warfarin (15), the presence of tissular factor, either thromboplastic (16), or phospholipid (17) in postoperative period and in various cardiovascular diseases. Of particular interest are hereditary states with increased factor VIII (18) and factor V (19), as well as with hyperclottable fibrinogen (20), which favour that at least partially excess of factors is a prothrombotic state and not only consequence of thrombosis. The increase of von Willebrand factor (vWf) is an excellent signal for suffering vessels, usually correlated to thrombosis. However this result is unspecific. In return very simple techniques (slide-test) could be available in general studies. Usually the level of vWf is correlated to VIII RA, this latter detected by immunological method.

(b) Detection of intravascular thrombin formation

-(1) Free thrombin in plasma split fibrinogen and left fp A to appear. This latter at high level exhibits the existence of free thrombin even if thromboses are few and unknown. Numerous actual works are in progress using radio-immunoassay of fp A (21) or immunoenzymatic assay (22). However difficulties persist concerning technology. From the clinical point of view the studies are obviously attractive (23, 24). Fibrinopeptide B and B 1 + 42 are also studied. The detection of prothrombin fragments, released by thrombin: F2 and F 1 + 2 (25), has been proposed recently.

-(2) Another approach is to detect fibrin monomers in the blood stream, related at least partially to thrombin. These products are able to gelify with ethanol (ethanol gelation test). It is also possible to detect their relation to fibrinogen using affinity chromatography on fibrinogen agarose (26). Also plasma fibrin chromatography can exhibit H M W F C (high molecular weight fibrin complexes) related to thrombin formation (27). It must be noted however that these two techniques are difficult to set up routinely and that the studied products are partially related to plasmin activity.

Finally the study of the kininogen-kinin system is of some interest in prethrombotic state, prekallikrein being consumed at the onset of the activation (28). However the decrease of this product is unspecific especially during stress.

(c) Study of the decrease in inhibitory system

AT III checking is very interesting. Several techniques have been used: biological related to show an antithrombin action (von Kaulla) or anti Xa effect; or immunological, detecting the weight of the circulating protein. The use of synthetic substrates (amidolytic method) is very attractive but expensive. This research is actually in progress (7, 8, 9) in numerous diseases, (inherited syndrome, Blood group A, oestrogen ingestion) and usually the decrease in AT III, is associated with an increase of factors. Further we have to keep in mind the other inhibitors. Particularly α 2 M and α 1 AT are able to neutralize thrombin and their variations are also important.

(d) Detection inhibitor complexes (neoantigens)

Recently it has been shown that circulating complexes between thrombus and AT III (or plasmin and antiplasmin) are detectable in blood. These complexes exhibit neoantigens and specific antibodies can be used (29). But the half life of these products is very short.

(e) Isotopic study of clotting factors

The turnover rate of certain factors appears modified in thrombosis. Prothrombin and fibrinogen are concerned. Particularly the Kakkar method, as we said, is attractive.

INTERPRETATION OF THE VARIATIONS OF CLOTTING TESTS IN PRETHROMBOTIC STATES

Three difficulties appear in view of the interpretation either in populations or in patients.

(a) Unspecificity of coagulation disturbances

It must be noted first that variations of factors are not always related to hypercoagulability (Table II). Thus the defect in AT III must possibly be related to an hepatic lesion. The increase in α 2 M

Table II. Unspecificity of coagulation disturbances: many clinical disorders are able to modify the clotting factors.

Disorders acting on: fibrinogen, factor VIII, AT III, α 2 A, α 1 AT and von Willebrand factor

Hypercoagulability	Various clinical disorders
Hereditary (Blood group A)	Inflammation
Smoking	Systemic Lupus E
Oestrogens	Cancers
Age	Haemopathias
Vessel wall alteration	Dyslipaemias
Homocystinuria	Liver diseases (Hepatitis, Cirrhosis)
	Diabetes
	Immun-complexes
	Kinin-system changes
	DIC (compensated or not)

and α 1 AT levels is quite frequent, especially in cancers, where fibrinolysis is less effective. The decrease of VIII C exists in haematological disorders. Finally the increase of VIII RA, vWf and fibrinogen are observed in all inflammatory states. It must be pointed out however that increase in vWf appears mainly in vascular diseases and changes.

(b) Multifactorial mechanism in thrombogenesis

The second difficulty arises from the numerous factors acting on a given vascular occlusion (Table III). Coagulation (and so it is for platelets and fibrinolysis) is only partially concerned. Not only general factors are important but also local conditions (stasis, vortices, turbulences) and finally one special event occurs leading to a special vascular damage. That is especially true in arterial thrombosis. In venous thrombosis environemental factors are even more important (4). Nevertheless, this multifactorial mechanism explains the variability of histology in occurring thrombi. Proportions of fibrin, platelets, WBC and RC are variable from one thrombus to another and from one lesion to another.

The role of blood cells is certainly important, either the WBC able to secrete thromboplastin, or RC becoming rigid when they are in close relation to the altered vessels and the inflammatory lesions.

Table III. Variability in the genesis of thrombus in arterial thrombosis.

For a given patient variable action of:	
Hereditary factors	
Risk factors	Overweight Diet Smoking
General Conditions	Diabetes HTA Stress Malignant disease Chronic inflammation
Coagulation disorders	High level of factors Defect in AT III
Local conditions	Stasis, turbulence Blood cells behaviour
Special event	Immun-complexes Mechanical damage

Variable thrombus obtained:

Fibrin
Fibrin + platelets
Fibrin + R cells + platelets
Fibrin + W B cells

Therefore they can increase the surface of the anoxic area and the thrombus (30).

(c) Management and cost of tests

The last difficulties we have to take into account are the problems of reproducibility, standardization and necessarily of low cost price. This point is fundamental and has to be resolved before starting in population or large patients groups studies.

CLOTTING TESTS AND EPIDEMIOLOGY OF CAD

On the whole it is obvious that difficulties exist to use clotting tests in the prethrombotic state and especially in coronary artery disease (CAD).

Here are concerned (a) normal values and their distribution in populations, as the published works of Meade pointed out (6). But it must be noted that a given people, with variations in the normal range, could have a risk if factors move to high level and AT III to the low value (5). Meade also showed the relationship between risk factors and variations of the coagulation factors, which in fact favours this kind of works. (b) the general situation of patients beside the question of thrombosis. It is absolutely necessary to know all about any disease they could present. Thus the variation of the factors or clotting tests cannot be related to arterial vessels, before all other parameters have been carefully excluded.

Two situations finally can be considered:

(1) Study in a large population (primary prevention)

In this case the chosen tests are: AT III (biological method) and vWf level determination (slide test). Decrease of AT III and increase of vWf are able to give the alarm in a group of individuals. This group has thus to be submitted to a complete and careful analysis (age, blood group A, clinical, cardiological examinations). From this group a second one can be so selected in view of an accurate study of haemostasis and perhaps angiocardiography.

(2) Study on selective patients

In a given group of patients (genetic, risk factors, blood groups or secondary prevention after primary accident) the clinical study has to be first processed. After several diseases have been discarded: malignant growth, inflammatory states, immune disease, etc..., an haemostasis study should be done. Here are concerned platelets, coagulation and fibrinolysis. In coagulation the chosen tests should be: fibrinogen, factor VIII (several methods), fp A and AT III. Further management and control are the same as above.

CONCLUSION

Detection of prethrombotic states does not only concern haemostasis which represents a part of the necessary investigations. At the limit a general study of individuals is necessary but impossible to do. Thus actually the use of simple tests, well correlated to the modern concepts of hypercoagulability, is only justifiable. If they do not provide any success in this research, the concepts will be discussed again and other tests included.

That will be perhaps the case for rheological investigations, the variations of which are not frequently used in prethrombotic states, as for example the viscosity (30) or the red cell behaviour (31).

REFERENCES

1. H.L. Nossel, J. Yudelman, R.E. Canfield, V.P. Butler, K. Spanondis, G.D. Wilner and G.D. Quershi, Measurement of fibrinopeptide A in human blood. J. Clin. Invest. 1:43-53 (1974).
2. O. Egeberg, Inherited antithrombin deficiency causing thrombophilia. Thromb. Diath. Haemorrh. 13:616-530 (1965).
3. J.R. O'Brien, The prothrombotic state. In: Recent advances in blood coagulation. p 241-266, Elsyver Ed, 1979.
4. J.J. Sixma, Techniques for diagnosing prethrombotic states. A review. Thrombos. Haemostas. (Stuttg.) 40:252-259 (1978).
5. H. Stormorken, The thrombo-haemorrhagic balance. Acta Med. Scand. (Suppl.) 642:131-140 (1980).
6. T.W. Meade and W.R.S. North, Population-based distributions of haemostatic variables. Br. Med. Bull.33, 3, 283-288 (1977).
7. H. Stormorken and J. Erikssen, Plasma antithrombin and factor VIII antigen in relation to angiographic findings, angina and blood groups in middle-aged men. Thrombos. Haemostas. (Stittg.) 38:874-880 (1977).
8. S. Sagar, J.D. Stamatakis, D.P. Thomas and V.V. Kakkar, Oral contraceptives, antithrombin III activity, post operative deep vein thrombosis. Lancet 1: 509-511 (1976).
9. E. Marciniak, C.H. Farley, P.A. de Simone, Familial thrombosis due to antithrombin III deficiency. Blood 43:219-221 (1974).
10. V.V. Kakkar, A.N. Nicolandes, Low doses of heparin in the prevention of deep vein thrombosis. Lancet 2:7726-7728 (1871).
11. D.J.S. Hunter, A.B.M. Anderson and M. Haddon, Changes in coagulation factors in postmenopausal women on ethinil oestradiol. Br. J. of Obst. and Gyn. 86:488-490 (1979).
12. I.M. Nilsson and S. Isacson, New aspects of the pathogenesis of thromboembolism. Progress in Surgery 11:46-68 (1973).
13. K.W.E. Denson, The ratio of factor VIII. Related antigen and factor VIII biological activity as an index of hypercoagulability and vascular clotting. Thrombosis Res. 10:107-119 (1977).
14. L. Poller, Factor VII and thrombosis. J. of Clin. Pathol. 10: 348-350 (1957).
15. J.A. Penner, Hypercoagulation and thrombosis. Symposium on advances in haematology. Med. Clinics of North America 64: 743-759 (1980).
16. Y. Sultan, Hypercoagulabilité et thrombose. Ann. Méd. Int. 131, 3, 137-140 (1980).
17. M.L. Boffa, Evaluation of the phospholipid-related procoagulant

activity in plasma. A new clue for detecting tendency of thrombosis? Thrombosis Res. 17:567-572 (1980).
18. P.D. Penick, H.R. Roberts and I.I. Dejanov, Covert intravascular clotting. Fed. Proc. 24:825-827 (1965).
19. L.W. Gaston, Studies on a family with elevated plasma level of factor V and a tendency to thrombosis. Pediatrics 68:376-378 (1966).
20. O. Egeberg, Inherited anti-thrombin deficiency causing thrombophilia. Thrombos. Diathes. Haemorrh. 13:176-178 (1967).
21. C. Kockum, Radioimmunoassay of fibrinopeptide A: clinical applications. Thrombosis Res. 8:225-227 (1976).
22. J. Soria, C. Soria, and J.J. Ryckewaert, Competitive radioimmunoassay for fibrinopeptide A. Clinical Applications. In: Abstract book Six. Int. Congress on Thrombosis of the Mediterranean League against thromboembolic disease. Monte Carlo 23-25 October 1980.
23. M. Cronlund, J. Hardin, H.J. Burton, L. Lee, E. Haber and K.J. Bloch, Fibrinipeptide A in plasma of normal subjects and patients with disseminated intravascular coagulation and systemic lupus erythematosus. J. Clin. Invest. 58:142-147 (1976).
24. F.W. Peuscher, W.G. van Aken, O.Th.N. Flier, E.A. Stoepman-van Dalen, T.M. Cremer-Goote and J.A. van Mourik, Effect of anticoagulant treatment measured by fibrinopeptide A (fp A) in patients with venous thrombo-embolism. Thrombosis Res. 18:33-43 (1980).
25. K.H. Lau, J.S. Rosenberg, D.L. Beeler and R.D. Rosenberg, The isolation and characterization of a specific antibody population directed against the prothrombin activation fragments F_2 and F_{1+2}. J. Biol. Chem. 254, 18, 8751-8761 (1979).
26. D.L. Heene, F.R. Mathias, Adsorption of fibrinogen derivatives on insolubilized fibrinogen and fibrin monomer. Thrombosis Res. 2:137-139 (1973).
27. N. Alkjaersig, A. Fletcher and R. Bursten, Association between oral contraceptive use and thromboembolism: a new approach to its investigation based on plasma fibrinogen chromatography. Am. J. Obstet. Gynecol. 122, 2, 189-211 (1975).
28. J. Soria, C. Soria, J.J. Rykewaert, F. Alhens-Gelas, P. Hourdille and M. Boisseau, Kallikrenin-kinin system as a model of proteolytic regulation in normal and some pathological situations. In; Proteases and hormones, M.K. Agarwal Ed.1979. Elsevier p 67-83.
29. D. Collen, F. De Cook, M. Verstraete, Quantitation of thrombin-antithrombin III Complex in human blood Europ. J. of Clin. Invest. 7:407-409 (1977).
30. M.F. Lorient, M.R. Boisseau, H. Bricaud, J.P. Manuau and C. Alliere, Réduction de la filterabilité érythrocytaire et accidents vasculaires cérébraux. Etude chez 80 patients. Sem. Hôp. Paris 55:27-30 (1979).

31. G.D.O. Lowe, M.M. Drummond, C.D. Forbes, C.R.M. Prentice and J.C. Barbenel, Blood and plasma viscosity in prediction of venous thrombosis. In: Abstract book Six. Int. Congress on Thrombosis of the Mediterranean League against thromboembolic diseases. Monte Carlo 23-25 October 1980.

PLATELET FUNCTION TESTS AND CORONARY HEART DISEASE

A. Strano and G. Davì

Institute of Clinical Medicine and Medical Therapy
University of Palermo
Piazza delle Cliniche, 2
90127 Palermo - Italy

It is well known that the formation of a platelet aggregate is the first step in an arterial thrombotic process.

The changes of platelet metabolic activity, particularly thromboxane A_2 release and intraplatelet c-AMP changes, are determining manifestations for platelet aggregation and platelet sensitivity to aggregating agents.

Besides a possible primitive platelet disturbance an increased platelet activity can be secondary to an activation of coagulation caused by the presence of small concentrations of thrombin or activated factor X; furthermore, changes of the plasmatic environment can induce thrombophilia through an increased platelet activity and particularly the conversion of arachidonic acid into thromboxane is significantly influenced by plasmatic cholesterol levels (1, 2, 3). An increase of shear stress (hypertension) (4, 5) can be responsible for platelet hyperaggregability; finally an increased platelet aggregation can also be due to the loss, also if partial, of endothelium athrombogenic properties.

Several prethrombotic states have, as main cause factor, a platelet activation (Fig. 1). Platelet micro-thrombi are responsible for some cases of T.I.A. carotid or vertebral; fatal and non-fatal arrhythmias (sudden death) can find in their pathogenesis the microvessels of the cardiac conduction occluded by platelet microemboli; one can postulate that some cases of non transmural myocardial infarction, not associated with coronary thrombosis, can be caused by platelet microthrombi; the release of thromboxane by platelets can influence the genesis of cerebral or coronary spasm that has a notable importance in some kinds of coronary pathology as Prinzmetal's angina or some cases of myocardial infarction arisen without a preexisting coronary stenosis. Important is also the role played by

PRETHROMBOTIC STATES AND PLATELETS
PLATELET MICROTHROMBI
T.I.A.
SEVERE BUT NON FATAL ARRYHYMIAS
SEVERE AND FATAL ARRHYTHMIAS (SUDDEN CARDIAC DEATH)
NON TRANSMURAL MYOCARDIAL INFARCTION NOT ASSOCIATED WITH CORONARY THROMBOSIS ?
MICROCIRCULATION WORSENING IN PERIPHERAL ARTEROPATHIES ?
PLATELET AGGREGATION WITH THROMBOXANE A2 RELEASE AND PROSTACYCLIN DEFICIT
CORONARY SPASM ?
ACTIVATION OF BLOOD COAGULATION ASSOCIATED WITH HYPOFIBRINOLYSIS AND PLATELET ACTIVATION
ATHERO-THROMBOTIC BRAIN INFARCTION
MYOCARDIAL INFARCTION WITH THROMBOSIS
ACUTE PERIPEHRAL ARTIERY OCCLUSION

Fig. 1

CORONARY ATHEROSCLEROSIS
INCREASED PLATELET ADHESION ON SUBENDOTHELIUM
THROMBOXANE A2 RELEASE
LDL
SMOKE
15 HPAA
INHIBITED GENERATION OF PROSTACYCLIN
CORONARY SPASM

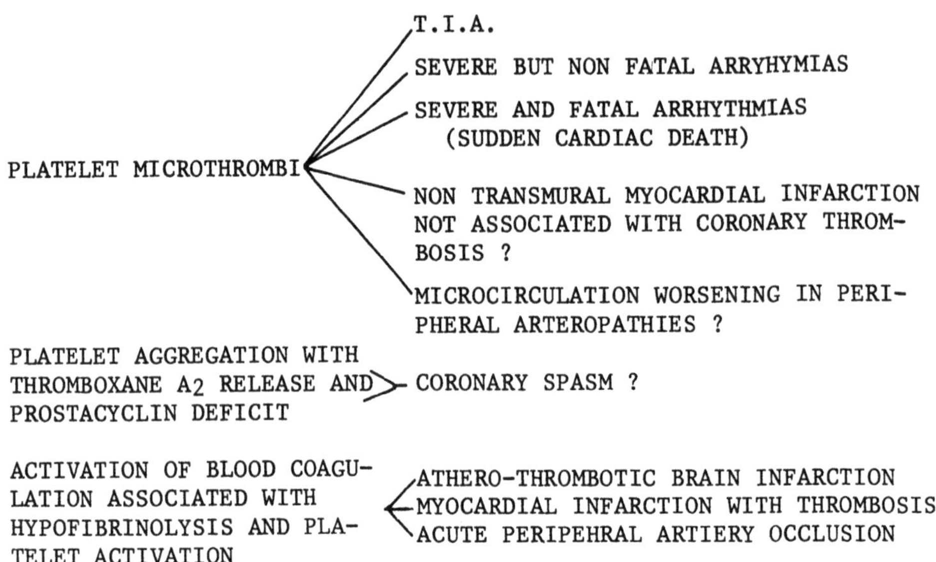

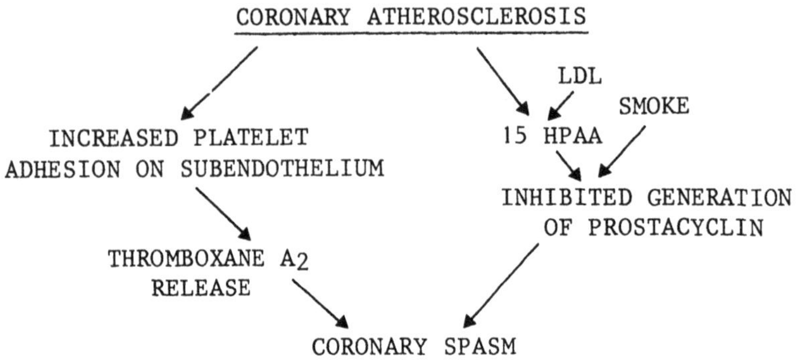

Fig. 2

platelets, together with a coagulative activation or a hypofibrinolysis, in some acute vascular events as brain infarction, myocardial infarction with thrombosis and acute peripheral occlusion.

A coronar vascular spasm can be induced by the concomitance of two phenomena: an increased release of thromboxane caused by an excited platelet adhesion to endothelial structures which have lost their characteristics of athrombogenic properties because of the presence of atherosclerosis; a reduced prostacyclin formation caused by the formation of lipid peroxides (15 HPAA) or by the action of cigarette smoke at pulmonary or endothelial level (Fig.2).

In most transmural myocardial infarctions a thrombus is present and hence a "dilemma" long debated by clinicians and anatomopathologists: (6, 7, 8, 9, 10) does the thrombus precede or follow the acute event? Whatever may be the answer to this question it is sure that the thrombus plants itself in the site of a stenosis; the number of reinfarctions can be reduced with a good anticoagulant therapy; an activated coagulation is often to be found in myocardial infarction.

Non-transmural or subendocardial myocardial infarction is usually without thrombosis; its pathogenesis can be ascribed to a sudden and persistent increase of oxygen demand or to one of the causes mentioned above, like the formation of reversible platelet thrombi, that have been found in post mortem examinations by Haerem (10) more frequently in subjects who had died of infarction than of other causes, or of a persistent coronary spasm.

It is thus certain that platelets play a key role in the formation of an arterial thrombus and for this reason it is very important to document a state of platelet activation; unfortunately, though several methods are available, such documentation can not be left to only one of them, because none of them is capable of demonstrating in vitro what really happens in vivo.

The study of platelet function implies the evaluation of the different activities carried out by platelets (Table I).

A. Platelet adhesiveness can be carried out with Baumgartner's method (11) that allows us to evaluate the capacity of platelets to adhere to subendothelium, but such a method involves too much investigation for clinical studies on large samples.

Other methods allow us to evaluate platelet tendency to adhere to artificial surfaces such as glass.

Chadhuri (12) and Sharma (13) have noticed an increased platelet adhesiveness in patients with acute myocardial infarction.

B. Platelet aggregation can be evalued with several methods: platelet aggregation in vitro according to Born's or Breddin's method, the research of the circulating platelet aggregates with Wu and Hoak's (14) method and with Hornstra's (15) filtragometer, spontaneous platelet aggregation (16), fibrinogen binding platelets (17) and the research of platelet sensitivity to prostacyclin (18).

Born's method, among the most studied, implies the evaluation in vitro of platelet aggregation to various aggregating agents such as ADP, adrenaline, collagen, etc. Plasma manipulation, the inevi-

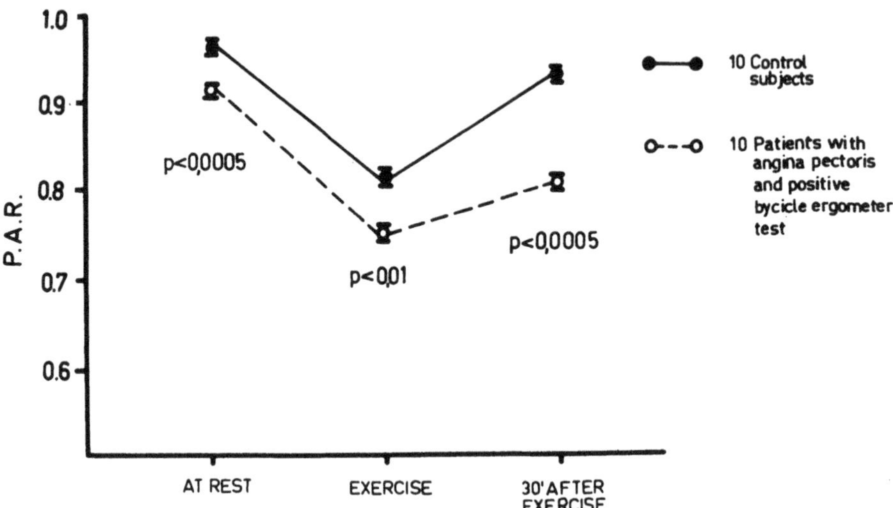

Fig. 3. Changes of platelet aggression ratio (PRA), during and after exercise, in 10 patients with stable angina and in 10 control subjects of equivalent age; mean ± 1 SD.

table delay with which the assay is carried out, the addition of aggregating substances at non-physiological concentrations, do not ensure that a hyperaggregability verified in vitro reflects the behaviour of platelets in vivo.

Gormsen (19) has recently reported how in patients with acute myocardial infarction the threshold concentration for an irreversible aggregation was higher than normal (that is, platelets were hyporeactive) during the first three days, while from the 4th - 5th day following the acute event there is a progressive reduction of the aggregating agent (ADP, adrenaline and collagen) necessary to obtain platelet aggregation (thus a condition of hyper-aggregability).

Also Breddin's method can show a hyperaggregability, as our group has proved in 1976 in patients with ischaemic heart disease, who, in over 50% of cases, had a pathological grade of aggregation - 3, 4 or 5 (20).

Metha (21) has found a noticeable increase of circulating platelet aggregates in the first day after acute myocardial infarction, with persistence of the increase of aggregates also at the 7th day in comparison with normal controls.

Our group (22) also has found a noticeable increase of platelet aggregates, significantly increased at stress peak, in patients suffering from angina and with a positive bicycle ergometer test (Fig. 3).

Wu and Hoak (16) have also proposed the study of spontaneous platelet aggregation in vitro, using Born's aggregometer without

Table I. PLATELET FUNCTION TESTS

1. STUDY OF PLATELET ADHESIVENESS

2. EVALUATION OF PLATELET AGGREGATION

A. Born's and Breddin's method
B. Spontaneous platelet aggregation
C. Circulating platelet aggregates
D. 125-fibrinogen binding in platelets
E. Platelet sensitivity to exogenous prostacyclin

3. MEASUREMENT OF PLATELET TURNOVER

A. Platelet survival time
B. Platelet regeneration time
C. Megathrombocytes count

4. DOSAGE OF PLATELET ACTIVATION PRODUCTS

A. Betathromboglobulin
B. Platelet factor 4
C. Platelet factor 3
D. Serotonin
E. Heparin neutralizing activity

The simultaneous measurements of plasmatic and intra-platelet levels reflect more accurately platelet activation and/or exaustion

5. INVESTIGATION OF PLATELET ARACHIDONIC ACID PATHWAY

A. MDA and thromboxane formation by platelets after stimulation with aggregating agents
B. Thromboxane B_2 detection in plasma or serum
C. Intraplatelet AMP-cyclic levels

6. STUDY OF CIRCULATING PROSTACYCLIN

Parallel to the study of intra-platelet arachidonic acid metabolism, an increasing interest is being given to the study of circulating prostacyclin, with biological methods or through the dosage of its main metabolite: 6-Keto-$PGF_{1\alpha}$

adding aggregating agents; such spontaneous aggregation, if present, can be seen only 20 minutes - 1 hour after blood sampling, fading after the 2nd hour and then disappearing.

Recently Caen's group (17) has studied fibrinogen binding platelets (fibrinogen is the necessary element for ADP aggregation and platelets have a specific receptor for fibrinogen). Such binding is increased in diabetic patients and is more evident in diabetics with retinopathy; of interest is the fact that such bond is indipendent from aggregation to ADP.

Metha and Metha (18) have prospected the study of platelet sensitivity to exogenous prostacyclin that could be one of the mechanisms implied in the genesis of an increased platelet aggregation. It is evident, in fact, that a reduced platelet sensitivity to prostacyclin, a part from a lower production of prostacyclin, means that less endogenous thromboxane is necessary to trigger a platelet aggregation.

The study of disaggregation with prostacyclin in patients with acute myocardial infarction (23) has allowed us to point out how sensitivity to prostacyclin is noticeably reduced in the days following the acute event, beacuse, in order to obtain a disaggregation of 50%, notably higher doses of prostacyclin than those needed by controls are necessary.

C. Platelet survival. A platelet hyperaggregability is permanent and irreversible and thus an expression of a thrombophilic condition, if associated with a reduced platelet survival. There are three main methods proposed for such a study: platelet survival time after platelet labelling with ^{51}Cr, platelet regeneration time (24, 25) and the per cent calculation of circulating megathrombocytes (26).

Platelet survival time is reduced in patients with myocardial infarction (27) and is still more reduced in patients that at coronary examination showed normal arteriograms, as if the presence of platelets in the infarct process (spasm? platelet microemboli?) was relevant.

The count of megathrombocytes is a good index of reduced platelet survival as shown by Neri Serneri (28) in patiens with a history of myocardial infarction, in correlation with circulating platelet aggregates.

Platelet regeneration time allows, through the administration of 500 mg of aspirin, an irreversible inhibition of platelet ability to synthetize endoperoxides, blocking the production of malondialdehyde; the time necessary to malondialdehyde formation to return to the values previous to aspirin administration, indicates the time necessary for a new population of platelets to substitute that whose cyclooxygenase has been inhibited. Such a method is equivalent to platelet survival time with radioactive methods.

Our group (29) has studied platelet regeneration time in diabetic patients who showed electrocardiographic signs of myocardial ischemia; this time was significantly reduced in diabetics compared to controls (Fig. 4).

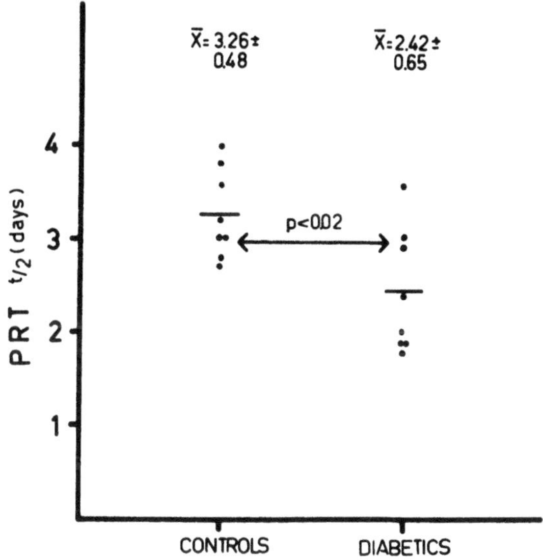

Fig. 4. Platelet regeneration time (PRT) in 8 diabetic patients with ECG. findings of myocardial ischemia in comparison with 8 healthy subjects of equivalent age; mean $\pm$ 1 SD.

A strong correlation between platelet half life and circulating platelet aggregates (30) has been found in patients with acute myocardial infarction.

D. Platelet release products. If platelets in vivo are stimulated in such a way that they go towards a release reaction, specific substances, whose concentration expresses the grade of platelet activation, can be looked for in plasma.

These specific platelet products (31) are: betathromboglobulin (32, 33), platelet factor 4 (34) and growth factor (35) released by alpha granuli, and whose release can occur without platelet aggregation and for much lower concentrations than those necessary for ADP release from dense bodies.

BTG seems to have an inhibiting action on prostacyclin production (36); platelet factor 4 has the property of neutralizing heparin. It is comparable to the so called activity neutralizing heparin, studied among others by O'Brien (37); though the basic method to dose such protein remains the radioimmunologic one. Of a certain importance is the fact that higher levels of BTG and PF4 are found in the old more than in the young and middle aged people (38).

Like ADP, serotonin is released from dense bodies, while the so called platelet factor 3 (39) is the expression of a state of platelet activation, because during the aggregation there is an exposure

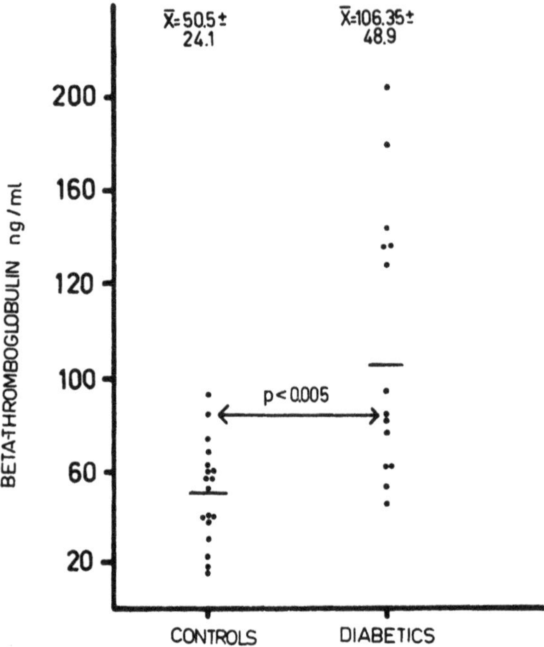

Fig. 5. Plasmatic levels of beta-thromboglobulin in 14 diabetic patients with ECG. findings of myocardial ischemia in comparison with 14 healthy subjects of equivalent age; mean ± 1 SD.

of membrane phospholipids which form a reaction surface for some coagulative reactions, particularly for prothrombin activation. This strengthening of coagulation by platelets is considered as platelet factor 3.

Recently O'Brien has proposed to consider simultaneously plasmatic and intraplatelet levels of BTG, PF4 and serotonin because they would reflect more accurately a state of platelet activation or platelet exaustion (40), expression of a previous platelet involvement in a thrombotic event, as can happen in the very first days after an acute event.

We have dosed PF4 in the days after myocardial infarction (23); we have found much higher mean values than normal and this demonstrates a state of platelet activation also in the very first days after infarction, even if the platelet aggregation index shows an "exaustion" of the platelet function.

Also in diabetics with electrocardiographic signs of myocardial ischemia (29) we have found high levels of betathromboglobulin in comparison with controls (Fig. 5).

Heparin/thrombin time indicates something similar to platelet factor 4 (factor neutralizing heparin) and has been found higher by O'Brien (36) in patients with acute myocardial infarction and with intermittent claudication.

E. Platelet metabolism in relation to aggregation. Platelet aggregation is linked both to the production of energy and to the formation of substances active on platelet aggregation, like cyclic endoperoxides and thromboxane A_2 (41, 42, 43).

A useful information on the metabolism of intraplatelet arachidonic acid is given by the study of thromboxane B_2 formation, stable transformation product of intraplatelet arachidonic acid metabolism (Fig. 6).

Platelet aggregation is then modulated by inhibiting activities represented by intraplatelet concentration of cyclic AMP (44, 45). The study of the dosage of cyclic AMP both in basal conditions, that is in non stimulated platelets, and after platelet stimulation with prostacyclin, is able to give useful informations on the cyclic AMP formation capacity and on the sensitivity to prostacyclin of the adenilcyclase which is the specific platelet receptor.

In patients with atherosclerosis obliterans of the lower limbs (2nd and 3rd stage according to Fontaine) our group (46) has found an increased thromboxane formation by platelets after thrombin stimulus (Fig. 7).

In patients with II-type hyperlipoproteinemia, thromboxane B_2 formation by platelets is markedly higher (3, 47); this is probably to correlate to the fact that hypercholesterolemia induces significant changes in the cholesterol/platelet membrane phospholipids ratio, with a stronger disposition to arachidonic acid release by membrane phospholipids (2, 48, 49).

Another important fact is that LDL are very rich in lipid peroxides and for this reason reduce prostacyclin production (50); HDL do not change it because they do not have lipid peroxides.

Smith's group (51) has recently proposed the study of circulating thromboxane in particular clinical or experimental situations, in which there is a suspect of a possible intervention of such factor in the genesis either of a spasm or of hyperaggregability. In fact, in patients with variable angina, in repeated checkings during the spontaneous angina crisis, there are higher levels of circulating thromboxane B_2 than in control subjects. The effects of pacing on lactate and thromboxane B_2 concentrations, both in the coronary sinus and in the peripheral vessels, have also been proven (52); during pacing there is a notable increase of thromboxane in the coronar sinus and, also if to a lesser extent, of peripheral circulating thromboxane B_2 together with a marked reduction of lactate extraction.

F. Prostacyclin. Besides the studies on the intraplatelet metabolism of arachidonic acid, in recent years particular attention has been given to circulating prostacyclin, either with biological method or through the dosage of its main metabolite, 6-keto $PGF_{1\alpha}$.

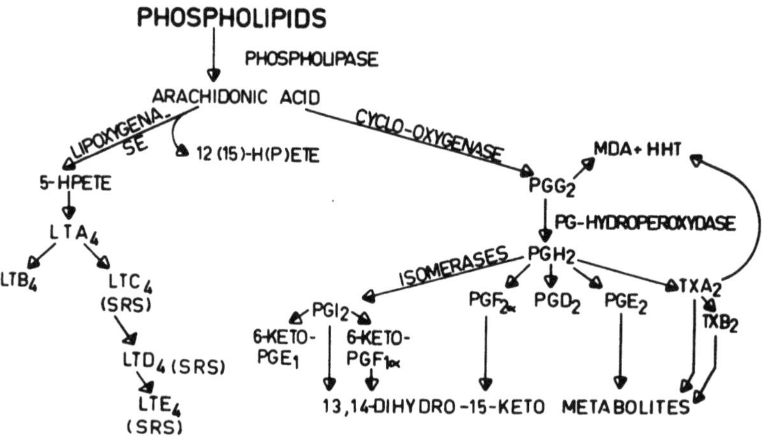

Fig. 6. Pathways of arachidonic acid metabolism.

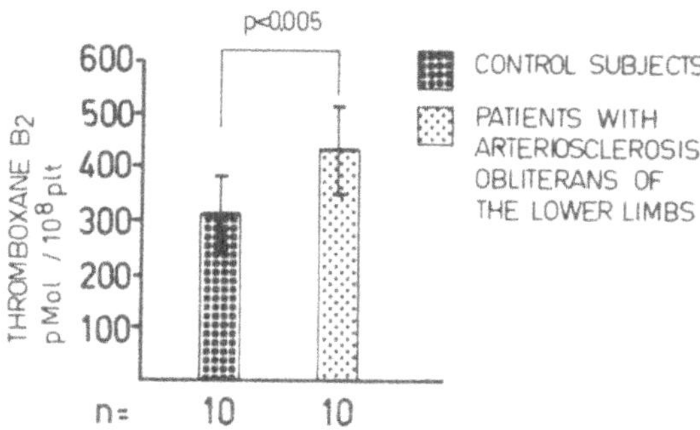

Fig. 7. Thromboxane B_2 formation by platelets, after thrombin stimulation (5U N.I.H.), in 10 patients with atherosclerosis obliterans of the lower limbs (2nd and 3rd stage according to Fontaine) and in 10 healthy subjects of equivalent age; mean $\pm$ 1 SD.

Neri Serneri's group (3) has pointed out how circulating prostacyclin is reduced, in comparison with age matched controls, in patients with ischaemic heart disease, both with angina and infarction.

Our group has studied 6-keto $PGF_{1\alpha}$ levels in patients with atherosclerosis obliterans of the lower limbs compared to controls (46). In basal conditions such values, though slightly reduced in comparison with controls, did not show a significant difference. After 3 minutes of arterial occlusion with strain-gauge plethysmography there is a notable increase of 6-keto $PGF_{1\alpha}$ production in the controls compared to the patients with atherosclerosis obliterans of the lower limbs.

G. Finally something must be said about the studies on the endothelium and on the platelet/vessel wall interaction. A lot of information, in fact, has been gathered on these two subjects in recent years.

The evidence of congenital and acquired deficiencies of the endothelium will allow a better understanding of the mechanisms acting at cellular level and therefore to adopt more rational and effective therapies than those used now.

Hoak (54) has recently studied the effects of thrombin in a vascular endothelium; thrombin stimulates the release of prostacyclin (evalued through the production of 6-keto $PGF_{1\alpha}$) and is still able to produce this effect when the endothelium has been treated with acetylsalicylic acid at concentrations that inhibit thromboxane B_2 formation by platelets. Of particular interest is the fact that an active product of coagulation like thrombin, highly thrombogenic, is able to strongly stimulate the release of the strongest inhibitor of platelet aggregation.

After a first exposure to thrombin, endothelial cell cultures are unable to respond to a second thrombin stimulus with a release of prostacyclin; it would be of particular importance to see if such a refractory state is verified also in vivo.

CONCLUSION

There are several methods available for the evaluation of platelet function; but there still is no ideal method to evalue the polyhedric effects of platelets and that at the same time can inform us precisely about what really happens in vivo.

Thus an investigation on platelet aggregation must necessarily include the simultaneous examination of different methods that evalue the different aspects of platelet function in order to diagnose a prethrombotic state with more certainty than with only one examination.

The simultaneous observation of the different aspects of platelet function allows us to point out some peculiar aspects, like platelet "exhaustion" (that is, hyporeactive platelets not because such but because they have taken part in a thrombotic process, exhausting thus their capacity to produce specific substances - BTG, PF4, etc. - or the capacity to produce cyclic endoperoxides - MDA, thromboxane).

In the choice of such methods we must prefer those that are highly specific and that do not involve too much plasma manipulation or technical devices, but that allow a standardization of methods in the different laboratories.

We would therefore be able to recognize those "high risk" patients who need a pharmacological prevention based on platelet antiaggregating drugs (55, 56, 57, 58).

REFERENCES

1. R.S. Lees, A.C.A. Carvalho, Hypercholesterolemia and platelets. Adv. Exp. Med. Biol. 104:301 (1978).
2. S.J. Shattil, R. Anaya-Galindo, J. Bennet, R.W. Colman, R.A. Cooper , Platelet hypersensitivity induced by cholesterol incorporation . J. Clin. Invest. 55:636 (1975).
3. G. Davi, M. Averna, F.P. Riolo, S. Novo, G. Mendola, M. Fiore, A. Strano, Increased thromboxane and malondialdehyde production by platelets from patients with hyperlipoproteinemia. In: VI Int. Cong. on Thrombosis of the Med. League against Thromboemb. Dis. Montecarlo, October 23-25 (1980).
4. D.E. Stevens, J.H. Joist, S.P. Sutera, Role of platelet-prostaglandin synthesis in shear-induced platelet alterations. Blood 56:753 (1980).
5. G. Davi, S. Novo, F.P. Riolo, A. Pinto, G. Mendola, A. Mazzola, M. Fazio, Formazione di malondialdeide piastrinica in pazienti ipertesi sottoposti a prova da sforzo al cicloergometro. In: Atti del Congresso Nazionale di Cardiologia, Firenze, Maggio 1980.
6. G. Baroldi, Coronary thrombosis: Facts and Beliefs. Am. Heart J. 91:683 (1976).
7. A. Strano, G. Davì, S. Novo, G. Avellone, Trombosi coronarica ed infarto del miocardio. Min. Angiol. 4:103 (1979).
8. W.C. Roberts, I.M. Buja, The frequency and the significance of coronary arterial thrombi and other observations in fatal acute myocardial infarction: a study of 107 necropsy patients. Am. J. Med. 52:425 (1972).
9. A.B. Chandler, I. Chapman, L.R. Erhardt, Coronary thrombosis in myocardial infarction: report of a workshop on the role of coronary thrombosis in the pathogenesis of acute myocardial infarction. Am. J. Cardiol. 34:823 (1974).
10. J.W. Haerem, Myocardial lesions in sudden unexpected coronary death. Am. Heart. J. 90:562 (1975).
11. H.R. Baumgartner, platelet interaction with vascular structures. Thromb. Diath. Haemorrh. Suppl. 51:161 (1972).
12. S. Chaudhuri, Platelet adhesiveness in the assessment of ischaemic heart disease. Thromb. Res. 6:208 (1975).
13. S.C. Sharma H.N. Seth, Platelet adhesiveness, plasma fibrinogen and fibrinolytic activity in acute myocardial infarction. Brit. Heart. J. 40:526 (1978).
14. K.K. Wu, J.C. Hoak, A new method for the quantitative detection of platelet aggregates in patients with arterial insufficiency. Lancet 2:924 (1974).
15. G. Hornstra, F. Ten Hoor, The filtragometer: a new device for measuring platelet aggregation in venous blood of man. Thromb. Diath. Haemorrh. 34:531 (1975).

16. K.K. Wu, J.C. Hoak, Spontaneous platelet aggregation in arterial insufficiency: mechanisms and implications. Thromb. Haemost. 35:702 (1976).
17. R.C. Paton, H. Lee, A. Thomaidis, P. Passa, J. Caen, ADP-induced aggregation and fibrinogen binding in platelets from diabetic patients. In: VI Int. Cong. on Thrombosis of the Med. League against Thromboemb. Dis. Montecarlo, October 23-25 (1980)
18. P. Mehta, J. Mehta, Platelet function studies in coronary heart disease: VIII. Decreased platelet sensitivity to prostacyclin in patients with myocardial ischaemia. Thromb. Res. 18:273 (1980).
19. J. Gormsen, J.B. Knudsen, J.D. Nielsen, O. Amtorp, K. Skagen, Platelet function, coagulation, fibrinolysis, factor XIII and antithrombin III in acute transmural myocardial infarction. In: Proc. of Florence Int. Meet. on Myoc. Inf. May 8-12, 1979, p. 233, Excerpta Medica, Amsterdam-Oxford-Princeton (1979).
20. G. Davì, S. Novo, F.P. Riolo, G. Avellone, Platelet aggregation in subjects with ischemic heart disease. In: Strano, A. (ed.) Advances in Coagulation, Fibrinolysis, Platelet Aggregation and Atherosclerosis, p. 372, CEPI, Roma (1976).
21. P. Mehta, J. Mehta, Platelet function studies in coronary artery disease: Evidence for enhanced platelet microthrombus formation activity in acute myocardial infarction. Am. J. Cardiol. 43:757 (1979).
22. A. Strano, S. Novo, G. Davì, G. Avellone, A. Pinto, Platelet aggregation, coagulation and fibrinolysis at rest and after bicycle ergometer test in CHD. In: Selected topics in exercise cardiology and rehabilitation (eds. A. Raineri, J.J. Kellermann, V. Rulli), Plenum Publishingn p. 265 (1980).
23. G. Davì, M. Traina, S. Novo, V. Albano, G.L. Piraino, M.P.Muzzo, G. Marano, A. Raineri, A. Strano, Platelet function changes in acute myocardial infarction. In: II Eur. Symp. on Coagulation, Platelet Function, Fibrinolysis and Vascular Diseases, Palermo, 5-8 December 1980.
24. M.J. Stuart, S. Murphy, F.A. Oski, A simple non radioisotope technic for the determination of platelet life-span. New. Engl. J. Med. 292:1310 (1975).
25. R. Roncucci, R. Deperon, J. Destailleur, J. Doumont, G. Lambelin J. Lansen, M. Moriau, F. Van Stalle, R. Vernaegher, Measurement of platelet regeneration time in cardiovascular patients. Thromb. Res. 14:3 (1979).
26. S.K. Garg, E.L. Amorosi, S. Karpatkin, Use of megathrombocytes as an index of megakaryocyte number. New. Engl. J. Med. 284:11 (1971).
27. P. Steele, J. Rainwater, R. Vogel, Abnormal platelet survival time in men with myocardial infarction and normal coronary arteriogram. Am. J. Cardiol. 41:60 (1978).
28. G.G. Neri Serneri, G.F. Gensini, R. Abbate, D. Prisco, C.

Mugnaini, Soluble fibrinogen complexes and platelet aggregates in patients with history of myocardial infarction and chronic cerebrovascular disorders. A rationale for prophylactic therapy. In: Strano A. (ed.) : Advances in Coagulation, Fibrinolysis, Platelet Aggregation and Atherosclerosis, p. 227, CEPI, Roma (1976).

29. G. Davì, F.P. Riolo, S. Novo, A. Pinto, G. Mendola, M.P. Muzzo, M. Russotto, Malondialdehyde formation and Beta-thromboglobulin levels in patients with diabetes mellitus. In: VI Int. Cong. on Thrombosis of the Med. League against Thromboemb. Dis. Montecarlo, October 23-25 (1980).
30. H.H. Salem, J. Koutts, B.G. Firkin, Circulating platelet aggregates in ischaemic heart disease and their correlation to platelet life span. Thromb. Res. 17:707 (1980).
31. J. Zahavi, V.V. Kakkar, Beta-thromboglobulin - a specific marker of in vivo platelet release reaction. Thromb. Haemost. 44: 23 (1980).
32. S. Moore, D.S. Pepper, J.D. Cash, The isolation and characterisation of a platelet specific Beta-thromboglobulin and the detection of antiurokinase and antiplasmin released from thrombin-aggregated washed human platelets. Bioch. Biophys. Acta 379:360 (1975).
33. C.A. Ludlam, S. Moore, A.E. Bolton, D.S. Pepper, J.D. Cash, The release of a human specific protein measured by a radioimmunoassay. Thromb. Res. 6:543 (1975).
34. K. Gjesdal, Platelet factor 4: an electroimmunoassay for PF4 in human plasma. Scand. J. Haemat. 13:232 (1974).
35. L.D. Witte, K.L. Kaplan, H.L. Nossel, B.A. Lages, H.J. Weiss, S.G. De Witt, Studies of the release from human platelets of the growth factor for cultured human arterial smooth muscle cells. Circ. Res. 42:402 (1978).
36. J.R. O'Brien, Antithrombin III and heparin clotting times in thrombosis and atherosclerosis. Thromb. Diath. Haemorrh. 32:116 (1974).
37. G. Pearson, Plasma factors regulating prostaglandin biosynthesisand metabolism. In: Int. Symp. "Prostaglandins and the Cardio-vascular system", Wiilrijk, December 1-3 (1980).
38. J. Zahavi, N.A.G. Jones, J. Leyton, M. Dubiel, V.V. Kakkar, Enhanced in vivo platelet release reaction in old healthy individuals. Thromb. Res. 17:329 (1980).
39. R.M. Hardisty R.A. Hutton, The kaolin clotting time of platelet-rich plasma. A test for platelet factor 3 availability. Br. J. Haemat. 11:258 (1965).
40. R.D. Shuttleworth, J.R. O'Brien, Intraplatelet serotonin and plasma 5-hydroxyindoles in health and disease. In: VI Int. Cong. on Thrombosis of the Med. League against Thromboemb. Dis. Montecarlo, October 23-25 (1980).
41. P. Needleman, M. Minkes, A. Raz, Tromboxanes: selective biosynthesis and distinct biological properties. Science 193: 163 (1979).

42. S. Moncada, J.R. Vane, Unstable metabolites of arachidonic acid and their role in haemostasis and thrombosis. Br. Med. Bull. 34:129 (1978).
43. J.B. Smith, C. Ingerman, M.J. Silver, Persistance of thromboxane A_2-like material and platelet release inducing activity in plasma. J. Clin. Invest. 58:1119 (1976).
44. E.W. Salzman, J.N. Lindon, R. Rodvien, Cyclic AMP in human blood platelets VI. Relation to platelet prostaglandin synthesis induced by centrifugation or surface contact. J. Cyc. Nucl. Res. 2:25 (1976).
45. C. Malmsten, E. Gränstrom, B. Samuelsson, Cyclic AMP inhibits synthesis of prostaglandins endoperoxide in human platelets. Biochim. Biophys. Res. Commun. 68:596 (1976).
46. G. Davì, A. Pinto, S. Novo, F. Riolo, A. Strano, 6-keto $PGF_{1\alpha}$ and TxB_2 formation in patients with claudicatio intermittens before and after dipyridamole. In: Int. Symp. "Prostaglandins and the Cardiovascular System", Wiilrijk, December 1-3 (1980).
47. E. Tremoli, G. Folco, E. Agradi, C. Galli, Platelet thromboxanes and serum cholesterol. Lancet 1:107 (1979).
48. E. Tremoli, P. Maderna, C.R. Sirtori, Platelet aggregation and MDA formation in type IIa hypercholesterolemic patients. Haemostasis 8:47 (1979).
49. M.J. Stuart, J.M. Gerrard, J.G. White, Effect of cholesterol on production of thromboxane B_2 by platelets in vitro. New. Engl. J. Med. 302:6 (1980).
50. R. Gryglewski, A. Szczeklik, Prostaglandins and atherosclerosis. In: Int. Sym. "Prostaglandins and the Cardiovascular System", Wiilrijk, December 1-3 (1980).
51. R.I. Lewy, B. Smith, M.J. Silver, J. Saia, P. Walinsky, L. Wiener, Detection of thromboxane B_2 in peripheral blood of patients with Prinzmetal's angina. Prostaglandins and Medicine 5:243 (1979).
52. J.B. Smith, Thromboxane release during pacing-induced angina pectoris: possible vasoconstrictor influence on the coronary vasculature. Circulation 61:1165 (1980).
53. G.G. Neri Serneri, Aterosclerosi e stati trombofolici. Ed. Pozzi, Roma (1979), p. 93.
54. J.C. Hoak, G.L. Fry, R.L. Czervionke, J.B. Smith, Haemostatic changes associated with acute myocardial infarction. In: Proc. of Florence Int. Meet. on Myocardial Infarction, May 8-12, 1979, p.290, Excerpta Medica, Amsterdam-Oxford-Princeton, (1979).
55. A. Strano, S. Novo, G. Davì, Prevenzione farmacologica della trombosi. In: Atti del Corso Int. "Cardiologia Preventiva", Catanzaro 29 Settembre - 3 Ottobre 1977. Ed: Piccin, Padova, p. 209.
56. A. Strano, G. Davì, S. Novo, Gli antiaggreganti piastrinici nella prevenzione dell'infarto del miocardio. Giorn.Arterioscl. 2:58 (1978).

57. A. Strano, S. Novo, F.P. Riolo, Quando e come usare gli antiaggreganti e gli anticoagulanti in cardiologia. In: Progressi in Cardiologia, ed. Pozzi, Roma, p. 420 (1978).
58. A. Strano, S. Novo, Prospettive nell'impiego degli antiaggreganti nella prevenzione dell'arteriosclerosi. Giorn. It. Card. IX, I, I (1980).

IMPAIRMENT OF FIBRINOLYSIS AND VASCULAR DISEASE

E.J.P. Brommer and P. Brakman

Gaubius Institute TNO
Herenstraat 5d, 2313 AD Leiden
The Netherlands

Among the proteolytic enzymes capable of resolving fibrin deposits in the body, plasmin appears to be the most important. Leucocyte proteases probably contribute to the resolution of thrombi and fibrin-rich exudates, but as yet their relevance to the removal of fibrin is less clear than that of "classical" fibrinolysis. In this paper the relation between vascular disease and classical i.e. plasmin-mediated fibrinolysis will be examined.

It is interesting to consider the old concept of the haemostatic balance in the light of recent knowledge. In this concept, fibrin deposition (coagulation) and its removal (fibrinolysis), which should maintain a dynamic equilibrium, were generally regarded as separate processes, though perhaps initiated by the same disturbance of the "*milieu interieur*". The activation was supposed to proceed, via its own pathway, to an extent which could or could not meet the demand. The release of tissue thromboplastin on one side and of plasminogen activator on the other formed the two arms of the balance (Astrup, 1967). For clinical conditions where fibrinolysis was thought to overshoot the demand, the term "hyperfibrinolysis" was introduced. The insight that in these cases intravascular coagulation and subsequent dissolution of fibrin provided an explanation of high levels of fibrin degradation products and of the disappearance of fibrinogen, plasminogen and clotting factors, did not change the concept. Terms like "secondary fibrinolysis" and "hyperfibrinolysis" are firmly rooted in clinical medicine. Several theories were postulated to explain the relative specificity of plasmin generated during the fibrinolytic events, for its natural substrate fibrin.

We have now come to realize that the onset of the fibrinolytic process is closely linked to the formation of fibrin, as already postulated by Nolf (1908). Both (lys-)plasminogen (Thorsen, 1975) and the circulating plasminogen activator (Fearnley, 1953; Thorsen et al., 1972) have an affinity for fibrin. As soon as fibrin is being formed in the blood, plasminogen and its converting enzyme stick to the surface of fibrin where conditions are optimal for their interaction. At this site the plasmin will be formed and in this way fibrin initiates its own destruction. The breakdown of fibrin is tempered by inhibitors present in the blood, as for instance α_2-antiplasmin (Collen, 1980) or by extravascular inhibitors, such as those extractable from various tissues (Kawano, 1968; Uszynski & Abildgaard, 1971; Bernik & Kwaan, 1971). Plasmin generation depends on the presence of plasminogen and its activator, on the concentration of inhibitors present, and on the presence of a triggering surface, i.e. fibrin. Theoretically, changes of any of these factors in the blood could modify the survival time of fibrin in the body and thereby influence all processes involving fibrin depositions, among which are thrombosis and atherosclerosis.

Abnormalities of fibrinolytic factors

In the blood of a normal individual the plasminogen concentration is fairly constant. Fibrinolysis will be hampered when the plasminogen concentration is very low, that is in the order of 30% of normal or less. Apart from thrombolytic therapy, such levels occur in severe liver disease and during acute defibrination. In these conditions multiple changes occur in the plasma protein levels - including clotting factors and inhibitors - and no single abnormality can be incriminated for the ensuing disturbance, resulting in either thrombosis or bleeding.

Congenitally abnormal plasminogen molecules have been described in patients admitted for treatment of thrombosis (Aoki et al., 1978; Robbins, Wohl & Summaria, 1979). A casual relationship has been suggested.

A higher than normal concentration of inhibitors of fibrinolysis might contribute to the development of thrombosis. The rising antiplasmin level found after trauma is thought to be responsible for multiple pulmonary microemboli resulting in a respiratory distress syndrome (Saldeen, 1976). This inhibitor is probably identical to α_2-antiplasmin (Bagge et al., 1979). Other, ill-defined inhibitory substances detectable in the blood of patients with thrombosis (Brakman et al., 1966; Astrup & Brakman, 1970) and of patients with malignant diseases (Hisazumi et al., 1974) may promote thrombosis by interfering with fibrin dissolution. Inglesby et al. (1973) described abnormal fibrinolysis in familial pulmonary hypertension. In all members studied, "antiplasmin" levels were abnormally elevated and it was suggested that this was related to an impaired ability to lyse recurrent pulmonary microemboli.

Thrombosis in connection with factor XII-deficiency has been noted several times since the publication of the thromboembolic events complicating the terminal illness of Mr. Hageman (Ratnoff, 1968). This, together with the observation of thrombosis in patients with antibody against factor XII (Hedner & Nilsson, 1976) or with an inhibitor against this factor (Hedner, 1973) this might indicate that factor XII is more important for fibrinolysis than for coagulation.

Regulation of plasminogen activator level

The most erratic compound of the fibrinolytic system is the enzyme responsible for the conversion of plasminogen to plasmin. This so-called plasminogen-activator is not a single entity. Two types of activator activity are discernable in the blood. One is derived from vascular endothelium (extrinsic activator) and the other from inactive precursors in the blood (intrinsic system). The extrinsic activator is very closely related to an activator which is extractable from tissue as shown by Rijken et al. (1980). Their studies confirm earlier evidence that the greater part of the resting fibrinolytic activity in blood is derived from a circulating proenzyme (Kluft, 1978). Quenching of the extrinsic activator by means of an antibody also extinguished the intrinsic activity of euglobulin fractions (Rijken, 1980). Obviously, the intrinsic system is activated via the extrinsic activator and this effect occurs only in the presence of fibrin. Baseline levels in normal resting persons, expressed in arbitrary blood activator units (BAU), are 1-2 BAU/ml. In healthy individuals this activity increases two or three-fold during the day in a diurnal rhythm. After certain stimuli, e.g., strenuous exercise, venous congestion of the arm or certain vasoactive drugs, the extrinsic activator can increase to 150 BAU/ml (Kluft, 1979). Nevertheless, even in the presence of such high levels of plasminogen activator, plasminogen is not converted to plasmin in the circulating blood or in vitro unless fibrin is present. The intrinsic system can be activated by dextran sulphate (Astrup & Rosa, 1974). The maximum activity to be obtained from this system is fairly constant among different individuals and does not change during the day or after stimuli; it has been estimated to be about 100 BAU/ml (Kluft, 1979).

Impaired plasminogen activator release

We can only guess at the purpose which the high concentration of plasminogen activator serves in conditions of stress and physical exercise. In theory, the higher the concentration of the enzyme, the faster the removal of fibrin. Perhaps, the effect of local concentrations of inhibitors can only be overcome in this way. Cash (1968) drew attention to the possibility that lack of such a response was related to a tendency to develop thrombotic disease. Indeed, a subnormal response to various stimuli has been described in patients with thrombosis (Isacson & Nilsson, 1972; Johansson et al., 1978).

Since factor XII is involved in the activation of the intrinsic system of fibrinolysis, the aforementioned occurrence of thrombosis in factor XII-deficiency or in subjects with inhibitors against factor XII, suggests that an abnormal intrinsic system may also predispose to thrombosis.

Not only thrombosis but also atherosclerotic cardiovascular disease might be aggravated by a delay in the removal of fibrin. The thrombogenic theory on the pathogenesis of atherosclerosis, proposed by Rokitansky (1852) and Duguid (1949) has lately received support from an epidemiological study (Meade et al., 1980). Haemostatic function was found to correlate with cardiovascular disease even better than cholesterol levels. Likewise, too slow a removal of fibrin might increase the risk by allowing a mural thrombus to settle permanently. In the study of Meade et al. fibrinolytic activity was also measured. In those individuals who eventually died of cardiovascular causes, fibrinolytic activity was found to be lowest. However, the difference in the values between those patients and the survivors was not statistically significant. Though more pronounced abnormalities have been found by others studying atherosclerosis (Peabody et al-, 1974) in all these studies only the spontaneous fibrinolytic activity has been assayed and is known to be linked to the physical and mental condition of the subject under investigation and upon the time of day.

The reaction to the aforementioned stimuli or the diurnal variation would probably give more information about the functioning of the fibrinolytic system. In elderly people more often than in young healthy individuals a subnormal diurnal rise of fibrinlytic activity was demonstrated by Rosing et al. (1973). Measuring physiological diurnal variation of the fibrinolytic activity would probably be the most natural way to obtain insight into its regulation. However, it has never been widely used because of its practical disadvantages.

Among patients with hyperlipoproteinemia type IV, who are predisposed to contract cardiovascular disease, Epstein et al. (1970) found a low response after stimulation of the fibrinolytic system by strenuous exercise.

Several other stimuli have been used in patients with vascular disease as a means of determining the fibrinolytic capacity, i.e. the ability of the body to respond to a certain challenge with a rise of the plasminogen activator concentration. In our opinion, venous occlusion does not come up to the requirements of such challenge because too many apparently normal, healthy subjects respond poorly if at all.

Recently, a new agent has been introduced for the stimulation of the fibrinolytic system: 1-desamino-8-D-arginine-vasopressine (DDAVP, Minirin®). This vasopressine-analogue, used as a substitute for the antidiuretic hormone, appears to release both clotting factor VIII and plasminogen activator from the vascular endothelium (Aberg et al., 1979). Abnormally low responses have been described in patients suffering from von Willebrand's disease (Ludlam et al., 1980; Nilsson et al., 1980) and in patients with thrombosis (Johansson et al., 1978). We tested the fibrinolytic capacity of hyperlipoproteinemic patients with infusion of DDAVP: 9 patients out of 23 showed a subnormal response or no response, whereas among 12 normal volunteers only one poor responder was found (Brommer, Barret, Gevers Leuven, in preparation). There was no correlation between the response of the fibrinolytic activity, measured with the fibrin plate method (Haverkate & Brakman 1975), and the lipoprotein concentration, irrespective of the type of hyperlipoproteinemia. Interestingly, factor VIII concentration rose in all subjects tested with DDAVP, indicating an imbalance between coagulation and fibrinolysis under challenging conditions in the majority of the hyperlipoproteinemic patients.

Conclusion

The evidence is accumulating to confirm that tipping of the haemostatic balance to the side of coagulation, either by high levels of clotting factors or by a thwarted activation of fibrinolysis, promotes not only thrombosis but also atherosclerosis. As discussed already by Cash in 1968, a disequilibrium might arise in some people merely during mental anxiety or physical exercise, when the generation of plasminogen activator lags behind the increase of coagulability of the blood. These people might be predisposed to contract thrombotic diseases. With the aid of DDAVP this situation has now been documented by us during the investigation of patients with hyperlipoproteinemia and with recurrent, spontaneous thrombosis. A subnormal response to venous occlusion has been observed in patients with coronary artery disease (Gritsyuk & Schigelski, 1979).

Perhaps physical conditioning can decrease the risk of cardiovascular death by enhancing the fibrinolytic capacity (Williams et al., 1980). The use of stimulation tests in prospective studies will be of great help in unravelling the influence of fibrinolysis upon atherosclerosis.

REFERENCES

Aberg, M., Nilsson, I.M., Vilhardt, H. The release of fibrinolytic activator and factor VIII after injection of DDAVP. p. 92-97. In:Progress in Chemical Fibrinolysis and Thrombolysis, Vol.4, Eds.: Davidson, Cepezak, Samama, Desnoyers, Churchill Livingstone, 1979, Edimburgh/London/New York.

Aoki, N., Moroi, M., Sakada, Y., Yoshida, N, & Matsuda, M.1978, Abnormal plasminogen. A hereditary molecular abnormality found in a patient with recurrent thrombosis.J. Clin. Invest., 61: 1186-1195.

Astrup, T.Blood coagulation, fibrinolysis and the development of the thrombogenic theory of arteriosclerosis. In: Le rôle de la paroi artérielle dans l'athérogénèse. 1976. Centre. Nat. Rech. Sc.

Astrup, T., & Rosa, A.T. 1974. A plasminogen proactivator-activator system in human blood effective in absence of Hageman factor. Thromb. Res. 4: 609-613.

Bagge, L., Carlin, G., Hjelmstedt, A., Hogstorp, Jacobsson, H., Modig, J., Saldeen, T. 1979. Fibrinolysis inhibition after a standardized trauma, total hip replacement sur-

gery. Thromb. Haemost. 42: 278 (abstract).
Bernik, M.B. & Kwaan, H.C. 1971. Inhibitors of fibrinolysis in human tissues in culture. Am. J. Physiol. 221: 916.
Brakman, p., Mohler, E.R. & Astrup, T. 1966. A group of patients with impaired plasma fibrinolytic system and selective inhibition of tissue activator-induced fibrinolysis. Scand. J. Haematol. 3: 389-398.
Brakman, P. & Astrup, T. Selective inhibition of tissue plasminogen activator in thrombotic disease. In: Abstract volume XIII Intern. Congr. Haemat. Munich. p.173. (1970).
Cash, J. 1968. A new approach to studies of the fibrinolytic enzyme system in man. Am. Heart J. 75: 424-427.
Collen, D. 1980. On the regulation and control of fibrinolysis. Thromb. & Haemost. 43: 77-89.
Duguid, J.B. 1949. Pathogenesis of arteriosclerosis. Lancet 2: 925.
Epstein, S.E., Rosing, D.R., Brakman, P., Redwood, D.R., Astrup, T. 1970. Impaired fibrinolytic response in patients with type IV hyperlipoproteinemia. Lancet 2: 631-634.
Fearnley, G.R. 1953. Fibrinolysis by adsorption. Nature (London) 172: 544.
Gritsyuk, A.I. & Schigelsky, V.I. 1979. Evaluation of blood coagulation and prethrombotic state in patients with coronary atherosclerosis by application of controlled local venous blokade. Circ. 60: 220 A.
Haverkate, F. & Brakman, P. In: Progress in chemical fibrinolysis and thrombolysis. Eds.: Davidson, J.F., Samama, M.M. & Desnoyers, P.C. Raven Press NY, 1975, p.151. Fibrin Plate assay.
Hender, U. 1973. Studies on an inhibitor of plasminogen activator in human serum. Thromb. Diath. Haemorrh. 30: 414-424.
Hender, U. & Nilsson, I.M. Acquired anticoagulants against factors XI and XII in patients with severe thrombotic disease. In: XVI Intern. Cong. Haematol. Kyoto. Sept. 1976 Abstract 8-88, p. 341.
Hisazumi, H., Naoito, K., Misaki, T., Kosaka, S. 1974. Urokinase inhibitor in patients with bladder cancer. Urological Research 2: 137-142.
Inglesby, T.V., Singer, J.W., Gordon, D.S. 1973. Abnormal fibrinolysis in familial pulmonary hypertension. Am. J. Med. 55: 5-14.
Isacson, S. & Nilsson, I.M. 1972. Defective fibrinolysis in blood and vein walls in recurrent "idiopathic" venous thrombosis. Acta Chir. Scand. 138: 313.
Johansson, L., Hender, U., Nilsson, I.M. A family with thromboembolic disease associated with deficient fibrinolytic activity in vessel wall. Acta Med. Scand. 203: 477-480.
Kawano, T., Morimoto, K. & Vemura, Y. 1968. Urokinase inhibitor in human placenta. Nature 217: 253.
Kluft, C. 1978. Levels of plasminogen activators in human plasma:

new methods to study the intrinsic and extrinsic activators. In: Progress in chemical fibrinolysis and thrombolysis, Vol.3. Eds.: Davidson, Rowan, Samama & Desnoyers. Raven Press NY, p. 141-154.

Kluft, C. 1979. Studies on the fibrinolytic system in human plasma: Quantitative determination of plasminogen activators and proactivators. Thrombos. Haemostas. 41: 365-383.

Ludlam, C.A., Peake, I.R., Allen, N., Davies, B.L., Furlong, R.A., Bloom, A.L. 1980. Factor VIII and fibrinolytic response to deamino-8-D-arginine vasopressin in normal subjects and dissociate response in some patients with haemophilia and von Willebrand's disease. Brit. J. Haemat. 45:499-511.

Meade, T.W., North, W.R.S., Chakrabarti, S., Stirling, Y., Haines, A.P., Thompson, S.G., Brozovic, M. 1980. Haemostatic function and cardiovascular death; early results of a prospective study. Lancet 1: 1050-1054.

Nilsson, I.M., Holmberg, L., Aberg, M., Vilhardt, H. 1980. The release of plasminogen activator and factor VIII after injection of DDAVP in healthy volunteers and in patients with von Willebrand's disease. Scan. J. Haematol. 24: 351-359.

Nolf; P. 1908. Contribution à l'étude de la coagulation du sang. La fibrinolyse. Arch. Int. Physiol. 6: 306-359.

Peabody, R.A., Tsapogas, M.J., Kwang-Tzen, W. 1974. Altered endogenous fibrinolysis and biochemical factors in atherosclerosis. Arch. Surg. 109: 309.

Ratnoff, O.D., Busse, R.J. & Sheon, R.P. 1968. The demise of John Hageman. N. Engl. J. Med. 279: 760.

Rosing, D.R., Redwood, D.R., Brakman, P., Astrup, T. & Epstein, S.E. 1973. Impairment of the diurnal fibrinolytic response in man. Effects of aging, type IV hyperlipoproteinemia, and coronary heart disease. Circ. Res. 32: 752-758.

Rijken, D.C. 1980. Thesis Leiden. Plasminogen activator from human tissue.

Rijken, D.C., Wijngaards, G., Welbergen, J. 1980. Relationship between tissue plasminogen activator and the activators in blood and vascular wall. Thromb. Res. 18: 815-830.

Robbins, K.C., Wohl, R.C., Summaria, L. 1979. Variant plasminogens in patients with history of venous thrombosis. Thromb. Haemost. 42: 190. Abstract London.

Rokitansky, K. von. Über einige der wichtigsten Krankheiten der Arterien. Meidingen, Vienna, 1852.

Saldeen, T. 1976. The microembolic syndrome. Microvasc. Res. 11: 227.

Thorsen, S., Glas-Greenwalt, P. & Astrup, T. 1972. Differences in the binding to fibrin of urokinase and tissue plasminogen activator. Thromb. Diath. Haemorrh.28: 65-74.

Thorsen, S. 1975. Differences in the binding to fibrin of native plasminogen modified by proteolytic degradation. Biochim. Biophys. Acta 393: 55-65.

Uszynski, M. & Abildgaard, U. 1971. Separation and characterization of two fibrinolytic inhibitors from human placenta. Thromb. Diath. Haemorrh. 25: 580.

Williams, R.S., Logue, E.E., Lewis, J.J., Barton, T., Stead, N. W., Wallace, A.G. & Pizzo, S.V. 1980. Physical conditioning augments the fibrinolytic response to venous occlusion in healthy adults. N. Engl. J. Med. 303: 987-991.

PART 2

COAGULATION AND VASCULAR DISEASES

ANTITHROMBIN III AND ATHEROSCLEROSIS

J. Conard, M. Castel, and M. Samama

Laboratoire Central d'Eématologie - Hôtel Dieu
Place du Parvis Notre Dame, 1
75004 Paris, France

The mechanisms leading to the initiation of atherosclerosis are very complex. Since Duguid's modification of Rokitansky's theory, atherosclerosis has been related to thrombogenesis. Several investigators proposed the clumping of platelets to play a crucial role in the initiation of atheroma formation. When platelets are stimulated, they release polypeptide that is mitogenic to smooth muscle cells.

Apart from platelets, the role of blood coagulation has not been well defined. However, a theory has been developed by Kadish (1), proposing that mural fibrin in vivo may produce a disorganized endothelium which can act as a nidus for further fibrin deposition and platelet aggregation. In the presence of inadequate fibrinolysis, a prolonged endothelial lesion could occur, which may eventually result in atheromatous plaque formation.

As the formation of fibrin is related to the concentration in coagulation inhibitors, a decrease in these inhibitors, and specially in antithrombin III (AT III), could possibly play a role in atherosclerosis.

Antithrombin III is the main physiological inhibitor of blood coagulation, the congenital deficiency of which is usually associated with venous thromboses. Among the 40 families published, 123 subjects have experienced venous thrombosis and 4 patients only had arterial thrombosis: arterial occlusion of the limbs in 2, coronary thrombosis before 40 in another 2 (2).

AT III and risk factors for atherosclerosis

The following factors are generally accepted as risk factors for atherosclerosis:

- age
- sex (Males and coronary heart disease)

- hypercholesterolemia
- hypertension (particularly for cerebro-vascular disease)
- diabetes mellitus
- cigarette smoking
- family history
- obesity, physical activity...

Some studies are available concerning AT III and some of the risk factors.

1 - AT III and age. It is generally accepted that AT III decreases with increasing age (3,4) and this finding is observed in men only. Some discrepancies have been observed with the different methods used for AT III determination: Meade et al. (4) found a decrease in AT III protein with increasing age in men between 18 and 64, while there was no statistically significant modification of the AT III activity. In our group, the same type of results were observed in 30 subjects above 80: the plasma AT III determined by the Mancini method was decreased as compared to young subjects, but the decrease found with the amidolytic method was not statistically significant (Table I).

Table I. AT III in subjects over 80

	YOUNG SUBJECTS n = 26	OLD SUBJECTS n = 30
AGE (years)	26 ± 4	85 ± 6
AT III ACTIVITY (chromo ym TH)	103 ± 13	97 ± 13
AT III protein(mg/dl) (Mancini)	30.6 ± 2.5	26.5 ± 3.2*

Mean values ± S.D.
*Statistically significant difference ($p<0.05$)

2 - AT III and sex. At III is said to be lower in women in fertile age than in men (3), but men are more prone to artherosclerosis.

3 - AT III and hyperlipoproteinemia. Carvalho et al. (5) have evaluated AT III in 30 patients with type II or IV familial hyperlipoproteinemia. Half the patinets had clinical evidence of atherosclerosis. AT III measured by radial immunodiffusion, was increased in type II

(mean AT III = 136%) as well as type IV hyperlipoproteinemia (mean AT III = 126%). The authors suggested that the increase in AT III could be a response to an increased production of thrombin through a feedbeck mechanism which increased synthesis or decreased catabolism of AT III.

4 - AT III and diabetes mellitus. Conflicting results have been published. A decrease in AT III has been found by some authors in maturity onset diabetes (6,7). In contrast, an increase has been reported in children (8) and in adults (9,10). Moreover, according to Fuller et al. (10), diabetics with retinopathy have higher values than those without this vascular complication.

AT III in myocardial infarction

In acute myocardial infarction, an increase in AT III has been reported in the 3 to 5 days following the attack (11, 12, 13). However, in patients studied long after myocardial infarction, a decrease has been observed (6, 14) men only (14).

AT III, coronary heart disease and angiographic findings

Innerfield et al. (15) have measured serum AT activity in 69 patients with documented angina pectoris and have compared the results with coronary angiograms. They found a good correlation between normal AT III values and normal angiogram or with only one-vessel stenosis (in 30 of the 35 patients with normal AT). In contrast, AT activity was decreased in 24 patients and in 21 of them, a 2 or 3 vessel occlusion was observed on the angiogram.

Stormorken and Erikssen (16) have published the results of a prospective study on latent coronary heart disease (CHD) in 2.014 presumably healthy men. In 115 patients, there was strong clinical evidence of CHD, so that coronary angiography was performed in 105. In 80 of these 105 patients, plasma AT III activity was measured: it was significantly lower (mean AT III = 86.1%) in patients with positive angiography than in the normal controls. In addition, in the group of positive angiography, AT III was significantly lower in patients with angina pectoris (mean AT III = 80.0%) than without (mean AT III = 91.0%). It was suggested that the low level of AT III in patients with angina could reflect a slow ongoing intravascular coagulation with increased AT III consumption.

AT III and cardiovascular death

In an epidemiologic prospective study, Meade et al. (17) have measured different haemostatic parameters in 1,510 men; 27 of them died from cardiovascular disease. There was no statistical difference in the AT III level in the survivors (mean AT III = 98.1%) and in the 27 who died later from cardiovascular disease (mean AT III = 95.8%).

Another epidemiologic study was recently presented at the Monte Carlo Congress of thrombosis by Wahlberg et al. (18). In Edimburgh, where the mortality from ischemic heart disease is 3 times greater than in Stockholm, a tendency for higher levels of AT III was observed.

Conclusion

It is now well established that a congenital decrease in AT III is a predisposing factor for venous thrombosis, but the role of this inhibitor in atherosclerosis is not clear.

Decreases, as well as increases, in AT III have been reported in conditions associated with atherosclerosis. A decrease in AT III might be considered as a cause of thrombosis, or could be the result of an increased consumption. In contrast, an increase in AT III might be considered as a response to thrombosis. However, any modification of AT III might have some significance since its normal range is so narrow. Thus, although AT III does not seem, at first, to have a crucial role in atherosclerosis, more prospective studies are still needed.

REFERENCES

1. J.L. Kadish, Fibrin and atherosclerosis. A hypothesis. Atherosclerosis 33:409-413 (1979).
2. J. Conard, Congenital AT III deficiency. In: abstract book VIème Congrès International sur la Thrombose, p.94 (1980).
3. O.R. Odegard, M.K. Fagerhol, M. Lie, Heparin cofactor activity and antithrombin III concentration in plasma related to age and sex. Scand. J. Haematol. 17:258-262 (1976).
4. T.W. Meade, W.R.S. North, Population-based distributions of haemostatic variables. Brit. Med. Bull. 33:283-288 (1977).
5. A.C. Carvalho, R.S. Lees, R.A. Vaillancourt, R.B. Cabral, R.M. Weinberg, R.W. Colman, Intravascular coagulation in hyperlipidemia. Thrombos Res. 8:843-857 (1976).
6. R.N. Banerjee, A.L. Sahni, V. Kumar, M. Arya, Antithrombin III deficiency in maturity onset diabetes mellitus and atherosclerosis. Thrombos. Diathes. Haemorrh. 31:339-344 (1974).
7. G. Follea, Antithrombine III et diabète sucré. Thèse Doct. Méd. Montpellier 1976.
8. E. Corbella, G. Miragliotta, R. Masperi, S. Villa, A. Bini, G. De Gaetano, G. Chiumello, Platelet aggregation and AT III levels in the diabetic children. Haemostasis 8:30-37 (1979).
9. J. Conard, P. Barbier, M. Samama, Automated amidolytic method for AT III determination. Thrombos. Haemostas. 4:1350-1352 (1979).

10. J.H. Fuller, H. Keen, R.J. Jarret, T. Omer, T.W. Meade, R. Chakrabarti, W.R.S. North, Y. Stirling, Haemostatic variables associated with diabetes and its complications. Brit. Med. J. 2:964-966 (1979).
11. H.W. Pratt, Alterations in plasma antithrombin III activity in patients with myocardial infarction. In: abstract book Int. Soc. Thrombos. Haemostas. Washington D.C., p.404 (1980).
12. U. Hedner, I.M. Nilsson, Antithrombin III in clinical material. Thrombos. Res. 3:631-641 (1973).
13. R.H. Yue, M.M. Gertler, T. Staar, R. Koutrouby, Alteration of plasma antithrombin III levels in ischemic heart disease. Thrombos Haemostas. 35:598-606 (1976).
14. J.R. O'Brien, Antithrombin III and heparin clotting times in thrombosis and atherosclerosis. Thromb. Diathes. Haemorrh. 32:116-123 (1974).
15. I. Innerfield, J.D. Goldfisher, H. Reicherreiss, J. Greenberg, Serum antithrombin in coronary artery disease. Am. J. Clin. Pathol. 65:64-68 (1976).
16. H. Stormorken, J. Erikssen, Plasma antithrombin III and factor VIII antigen in relation to angiographic findings, angina and blood groups in middle-aged men. Thrombos. Haemostas. 38:874-880 (1977).
17. T.W. Meade, W.R.S. North, R. Chakrabarti, Y. Stirling, A.P. Haines, S.G. Thompson, M. Brozovic, Haemostatic function and cardiovascular death: early results of a prospective study. Lancet 1:1050-1054 (1980).
18. T.B. Wahlberg, M. Blomback, J. Cash, Risk factors for ischemic heart disease reflected by six blood coagulation variables. Population comparisons between males, aged forty, from Edimburgh and Stockholm. In: abstract book VIème Congrès International sur la Thrombose, Monte-Carlo, p. 229 (1980).

FACTOR VIII AND ANTITHROMBIN III IN ATHEROSCLEROSIS OBLITERANS OF THE LOWER LIMBS

G. Avellone, V. Mandalà, S. Novo, A. Pinto, F.P. Riolo, F. Cannioto, and G. Raneli

Institute of Clinical Medicine and Medical Therapy
University of Palermo
Piazza delle Cliniche, 2
90127 Palermo - Italy

In the multifactorial pathogenesis of atherosclerosis (the W.H.O. gives a list of about forty risk factors) recent acquisitions have allowed to determine in part the role carried out by the term "haemocoagulative disorders" (90) showing the possible connections between haematic components of haemocoagulation and vascular wall that up to now have been only hypothesised.

It is now well known that clinical manifestations of atherosclerosis are associated with a syndrome of haematic hypercoagulability characterized by a platelet hyperactivity, an increase of fibrin-formation processes and by a reduced fibrinolytic activity (3, 5, 9, 30, 34, 60, 61, 69, 75, 81, 82, 88, 89). This syndrome accounts not only for occlusive thrombotic events of the vascular lumen that often complicate the course of the vasculopathy, (21, 22, 35, 96) but also for the progressiveness of the parietal lesion characterized by thickenings of the vessel intima and atheromatous plaques (20, 21, 53, 80, 102).

The syndrome caused by the activation of fibrinogenic processes has its pathogenesis in the thrombinic effect. In fact, the changes that can be seen in association with the atherosclerotic vasculopathy are the result of a chronic activation of haemocoagulation with an increased thrombin formation. The latter generated by the action of F. Xa on prothrombin catalyzes the transformation of fibrinogen into fibrin (soluble), whose entity is related to the speed with which it is generated and the concentration reached. The physiological inhibitors of thrombin, antithrombins, carry out a limiting role on the thrombin/fibrinogen reaction, and, among these, antithrombin III represents the specific antiprotease apt to modulate not only the action of thrombin on fibrinogen but also to inhibit some factors above the activated factor X: F.XIa, F. IXa and F. VIIIa (10, 23, 77, 78). Other physiological antiproteases, like alpha-1-antitripsin have an anithrombinic action, but their major activity is for the plasmin substrate, though the possibility of their intervention in a situation of accelerated thrombin formation cannot be left out (2, 54, 63, 64).

From the moment that the thrombin formation speed/antithrombin activity ratio represents the physiopathological moment for the manifestation of acute and chronic haemocoagulative situations (thrombosis and/or hypercoagulability) it is possible to identify an increase of thrombin formation through the effects induced by thrombin on the kinetics of antithrombins, on the enzymatic activity of those coagulation factors sensible to the action of thrombin, and on platelet reactivity.

Thrombin, at very low concentrations, is able to render platelets hyper-reactive, (12, 82) stimulating the synthesis of endoperoxides with thromboxane A_2 formation which has an aggregating and vasoconstrictive action (66, 91, 94). It has also been shown that in atherosclerosis, together with this platelet hyper-reactivity, there is a platelet secretion caused by thrombin, with a release, in plasma, of the intraplatelet granuli content (39) constituted by antiheparin factor, beta thromboglobulin and the factor stimulating the growth of the subintimal smooth muscle fibres (50, 58, 59, 62, 79, 84, 104, 105). This factor is deemed responsible for the intimal thickenings and for the evaluation of the arterial wall damage (4, 20, 36, 80, 103, 106). This platelet component can be correlated to the haemorheological one of the arterial district, where high shear stresses push platelets against the endothelial surface determining a stronger stimulus to adhesiveness and aggregability with formation of parietal platelet/fibrin microthrombi and release of intraplatelet factors.

An acceleration of enzymatic kinetics with an increase of the coagulant activity of factors V, VIII and XIII (47) is provoked, and anyway only for very low concentrations, on the coagulation factors sensible to the action of thrombin. On fibrinogen, instead, low concentrations of thrombin cause a partial degradation of the molecule, through the detachment of fibrinopeptide A (50, 71) and the consequent release of fibrinmonomer. The latter for concentrations over 1/5 of total fibrinogen can give origin (8, 31, 51) to big molecular aggregates (68, 70) (soluble complexes of fibrinogen at high molecular weight HMWFC) that render the coagulative system unstable and interfere negatively on blood fluidity (31).

The increase of fibrinogen soluble complexes and of fibrinopeptide A has been reported in patients with clinical and angiographical signs of coronary atherosclerosis (67, 68).

Recent acquisitions have also enabled to identify in the "factor VIII" three subcomponents: F. VIII R:AG (secrete by vascular endothelium cells) (18, 43, 44, 45, 46, 64), F. VIII R:vW (produced by endothelial cells and responsible for platelet adhesiveness) (9, 14, 18, 37, 38, 73, 95), F. VIII R:C (subcomponent of hepatic synthesis and responsible for the coagulant activity of F. VIII)

(40, 65, 68). These, because of their site of synthesis and because of a different sensibility to thrombin (57, 92) (the first one is not sensible while the other two show an increasing sensibility respectively), constitute a diagnostic support to the identification of a state of activation of the coagulative system on a thrombin base and of a pathological alteration of the endothelial vascular surface (9, 16, 17, 29, 60, 59, 85). The determination of these subcomponents of F. VIII has, therefore, been proposed in order to evalue the entity of the endothelial damage in atherosclerosis and of the coagulation activation syndrome associated to the former.

Marked changes, characterized by an increase of the three subcomponents of F. VIII, have been found in patients suffering from coronary atherosclerosis (stable angina, unstable angina, history of myocardial infarction) (68).

To these actions of thrombin, which amplify the processes of fibrin formation, is opposed the action of thrombin inhibitors, and among these antithrombin III or heparin cofactor is able to inhibit (with a "slow" kind kinetics) (1, 2) rising formations of thrombin and of F. Xa (74, 103, 107). In the presence even of slight traces of heparin this antithrombin activity becomes "instantaneous" (76,77) constituting a compensatory mechanism among the most efficacious in preventing an excessive fibrin formation (93). In the states of coagulation activation on a thrombin base, like in atherosclerosis, platelet secretion with consequent release of platelet factor 4, while it inactivates the heparin/heparin co-factor system (19, 72, 93), imposes to antithrombin III a slow kind kinetics, with a reduction of its plasmatic concentration and of its enzymatic activity (5, 6, 7, 68).

In atherosclerosis in fact, reduced plasmatic levels of protein and of biological activity have been found and interpreted as an indirect index of the accelerated thrombin production and of the process leading to the formation of F. Xa (5, 6, 7, 68, 86, 87).

We have therefore carried out a survey on the behaviour of F. VIII and of its three components and also of the biological activity of antithrombin III in patients suffering from atherosclerosis obliterans of the lower limbs, evaluating at the same time the entity in relation to the clinical symptomatology and to the stage of the disease according to Fontaine.

MATERIALS AND METHODS

We have studied 92 patients (61 males and 31 females) suffering from atherosclerosis obliterans of the lower limbs. According to the clinical symptomatology and after flow examination (strain gauge) the patients were divided into three groups corresponding to the stages II, III and IV of the international clinico-functional classification of atherosclerosis obliterans of the lower limbs (Fontaine). In the II stage group were 38 patients aged between 40 and 58 years (average age = 46.2; in the III stage group 33 patients aged between 51 and 70 years (average age = 59.15) and in the IV stage group 21 subjects aged between 64 and 76 years (average age = 70.09); healthy controls of equivalent age and sex were matched to the above patients. Pharmacological treatment was suspended or reduced to the use of analgesics only in the immediate days before blood sampling (3.5 days on the average).

Blood samples, for all patients, have been taken after a fasting period of 12 hours, without having smoked, at rest, without stasis and with the double syringe technique. All the samples were taken with polypropilene syringes, using as anticoagulant sodium citrate 0.11 mol/l sterile (blood/anticoagulant ratio 9/1). All laboratory exams have been carried out within 4 hours of blood sampling and using polypropilene test tubes and containers.

On each sample we have determined F. VIII in its three subcomponents: F. VIII R:AG - F. VIII R:vW - F. VIII R:C, and the biological activity of antithrombin III.

For F. VIII R:C we have used the two time method described by Denson (25, 26, 27, 28); for F. VIII R:AG, immunoelectophoresis according to Laurell (32, 55, 56); for F. VIII R:vW, Weiss' method (101) preparing the platelet suspension with platelets washed according to Walsh's technique (99, 100). Antithrombin III, as antithrombin activity, has been determined, according to Von Kaulla's method (98), on serum obtained from 3 ml of whole blood set in a glass test tube and left to coagulate at room temperature.

For statistical calculations we have used Student's "t" test and the correlation index "r".

RESULTS

In all the patients suffering from atherosclerosis obliterans of the lower limbs the three subcomponents of F. VIII showed changes characterized by a constant increase, and particularly of F. VIII R:C (Fig. 1).

F. VIII R:AG showed an increase of 35.15% (arteriopathic patients $\bar{x}$ 232.45 S.D. 63.76 - controls $\bar{x}$ 171.97 S.D. 45.75); F. VIII R:vW showed an increase of 35.23% (arteriopathic patients $\bar{x}$ 169.08 S.D. 29.92 - controls $\bar{x}$ 125.03 S.D. 17.44); F. VIII R:C showed the highest increase, 89.60%, (arteriopathic patients $\bar{x}$ 330.55 S.D. 74.45 - controls $\bar{x}$ 174.34 S.D. 46.61). Dividing the patients in relation to the clinico-functional stages of the arteriopathy it becomes evident that the three subcomponents of F. VIII show a higher increase in the more advanced stages of the arteriopathy. F. VIII R:AG (Fig 2), in fact, in the patients at II stage, was on the average 214.18% (S.D. 53.62), 239.21% (S.D. 43.65) at III stage and 273.00% (S.D. 70.79) at IV stage, even though there is a certain overlapping of values in the single subjects, especially at III and IV stage. F. VIII R:vW (Fig. 3) showed, in the patients at II stage, a mean value of 154.36% (S.D. 16.85), of 172.06% (S.D. 13.99) at III stage and of 207.33% (S.D. 24.82) at IV stage, pointing out also a good discrimination

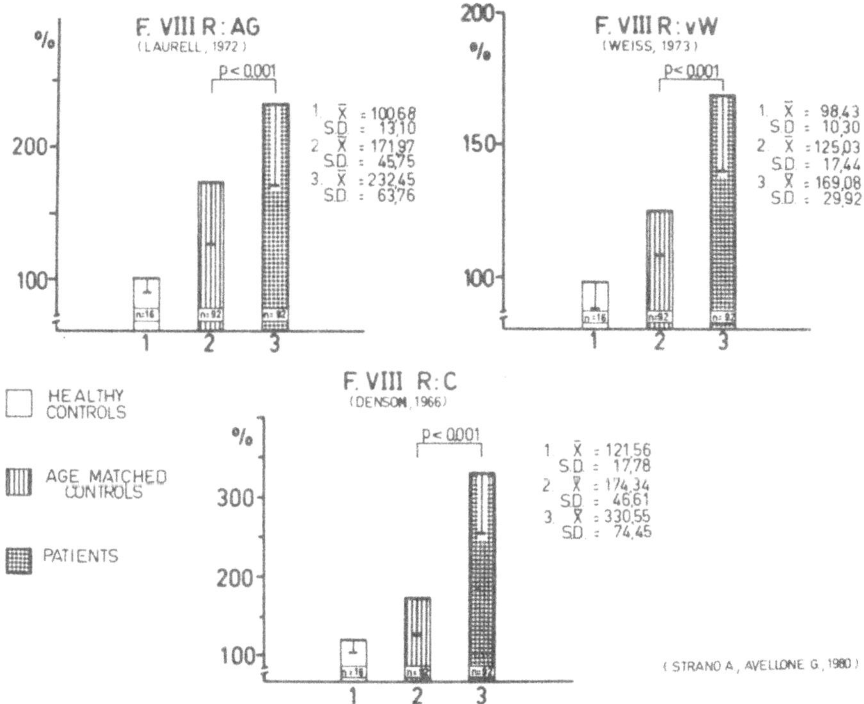

Fig. 1. F. VIII in patients with atherosclerotic vascular disease of the lower limbs.

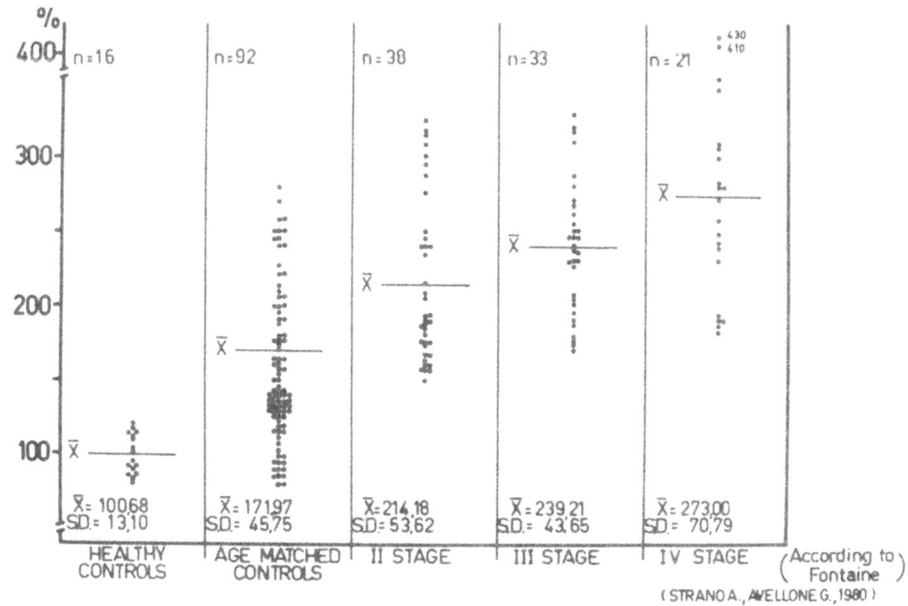

Fig. 2. F. VIII R:AG in patients with atherosclerotic vascular disease of the lower limbs.

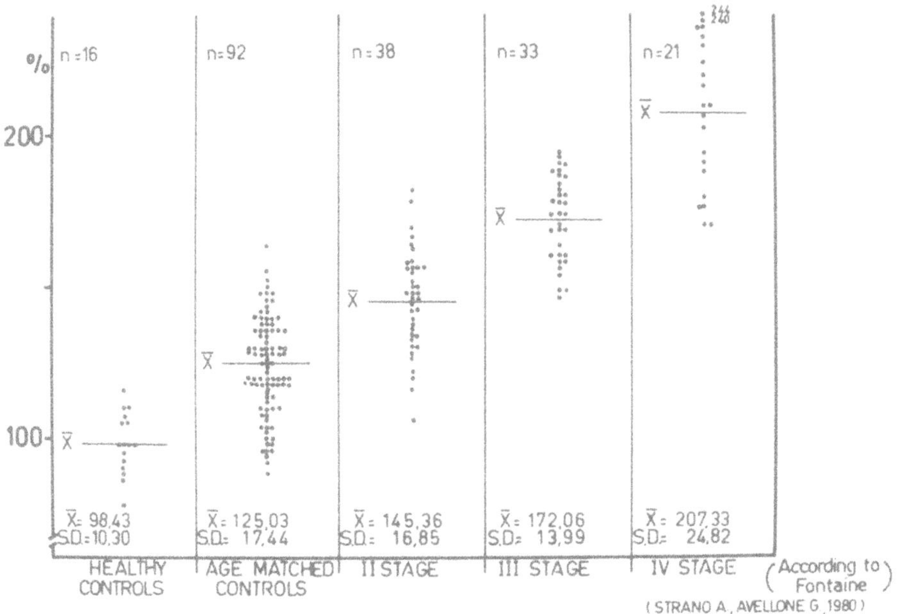

Fig. 3. F. VIII R:vW in patients with atherosclerotic vascular disease of the lower limbs.

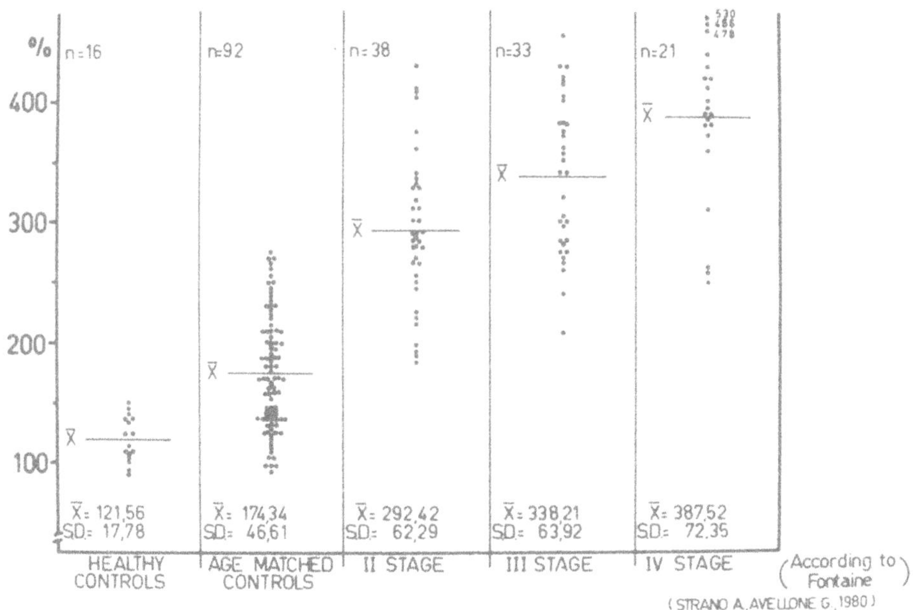

Fig. 4. F. VIII R:C in patients with atherosclerotic vascular disease of the lower limbs.

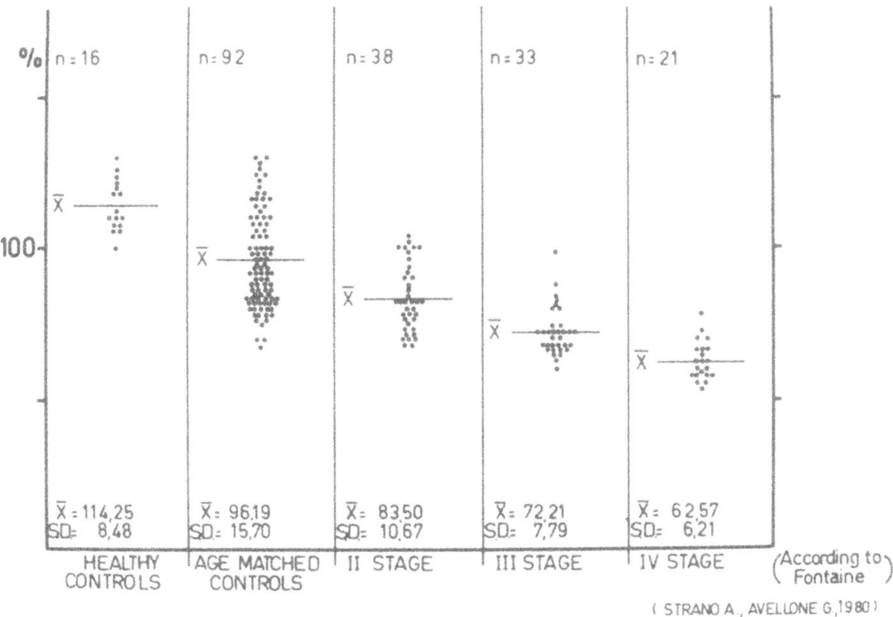

Fig. 5. AT III in patients with atherosclerotic vascular disease of the lower limbs.

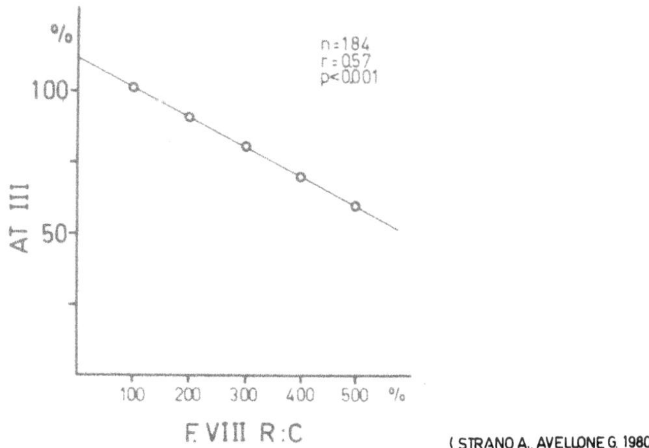

Fig. 6. Correlation between the activity of antithrombin III and that of F. VIII R:C.

between the activity of F. VIII R:vW and the stages of the arteriopathy. Also F. VIII R:C showed progressive increase of activity with the progression of the disease; in fact, (Fig. 4) from an average value of 292.42% (S.D. 62.69) at II stage we move over to a value of 338.21% (S.D. 63.92) at III stage and to a value of 387.52% (S.D. 72.35 at IV stage.

The increase observed for F. VIII R:C and for F. VIII R:vW, especially in relation to the clinico-functional stage, confirms the role played by F. VIII in this form of vascular pathology, and particularly of the two subcomponents involved (F. VIII R:vW - F. VIII R:C) in the pathogenesis of the arterial wall lesion through an increase of platelet adhesiveness and of hypercoagulability.

These changes are linked to a thrombin kind mechanism made evident by a constant reduction of the biological activity of antithrombin III, which decreases progressively with the increasing stage of the arteriopathy. In fact, the mean value at II stage (Fig. 5) was 83.50% (S.D. 1067), 72.21% (S.D. 7.79) at III stage and 62.57% (S.D. 6.21) at IV stage. This last value, so markedly reduced, can be an indirect index of a thromboembolic situation present in the microvascular district.

We have compared the values of F. VIII R:C with those of antithrombin III and we have obtained a correlation index of 0.57 ($p < 0.001$) (Fig. 6). This positive correlation confirms the close connection existing between antithrombin activity of antithrombin III and excited coagulant activity of F. VIII R:C, though we must suppose that other antithrombin proteases surely act to confine the action of thrombin.

An even higher correlation index resulted from the comparison of the stages of the arteriopathy and the reduction of antithrombin III ("r" = 0.69 - $p < 0.001$) (Fig. 7).

CONCLUSIONS

In atherosclerosis obliterans of the lower limbs there are changes of the coagulative system showing an acceleration of the enzymatic processes that lead to the formation of thrombin. The increase of F. VIII R:C and of F. VIII R:vW (subcomponents of F. VIII sensible to thrombin) and simultaneous reduction of antithrombin III activity confirm the formation of thrombin caused by an activation of coagulative factors above the F. Xa of the intrinsic pathway, partially inhibited by the physiological antiprotease. Furthermore, the positive correlation between the coagulant activity of F. VIII (F. VIII R:C) and the antithrombin activity of antithrombin III shows that parts of thrombin escape the action of the physiological inhibitor and that the long compensation phase that precedes an acute thromboembolic episode is linked to other plasmatic and/or tissue components able to confine the effect of thrombin. This haemocoagulative situation suggests that there is an automaintainance mechanism of the activation and a progressive increase with the evolution

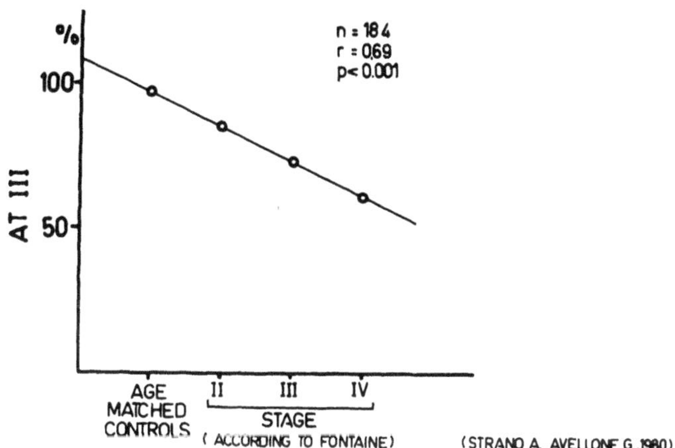

Fig. 7. Correlation between the activity of antithrombin III and the stages of the vasculopathy.

of the arteriopathy. The marked decrease of antithrombin III in patients with skin lesions of the lower limbs can be considered the expression of a thrombotic situation present in the microcircle district.

The increase of F. VIII R:AG (subcomponent of F. VIII not sensible to thrombin action) does not constantly go together with the entity of the clinico-functional symptomatology, being the latter correlated more strongly to the grade of arterial hypo-afflux.

The clinico-functional stage of atherosclerosis obliterans of lower limbs cannot therefore be separated from a clear picture of the haemocoagulative stiuation, in that it cannot be evalued only in terms of hematic output but also as activation of the coagulative system, being the latter a pathogenetic mechanism involved in the evolution of the arteriopathy.

The therapeutic implications that follow suggest the use of drugs that change positively the coagulation activation syndrome. We obtain thus a prophylaxis of the acute thrombotic events that occlude the vascular lumen and the evolution of the arteriopathy.

REFERENCES

1. U. Abilgaard, Inhibition of the thrombin-fibrinogen reaction by antithrombin III studied by N-terminal analysis. Scand. J. Clin. Lab. Inv. 20:205 (1967).
2. U. Abilgaard, Inhibition of the thrombin-fibrinogen reaction by alpha 2-macroglobulin, studied by N-terminal analysis. Thromb. Diath. Haemorrh. 21:173 (1968).
3. L.O. Almer, I.M. Nilsson, On fibrinolysis in diabetes mellitus. Acta Med. Scand. 198:101 (1975).
4. H.N. Antoniades, C.D. Scher, Growth factor derived from human serum, human platelets and human pituitary: properties and immunological cross reactivity. J. Natl. Cancer Institute p. 137 (1978).
5. G. Avellone, V. Mandalà, G. Raneli, Coagulazione, aggregazione piastrinica, fibrinolisi in pazienti affetti da arteriopatia ad evoluzione obliterante degli arti inferiori. In: Di Matteo G. & Pola P. (eds.): Atti I Congresso Nazionale della Società Italiana di Patologia Vascolare, p. 231, ERRE.DI.E., Roma, 1979.
6. G. Avellone, S. Novo, G. Davì, G. Abruzzese, Plasmatic fibrinogen, plasminogen and antithrombin III levels in atherosclerotic patients. In: Strano A. (ed.): Proceedings of European Symposium on advances in coagulation, fibrinolysis, platelet aggregation and atherosclerosis, p. 183, C.E.P.I., Roma, 1978.
7. G. Avellone, V. Mandalà, F.P. Riolo, A. Pinto, Antithrombin III in patients with atherosclerotic vascular disease. Abstracts of: First International "Colloquy" of Angiology, p. 271, Firenze, 1979.
8. N.U. Bang, M.L. Chang, Soluble Fibrin complexes. Sem. Thromb. Haemostas. 1:91 (1974).
9. D. Bensoussan, S. Levi-Toledano, P. Passa, Platelet hyperaggregation in increased plasma level of von Willebrand factor in diabetics with retinopathy. Diabetologia 11:307 (1975).
10. R. Biggs, K.W.E. Denson, N. Alkman, R. Barrett, M. Hadden, Antithrombin III, antifactor Xa and heparin. Br. J. Haematol. 19:283 (1970).
11. R. Biggs, The absorption of human F. VIII neutralising antibody by factor VIII. Br. J. Haematol. 26:259-268 (1974).
12. T.K. Bills, J.B. Smith, M.J. Silver, Metabolism of (^{14}C) arachidonic acid by human platelets. Biochim. Biophys. Acta 124: 303 (1976).
13. A.L. Bloom, J.C. Giddings, G.R. Peake, Low molecular weight factor VIII. Lancet 1:661-662 (1973).
14. A.L. Bloom, G.R. Peake, J.C. Giddings, The presence and reactions of high and lower molecular weight procoagulant F.VIII in the plasma of patients with von Willebrand disease after treatment; significance for a structural hypothesis for F.VIII. Thromb. Res. 3:389-404 (1973).

15. A.L. Bloom, S.C. Giddings, C.J. Wilks, Factor VIII on vascular intima: possible importance in hemostasis and thrombosis. Nature. New Biology 241:217 (1973).
16. B. Boneu, M. Abbal, J. Plante, R. Bierme, Factor VIII complex and endothelial damage. Lancet 1:1430 (1975).
17. B. Boneu, D. Durand, F. Counillan, J.P. Charlet, R. Bierme, J.M. Sue, Increased level of factor VIII complex in severe arterial hypertension. Haemostasis 7:332 (1978).
18. B.N. Bouma, J.M. Hordijk-Hoss, S. De Graaf, J.J. Sixma, J.A. Van Mourik, Presence of factor VIII related antigen in blood platelets of patients with von Willebrand's disease. Nature 257:510 (1975).
19. C. Busch, J. Dawes, D.S. Pepper, A. Wasteson, Binding of platelet factor 4 to cultured human endothelial cells. Thrombos. Haemostas. 42:43 (1979).
20. C. Cavallero, Modificazioni della parete arteriosa nell'arteriosclerosi. In: Cardiologia Oggi, vol. 1, p. 193, Ed. Med. Scient., Torino 1975.
21. A.B. Chandler, Thrombosis and the development of atherosclerosis lesion. In: Jones R. (ed.): Atherosclerosis, p. 88, Springer, New York, 1970.
22. A.B. Chandler, I. Chapman, L.R. Erhardt, W.C. Roberts, J.C. Schwartz, D. Sinapius, D.M. Spain, S. Sherry, P.M. Neiss, T.L. Simon, Coronary thrombosis in myocardial infarction. Report of a workshop on the role of coronary thrombosis in the pathogenesis of acute myocardial infarction. Am. J. Cardiol. 34:823 (1974).
23. P.S. Damus, M. Hicks, R.D. Rosenberg, A generalized view of heparin's anticoagulatnt action. Nature 246:355 (1973).
24. M.J. Davies, N. Woolf, J.W.P. Bradley, Endothelialisation of experimentally produced mural thrombi in the pig aorta. J. Pathol. 97:589 (1969).
25. K.W.E. Denson, Reagents and techniques. In: The treatment of haemophilia and other clotting disorders. Ed. by R. Biggs and R.G. Macfarlane, p. 337. Blackwell Scientific Publication, Oxford 1966.
26. K.W.E. Denson, Standardization of methods for the determination of factor VIII. Thrombos. Diathes. Haemorrh. Suppl. 43:99 (1971).
27. K.W.E. Denson, G.I.C. Ingram, Antigen/biologival-activity ratio for factor VIII. Lancet, 1: 1973.
28. K.W.E. Denson, In: Human blood coagulation, haemostasis and thrombosis. Ed. by: Biggs R., Blackwell Scientific Publications, Oxford-Edinburgh, 1976.
29. M. Ekberg, I.M. Nilsson, Factor VIII and glomerulonephritis. Lancet 1: 1111 (1975).
30. A.P. Fletcher, N. Alkjaersig, O. Owens, G. Wolff, J.R. Smith, Blood hypercoagulability, thrombosis and acute myocardial infarction. J. Lab. Clin. Med. 78:798 (1971).
31. A.P. Fletcher, N. Alkjaersig, Blood screening methods for the diagnosis of venous thrombosis. Milkbank Mem. Fund. Q. 50: 170 (1972).

32. A. Girolami, A. Sticchi, T. Barbui, G. Bareggi, Factor VIII immunological assay. An evaluation of several methods using whole plasma. Blut, Band XXIX:309 (1974).
33. H.L. Goldsmith, The flow of model particles and blood cells and its relation to thrombogenesis. In: Spet T.H. (ed.): Progress in haemostasis and thrombosis. Grune and Stratton, New York, 1972.
34. J. Gormsen, J.D. Nielsen, L.A. Andersen, ADP-induced platelet aggregation in patients with ischemic heart disease and peripheral thrombo-atherosclerosis. Acta Med. Scand. 201: 509 (1977).
35. J.W. Haerem, Platelets and sudden death. In: Neri Serneri G.G., Mason, D.T. (eds.): Myocardial Infarction. Excerpta Medica, Amsterdam, p. 30, 1979.
36. M.D. Haust, R.H. Moore, Development of modern theories on the pathogenesis of atherosclerosis. In: Wissler R.W., Geer J.C. (eds.): The pathogenesis of atherosclerosis, p. 1, Williams & Wilkins, Baltimora 1972.
37. E.J. Hershgold, A.M. Davison, M.E. Jansgen, Human F. VIII (antihemophilic factor): activation and inactivation by phospholipases. J. Lab. Clin. Med. 77:206 (1971).
38. E.J. Hershgold, A.M. Davison, M.E. Jansgen, Isolation and some clinical properties of human F. VIII J. Lab. Clin. Med. 77: 185 (1971).
39. H. Holmsen, Prostaglandin endoperoxide-thromboxane synthesis and dense granuli secretion as positive feedback loops in the propagation of platelet responses during "the basic platelet reaction". Thromb. Haemost. 38:1030 (1977).
40. P.W. Howie, C.B. Begg, D.W. Purdie, & coll. Use of coagulation tests to predict the clinical progress of pre-eclampsia. Lancet 2:323 (1976).
41. J. Hudson, W.T.E. McCaughy, Mural thrombosis and atherogenesis in coronary arteries and aorta. An investigation using antifibrin and antiplatelet sera. Atherosclerosis 19:543 (1974).
42. A. Huges, R.S. Tonks, The role of microemboli in the production of carditis in hypersensitivity experiments. J. Path. Bacteriol. 77:207 (1959).
43. E.A. Jaffe, L.W. Hoyer, R.L. Nachman, Synthesis of antiemophilic factor antigen by cultured human endothelial cells. J. Clin. Invest. 52:2757 (1973).
44. E.A. Jaffe, L.W. Hoyer, R.L. Nachman, Synthesis of von Willebrand factor by cultured human endothelial cells. Proc. Natl. Acad. Sci. USA, 7:190 (1974).
45. E.A. Jaffe, R.L. Nachman, Submit structure of factor VIII antigen synthetized by cultured human endothelial cells. J. Clin. Invest. 56:698 (1975).
46. E.A. Jaffe, Endothelial cells and the biology of factor VIII. Nature 296:377 (1977).
47. C.L. Janssen, W.M. van Leuwen, Behaviour of factors V and factor VII during the process of blood coagulation. Scand. J. Haemat. 9:531 (1972).

48. L. Jorgensen, T. Hovig, H.C. Roswell, J.F. Mustard, Adenosine diphosphate induced platelet aggregation and vascular injury in swine and rabbits. Am. J. Pathol. 61:161 (1970).
49. L. Jorgensen, M.A. Packham, H.C. Roswell, M.R. Buchanan, J.F. Mustard, Local aortic injury caused by cannulation: increased plasma protein accumulation and thrombosis. Acta Path. Microbiol.Scand. 82:637 (1974).
50. K.L. Kaplan, H.L. Nossel, M. Drillings, G. Lesznik, Radioimmunoassay of platelet factor 4 and beta-thromboglobulin: development and application to studies of platelet release in relation to fibrinipeptide A generation. Br. J. Haematol. 38:129 (1978).
51. M. Kazama, T. Abe, Change of the molecular mass of fibrinogen in circulating blood, as an index of hypercoagulable states. Thromb. Res. 8:(Suppl. II) 133 (1976).
52. P.E.A. Kernoff, Affinity of factor VIII clotting activity for antigen detectable immunologically. Nature. New Biology 244:148 (1973).
53. B.A. Kottke, M.T.R. Subbiah, Subject review pathogenesis of atherosclerosis, concepts based on animal models. Mayo Clin. Proc. 53:35 (1978).
54. J.L. Lane, P. Bird, C.R. Rizza, A new assay for measurement of total progressive antithrombin. Br. J. Haematol. 30:103 (1975).
55. C.B. Laurell, Quantitative estimation of proteins by elettrophoresis in agarose gel containing antibodies. Analitical Biochemistry 15:45 (1966).
56. C.B. Laurell, Electroimmuno assay. Scand. J. Clin. Lab. Invest. 29, suppl. 124:21 (1972).
57. E.C. Lian, R.R. Minej, D.R. Harnnes, In vitro and in vivo effects of thrombin and plasmin on human factor VIII (AHF). Am. J. Haemat. 1:481 (1976).
58. C.A. Ludlam, J.D. Cash, Studies on the liberation of beta-thromboglobulin from human platelets in vitro. Brit. J. Haematol. 33:239 (1976).
59. C.A. Ludlam, Beta-thromboglobulin. A new diagnostic tool in the diagnosis of hypercoagulability? In: Neri Serneri G.G., Prentice C.R.M. (eds.): Florence Conference on Haemostasis and Thrombosis. Academic Press, London 1977.
60. P.M. Mannucci, F.I. Pareti, L. Holmberg, I.M. Nilsson, Z.M. Ruggeri, Studies on the prolonged bleeding time in von Willebrand's disease. J. Lab. Clin. Med., October, 662 (1976).
61. E.E. Mayne, J.M. Bridges, J.A. Weawer, Platelet adhesiveness, plasma fibrinogen and factor VIII levels in diabetes mellitus. Diabetologia. 6:436 (1970).
62. S. Moore, D.S. Pepper, J.D. Cash, The isolation and characterization of a platelet specific release beta-globulin: beta-thromboglobulin and the detection of antiurokinase and antiplasmin released from thrombin aggregated washed human platelets. Bioch. Biophys. Acta 379:360 (1975).

63. M. Moroi, N. Aoki, Inhibition of plasminogen binding to fibrin by alpha-2-plasmin inhibitor. Thromb. Res. 10:851 (1977a).
64. M. Moroi, N. Aoki, On the interaction of alpha-2-plasmin inhibitor and proteases. Evidence for the formation of a covalent crosslinkage and non-covalent weak bindings between the inhibitor and proteases. Bioch. Biophys. Acta 482:412 (1977b).
65. R.L. Nachman, E.A. Jaffe, Subcellular platelet factor VIII antigen and von Willebrand factor. J. Exp. Med. 141:1101 (1975).
66. P. Needleman, P.S. Kulkarni, A. Raz, Coronary tone modulation: formation and actions of prostaglandins endoperoxides and thromboxanes. Science 195:409 (1977).
67. G.G. Neri Serneri, G.F. Gensini, R. Abbate, D. Prisco, C. Mugnaini, Soluble fibrinogen complexes and platelet aggregates in patients with history of myocardial infarction and chronic cerebrovascular disorders. A rationale for prophylactic therapy. Europ. Symp. on Platelet Aggregation, Coagulation Fibrinolysis and Atherosclerosis. (A. Strano ed.) p. 277, CEPI, Roma, 1976.
68. G.G. Neri Serneri, R. Abbate, G.F. Gensini, G. Masotti, Aterosclerosi e stati trombofilici. In: Atti dell'Ottantesimo Congresso della Società Italiana di Medicina Interna, p. 427, Pozzi L., Roma, 1979.
69. G.G. Neri Serneri, Relationships between system and ischaemic heart disease. In: Neri Serneri G.G., Mason T.D. (eds.): Myocardial Infarction. Excerpta Medica, Amsterdam, 1979.
70. G.G. Neri Serneri, High molecular weight fibrinogen complexes in the assessment of hypercoagulability. In: Neri Serneri G.G., Prentice C.R.M. (eds.) Haemostasis and Thrombosis, p. 211. Academic Press, London 1979.
71. H.L. Nossel, I. Yudelman, R.E. Canfield, Measurement of fibrinopeptide A in human blood. J. Clin. Invest. 54:43 (1974).
72. J.R. O'Brien, M.D. Etherington, S. Jamieson, P. Lawford, S.V. Lincoln, N.J. Alkjaersig, Blood changes in atherosclerosis and long after myocardial infarction and venous thrombosis. Thromb. Diath. Haemorrh. 34:483 (1975).
73. M. Pandolfi, L.O. Almer, L. Holmberg, Increased von Willebrand antiemophylic factor in diabetic retinopathy. Acta Ophtalmol. 52:823 (1974).
74. F. Panicucci, A. Sacripanti, E. Pinori, M. Vispi, B. Conte, L. Lecchini, Antithrombin III, heparin cofactor and antifactor Xa in relation to age, sex and pathological conditions. Thromb. Haemost. 42:127 (1979).
75. S. Renaud, K. Kuba, C. Goulet, Y. Lemire, C. Allard, Relationship between fatty-acid composition of platelets and platelet aggregation in rat and man. Circ. Res. 26:343 (1970).
76. R.D. Rosenberg, P.S. Damus, The purification and mechanism of action of human antithrombin-heparin cofactor. J. Biol. Chem. 248:6490 (1973).
77. J.S. Rosenberg P. McKenna, R.D. Rosenberg, Inhibition of human factor IX by human antithrombin-hepatin cofactor. J. Biol. Chem. 250:8883 (1975).

78. R.D. Rosenberg, G. Armand, L. Lam, Structure-function relationship of heparin species. Proc. Natl. Sci. USA 75:3065 (1978).

79. R. Ross, J. Glomset, B. Kariya, R. Harker, A platelet dependent serum factor that stimulates the proliferation of arterial smooth muscle cells in vitro. Proc. Natl. Sci. USA 71:1207 (1974).

80. R. Ross, J. Glomset, The pathogenesis of atherosclerosis. New Engl. J. Med. 295:369 (1976).

81. N. Salky, M. Dugdale, Platelet abnormalities in ischaemic heart disease. Am. J. Cardiol. 32:612 (1973).

82. S.C. Sharma, H.N. Seth, Platelet adhesiveness, plasma fibrinogen and fibrinolytic activity in acute myocardial infarction Br. Heart J. 40:526 (1978).

83. M.J. Silver, T.K. Bills, J.B. Smith, Platelets and prostaglandins: the key role of platelet phospholipase A_2 activity. In: De Gaetano G., Garattini S. (eds.): Platelets: A multidisciplinary approach. Raven Press, New York, 1978.

84. J.B. Smith, C. Ingerman, M.J. Silver, Persistence of thromboxane A-2 like material and platelet relase inducing activity in plasma. J. Clin. Inv. 58:1119 (1976).

85. J. Stibbe, Effect of exercise on F. VIII complex: proportional increase of Ristocetin cofactor (von Willebrand cofactor) and F. VIII AGN, but disproportional increase of F. VIII AHF. Thromb. Res., vol.10:163 (1977).

86. H. Stormorken, J. Herikssen, S. Nitter-Hange, A. Hellem, Antithrombin III and arterial thromboembolism. In: A. Strano (ed.) Proceedings of European Symposium on Advances in Coagulation, Fibrinolysis, Platelet Aggregation and Atherosclerosis. p. 19, C.E.P.I., Roma, 1978.

87. A. Strano, S. Novo, G. Davì, G. Avellone, A. Pinto, La sindrome trombofilica delle arteriopatie obliteranti degli arti inferiori. In: Atti dell'Ottantesimo Congresso della Società Italiana di Medicina Interna, p. 535, Pozzi L. Roma, 1979.

88. A. Strano, S. Novo, Prospettive sull'impiego degli antiaggreganti piastrinici nell'arteriosclerosi. Editoriale Giorn. Ital. Cardiol. 9:1 (1979).

89. A. Strano, S. Novo, G. Davì, G. Avellone, Fisiopatologia della coagulazione, dell'aggregazione piastrinica nella cardiopatia ischemica. In: Atti del XXXVIII Congresso Nazionale della Società Italiana di Cardiologia, suppl. Boll. Soc. Ital. Cardiol., p. 499, Roma, 1980.

90. T. Strasser, Atherosclerosis and coronary heart disease: the contribution of epidemiology. WHO Chron. 26:7 (1972).

91. J. Svensson, M. Hamberg, B. Samuelsson, Prostaglandin endoperoxides IX. Characterization of rabbit aorta contracting substance (RCS) from guinea pig lung and human platelets. Acta Physiol. Scand. 94:222 (1975).

92. M.E. Switzer, P.A. McKee, Some effects of calcium on the activation of human factor VIII: von Willebrand factor protein by thrombin. J. Clin. Invest. 60:819 (1977).

93. A. Teien, V. Abildgaard, M. Höök, The anticoagulant effect of heparin sulphate and dermatan sulphate. Thromb. Res. 8: 859 (1976).
94. Z.I. Terashita, H. Fukui, K. Nishikawa, M. Hirata, S. Kikuchi, Coronary vasospastic action of thromboxane A_2 in isolated working guinea pig hearts. Europ. J. Pharmacol. 53:94 (1978).
95. C. Thomson, C.D. Forbes, C.R.M. Prentice, Relationship of factor VIII to Ristocetin induced platelet aggregation: effect of heterologous and acquired factor VIII antibodies. Thromb. Res. 3:363 (1973).
96. J.F. Toole, R. Janeway, K. Choi, R. Cordell, F. Johnston, H.S. Muller, Transient ischemic attacks due to atherosclerosis: a prospective study of 160 patients. Arch. Neurol. 32:5 (1975).
97. V.T. Turitto, H.R. Baumgartner, Platelet interaction with sub-endothelium in a perfusion system: physical role of red blood cells. Microvasc. Res. 9:335 (1975).
98. E. von Kaulla, K.N. von Kaulla, Antithrombin III and disease. Am. J. Clin. Pathol. 48:69 (1967).
99. P.N. Walsh, Albumin density gradient and washing of platelets and the study of platelet coagulant activities. Br. J. Haemat. 22:205 (1972).
100. P.N. Walsh, Platelet coagulant activities and haemostasis: a hypothesis. Blood 43:597 (1974).
101. H.J. Weiss, L.W. Hoyer, R.F. Rickles, A. Varma, J. Rogers, Quantitative assay of a plasma factor deficient in von Willebrand disease that is necessary for platelet aggregation: relationship to decrease F. VIII procoagulant activity and antigen content. J. Clin. Invest. 52:2708 (1973).
102. R.W. Wissler, Overview of problems of atherosclerosis. In: Scheinberg P. (ed.): Cerebrovascular disease, p. 56, Raven Press, New York, 1976.
103. S. Wessler, E.T. Yin, On the antithrombotic action of heparin. Thromb. Diath. Haemorrh. 32:71 (1974).
104. J.C. White, Electron microscopic studies of platelet secretion. Prog. Haemostas. Thromb. 2:49 (1974).
105. L.D. Witte, K.L. Kaplan, H.L. Nossel, B.A. Lages, H.J. Weiss, S.G. De Witt, Studies of the release from human platelets of the growth factor for cultured human arterial smooth muscle cells. Circ. Res. 42:402 (1978).
106. N. Woolf, K.C. Carstairs, Infiltration and thrombosis in atherogenesis. A study using immunofluorescent technique. Am. J. Pathol. 51:373 (1967).
107. E.T. Yin, L.C. Guidice, S. Wessler, Inhibition of activated factor X-induced platelet aggregation: the role of heparin and the plasma inhibitor to activated factor X. J. Clin. Med. 81:298 (1973).

ADVANCES IN THE PREVENTION OF VENOUS THROMBOEMBOLIC DISEASE

P.G. Bentley and V.V. Kakkar

Thrombosis Research Unit and Department of Medical Physics
King's College Hospital Medical School
Denmark Hill
London SE5 8RX, UK

Before outlining the possible advances in the prevention of thromboembolism, may we draw your attention to the size of the problem.

Figures from the United States of America indicate the epidemic of thromboembolism, being the sole cause of 50,000 deaths and contributing to three times that number per year. In addition of course there is the cost of hospitalisation and the subsequent treatment of the post-phlebitic limb. We might point out that although the association between surgery and thromboembolism is well known, approximately half the pulmonary emboli that we see occur in patients who did not undergo surgery. Perhaps some of our efforts should be directed towards these patients in our medical wards. An advance in prevention may well be the use of prophylaxis in patients acutely hospitalised regardless of whether or not they have surgery.

In the late nineteenth century, Rudolph Virchow suggested the three main causes of coagulation of the blood. It is against the first and third of these, that most of our efforts have been directed. There seems to be little that we can do at present to prevent venous intimal damage. More than 20 years ago, Sevitt and Gallagher, showed that the incidence of thromboembolism was drastically reduced by fully anticoagulating their patients. However, both they and others have shown an unacceptably high incidence of haemorrhagic complications - between eleven and thirty five percent. A regimen of low doses of heparin, administered subcutaneously has been shown in many trials to reduce the incidence of thrombosis, and with this, the incidence of fatal pulmonary embolus has also been significantly reduced. However, the price to be paid for this reduction in deaths from pulmonary embolus is a small increase in the number of wound haematomas following surgery. A benefit risk/ratio has been calculated showing an 88% reduction of fatal pulmonary emboli with a 2.1% increase in wound haematoma. In our research we aimed at improving on these figures.

We took as our starting point, the suggested mechanism of action of low dose heparin. It appears to increase the activity of an alpha-two globulin, anti-Xa (also known as antithrombin three and heparin co-factor). There are probably four points of action in addition to a very weak effect on thrombin. I prefer to simplify the coagulation cascade, showing anti-Xa as the modulator of hyperthrombotic tendency by limiting the critical activation of factor X, through which all the thrombogenic stimuli must pass. Our search has been for an agent with a selective ability to potentiate anti-Xa, without altering the overall coagulation mechanism.

One promising substance, is the semi synthetic heparin analogue A73025. This is a glicosaminoglycan polysulphate prepared from beef lung. It is not a true heparin, containing mostly galactosamine, with little glucosamine and has half the molecular weight of commercial heparins. We have assessed its anticoagulant effect by Kaolin Cephalin Clotting Time (Activated Partial Thromboplastin Time) and its antithrombotic effect by the increase in activity of anti-Xa. In studies with volunteers we found that 10,000 units of the analogue produced the same prolongation of KCCT as calcium heparin 5,000 units, but three times the increase in activity of anti-Xa. A clinical trial was set up to compare the analogue with the calcium heparin. Two hundred consecutive patients, over the age of 40, undergoing major abdominal surgery were randomly allocated to receive either heparin or analogue. The dose of analogue was reduced slightly to 7,500 units in the hope of reducing haemorrhagic side effects whilst maintaining the improved protection against thromboembolism. Assessment was by I^{125} fibrinogen test, backed up by phlebography. Twelve of the heparin group and six of the analogue group developed deep vein thrombosis. Although the trend is exciting the differences are not statistically significant. The blood loss, transfusion requirements and wound haematoma rate appeared to be the same in each group.

We concluded that the semi synthetic heparin analogue A73025 was at least as effective as heparin, with a similar complication rate. A major multicentre trial has been set up to test this substance in a large number of patients, to find out whether it is better than heparin at prevention of deep vein thrombosis with fewer haemorrhagic complications. We hope to be able to give you the answer to this question in two years time.

You may have noticed that the molecular weight of A73025 was approximately half that of normal heparin, which is a heterogenous mixture of different mucopolysaccharides. We have been dividing commercial heparins into fractions of different molecular weights by gel filtration. The fractions have been evaluated in three molecular weight bands. The highest band, between 22,000 and 35,000 contains much low activity and unreactive substances, the middle band between 10,500 and 22,000 behaves very much like the parent heparin, but the low molecular fraction is of great interest. It has very slightly more KCCT activity than unfractioned heparin. Here the prolongation is never more than 10 seconds, but there does appear to be a real difference although there is some variability between different commercial heparins. When the anti-Xa assay is considered , however, the low molecular weight heparin fraction is found to have a very much enhanced activity and this activity lasts more than the usual 6 hours, being significant often at twelve hours.

A preliminary pilot study with 46 consecutive patients undergoing major surgery suggests that it may be an effective prophylactic agent. None of the patients developed deep vein thrombosis as assessed by the fibrinogen test, although 21 had malignancy and 9 active infection. Although these numbers are low they certainly suggest that more clinical work is needed to determine the place of low molecular weight heparin.

Finally, may I mention the third of Wirchow's triad of factors, the stasis of blood. The helpful effect of compression stockings and various mechanical methods of increasing flow in the deep veins has promoted a review of the drug dihydroergotamine. It acts by increasing the venomotor tone, decreasing the venous capacitance and increasing the velocity of flow in the deep veins. Trials of the addition of dihydroergotamine to twice daily low dose heparin have shown a significant reduction of deep vein thrombosis and pulmonary embolus. Furthermore, halving the dose of heparin and adding dihydroergotamine still produced a better effect than heparin alone. This suggests that dihydroergotamine may well be a valuable adjunct to our prophylactic agents and may obviate the need for cumbersome stockings and other apparatus.

In conclusion, therefore, I feel that advances in the prevention of thromboembolism may be made in three ways. First by halving the dose of heparin and adding dihydroergotamine, second, the use of the semi synthetic heparin analogue, and thirdly, the low molecular weight fractions of heparin.

CURRENT STATUS OF ANTICOAGULANT TREATMENT

L. Poller

Department of Haematology
Withington Hospital
Manchester M20 8LR
England

Heparin and oral anticoagulant drugs are widely used for prophylaxis and treatment of venous thrombosis. Anticoagulant administration in arterial thrombosis is less successful probably due to the different morphology of the arterial thrombus with proportionately less fibrin.

Although anticoagulants fell from favour in the 1960's because of reservations on their value after myocardial infarction, in the past decade there has been a dramatic increase in their use. The increased recognition of the high incidence of venous thrombosis has been a governing factor in the trend. Recent trials of anticoagulant prophylaxis have been able to use the ^{125}I fibrinogen technique as the end-point for the diagnosis of thrombosis and have established the true clinical extent of the need for prophylaxis.

The usual clinical indications for anticoagulants are shown in Tables 1 and 2. Then we will consider, in view of the very brief time allotted, three situations:
i) treatment of established venous thrombosis; ii)prophylaxis of venous thrombosis; iii) myocardial infarction. In venous thrombosis and pulmonary embolism, which we shall consider together, oral anticoagulant administration with heparin cover, until a therapeutic level is reached, is the routine treatment. The clinical acceptance of this regime antedated modern methods of statistical evaluation. Table 3 gives the results of these early studies in venous thrombosis and pulmonary embolism.

The controlled trial of the anticoagulant treatment of established pulmonary embolism by Barrie and Jordan (1960) was abandoned on moral grounds because of the obvious high risk to the untreated control group. Although the design of this trial has been criticized, the evaluation of anticoagulants with an untreated control group in

Table 1. Indications

1. <u>Short-term</u>	up to 6 weeks
Prophylaxis in medical and surgical patients	
Prophylaxis post-partum	
Conversion of atrial fibrillation	

Table 2. Indications

3. <u>Long-term</u> over one year

Recurrent venous thrombosis
Recurrent pulmonary embolism
Prophylaxis in rheumatic heart disease
Prophylaxis in mitral valve prostheses
Prophylaxis in atrial fibrillation

<u>Cerebral artery syndrome</u>

Transient ischaemic attacks
Progressively evolving strokes
? basilar and vertebral artery syndrome
Myocardial infarction in males under 55
? acute coronary insufficiency
? angina pectoris

Table 3. Pulmonary Embolism

Series	Country	Treated	Control	Complications percentage		Deaths percentage	
				Treated	Control	Treated	Control
Ziliacus 1946	Sweden	103	64			0.4	18
Sise and others 1975	USA	26		11.6		15.4	
Coon and others 1958	USA	152		7.9		5.7	
Barrit and Jordan 1960	Britain	54	19		5	3.3	27

Table 4

	Total	DVT
Low-dose heparin	35	9
Oral anticoagulant	33	0

pulmonary embolism has never since been thought to be justified on ethical grounds. Firm statistical support for the effectiveness of oral anticoagulation in the treatment of the acute phase of deep vein thrombosis, however, has come only recently from the study of the McMaster workers (Hull et al. 1979)(Table 4). All patients were treated with intravenous haparin for 14 days in conventional dosage and then changed either to oral anticoagulants or to subcutaneous heparin (a low dose regime) of 5,000 units twice dayly. Nine of the 35 patients who received low-dose heparin had a venographically-proved recurrence of DTV whereas none of the 33 Warfarin-treated patients suffered a further episode. This well-conducted study leaves little doubt as to the effectiveness of short-term oral anticoagulant administration in the prevention of recurrence of established venous thrombosis whilst showing the lack of protection by low-dose heparin in this situation.

The value of oral anticoagulants in calf vein and thigh vein thrombosis is not now questioned but their application is isotopically-diagnosed DTV and superficial venous thrombosis is arguable. As the main effectiveness of oral anticoaglulants is in prophylaxis, it would, however, seem illogical to deny such treatment to these latter two groups.

The tendency is to give coumarin drugs for up to six months after deep vein thrombosis and up to nine months after a pulmonary embolism provided that there are good facilities for anticoagulant control. The long duration of anticoagulant administration is because the incidence is higher in the first few months after the episode.

Prophylaxis of venous thrombosis

The outstanding benefit conferred by oral anticoagulants in prophylaxis of venous thromboembolism in high risk groups particularly in patients undergoing surgical operations. Sevitt and Gallagher (1959) showed that pulmonary embolism was responsible for the death of up to 50% of elderly patients with fractures of the pelvis and lower limbs. the incidence of deep vein thrombosis was reduced to less than one-tenth with oral anticoagulant administration. No pulmonary embolism occurred during anticoagulant prophylaxis. Unfortunately, oral anticoagulation, shown to be effective and safe by the Birmingham Accident Hospital studies, has not proved popular because of the reputation of oral anticoagulants to produce bleeding.

Attempts have, therefore, been made to arrive at successful prophylaxis during surgery using a variety of approaches. The main one in the last few years has been to use heparin in a low dose of 5,000 units subcutaneously twice daily or three times daily to achieve protection without excessive haemorrhage. The success of the regime in moderate risk cases is now firmly established (see Table 5).

The results of our own controlled study (Taberner et al. 1978) (Table 6) indicated that, while less trouble from oral anticoagulants, the use of low-dose subcutaneous heparin was as effective as oral anticoagulants in patients undergoing gynaecological surgery for non-malignant conditions.

Table 5. Low-Dose Heparin and General Surgery

Author	Dose	Total no. patients	Control Group incidence DVT	Control Group incidence DVT
Kakkar et al. (1972)	5000 u bd	78	42%	8%
Gallus et al. (1973)	5000 u tds	236	16%	2%
International multicentre trial	5000 u tds	1292	25%	8%

Table 6. Incidence of DVT

Group	Oral anticoagulant	Heparin	Saline
DVT	3	3	11
Total	48	49	49

P using Chi squared test with Yates Correction

Oral anticoagulant v Saline	<0.05
Heparin v Saline	<0.05

It is the high risk cases, i.e. hip surgery, hip fractures and patients with malignancies, where the real need for prophylaxis exists and it is in this group that the low-dose heparin regime is not so successful. In these patients oral anticoagulants remain the most effective prophylaxis.

Myocardial infarction

Although many hundred reports have been published, few fulfil the basic requirements of clinical trials. The shortcomings of the early enthusiastic studies are now well recognised. The enthusiastic early reports were qualified by later studies. Some of these, e.g. the Medical Research Council Study (1969), aimed at a very slight coagulation defect (i.e. 15% Thrombotest) which may partly explain some difference from the previous Medical Research Council report which had shown long-term benefit from oral anticoagulants but using a conventional dosage based on the Quick test.

The long term trials were reviewed by Douglas and McNicol (1976) who concluded that 40 to 50 lives would be saved for every 1,000 patients treated. Greater benefit may be achieved if the patients were divided by age and sex, more benefits arising in males and younger age groups. Opinions, however, may be changing to a more favourable view of the role of anticoagulants. The latest report is the Netherlands randomised double-blind study (de Vries et al. 1979) of a large series of patients over the age of 60. There was a highly significant reduction of recurrent infarction and a significant reduction in mortality (see Table 7). The intensity of treatment was of the order of 5 to 10% Thrombotest equivalent to a prothrombin ratio of 2.5 to 4.5 with British Comparative Thromboplastin. The

Table 7

		Controls		Treated	
		Total	Deaths	Total	Deaths
Bjerkelund	1957	118	48	119	30
MRC	1959 1964	188	35	195	25
Harvald et al.	1962	170	26	145	14
Aspenstrom and Korsan-Bengtsen	1964	113	50	118	39
Veterans Administration	1965	359	97	388	87
Loeliger et al.	1967	122	12	122	8
Lovell et al.	1967	178	39	172	33
* de Vires et al.	1979	-	49	-	28

Dutch workers were very successful in controlling their patients, over 70% of results being at therapeutic levels. The results of this well-designed study appear convincing and suggest that it may be time for a re-appraisal of the tendency over the last decade to regard the use of anticoagulants after myocardial infarction as not worthwhile. As in other clinical situations, the possible benefits of treatment must be set against the risks. The availability of good facilities for the laboratory control and drug dose supervision must be an important factor in the decision to discontinue or administer long-term anticoagulants. The safety and good results obtained with laboratory control based on the European-type range with BCT and Thrombotest cannot be transposed to the USA and other parts of the world where more intense and hence more dangerous coagulation defects result from the use of animal tissue thromboplastin in the prothrombin time test.

Laboratory control

The all-important question which appears to explain discrepancies above, is the laboratory control of anticoagulants. Oral anticoagulant treatment must be regularly and frequently controlled by laboratory tests to ensure adequacy of treatment without over-anticiagulation. The therapeutic range with a method of laboratory control is established by clinical trials. Alternatively, correlation of results of a new technique with a previously established method of control provides an approximate guide. Recently the introduction of the ^{125}I fibrinogen isotope diagnosis has allowed non-ivasive monitoring of the effectiveness of a given therapeutic range.

The prothrombin time introduced by Quick in 1935 is still the most popular method of laboratory control and the most extensively used (Lam-Po-Tang and Poller 1975). The lack of standardization of its methodology, particularly in relation to the type of thromboplastin reagent used, has led to great discrepancies. In addition, different methods of expression of prothrombin time results, e.g. the prothrombin time, the prothrombin percentage activities from a variety of types of dilution curve, the prothrombin ratio, have led to vast confusion and varying intensities of treatment. In some centres the coagulation defect thought to be therapeutic on the basis of percentage activity, ratio or activity results, is homeopathic, whereas at others, a seemingly similar safe result causes dangerous over-dosage.

In the UK, a national reagent, designated the British Comparative Thromboplastin (BCT), was introduced in 1969 with a national system of reporting the prothrombin time, termed the British Ratio. The therapeutic range normally recommended is a prothrombin ratio of 2.0 to 4.0 but for prophylaxis, a less intensive regim of 2.0 to 2.5 has been shown to be adequate (Taberner et al. 1978) (Table 8). In the USA and elsewhere commercial reagents which are necessarily of animal origin, are usually rabbit brain extracts or rabbit brain-lung mixtures. Because of the problems of species-specifity of human clot-

Table 8

Thromboplastin	Mean ratio
British Comparative Thromboplastin	2.96
Thrombotest	2.47
Tromborel	1.91
Diagen (phenolised)	1.87
Simplastin A	1.83
Diagen (freeze-dried)	1.74
Ortho	1.63
Dade thromboplastin 'C'	1.61
Boehringer	1.57
Hyland	1.55
Simplastin	1.52
Dade activated (liquid)	1.48
Dade (freeze-dried)	1.47

Table 9. Therapeutic Ranges with Other Reagents Equivalent to the Conventional Range with BCT (Ratio 2.0 - 4.0)

BCT	2.0	4.0
Boehringer	1.35	1.8
Dade	1.4	1.8
Dade FS	1.7	2.66
Diagen	1.4	2.05
Hyland	1.25	1.8
Ortho'	1.3	1.8
Simplastin	1.3	1.7
Simplastin A	1.5	2.1
Thromborel	1.55	2.35
Thrombotest	2.0 (16%)	3.5 (7%)

Ratios with commercial reagents corresponding to extremes of therapeutic scale (ratios 2.0 and 4.0) with BCT based on correlation performed in 1979 at the National (UK) Reference Laboratory for Anticoagulant Reagents and Control, using the recommended procedure (Assiciation of Clinical Pathologists' Broadsheet No. 71).

Table 10

	%	
	35	
Geigy		Human Brain (Acetone 1)
Phenolised		Simplastin
Human brain (Acetone 2)	30	
		Difco
Stayne		
	25	Human brain (Saline)
Dade		
	20	
		2.7.10
	15	
Thrombotest (Owren)		

ting factors, these preparations give shorter prothrombin times than human brain in patients on anticoagulant therapy. Their prothrombin ratios are, therefore, much shorter than with BCT on a given plasma sample from a coumarin treated patient (Table 9). The tendency in clinical practice has been to use therapeutic ranges of 15 to 30% prothrombin activity from saline dilution curves (Table 10) or two or three times prolongation of prothrombin ratio, irrespective of the type of thromboplastin reagent used. The intensity of treatment when controlled by commercial reagents tends to be far greater and there is a tendency to have an increased number of bleeding complications. A recent example of this was the McMaster venous thrombosis trial (Hull et al. 1979) where the target prothrombin ratio was a modest 2.0 with Simplastin reagent. The BCT correlation shows that with 2.0 with simplastin which is a shorter ratio than often employed with this reagent, the patients may be at dangerous levels of anticoagulation (Fig. 1). (The bleeding level with BCT is $<$ 5.0 ratio.) As the BCT-type range has been validated in the prophylaxis of venous thrombosis (Hume et al. 1971, Taberner et al. 1978), it is possible that the incidence of haemorrhagic complications may be reduced using less-intensive dosage regimes with the commercial reagents of animal origin. The therapeutic range with commercial reagents corresponding to the BCT range is given in Table 9.

The use of BCT reference preparation on a world scale in recent years has helped to elucidate these problems of calibration of reagents. The availability from WHO and EEC of BCT preparations and other well-characterised reference thromboplastin preparations should

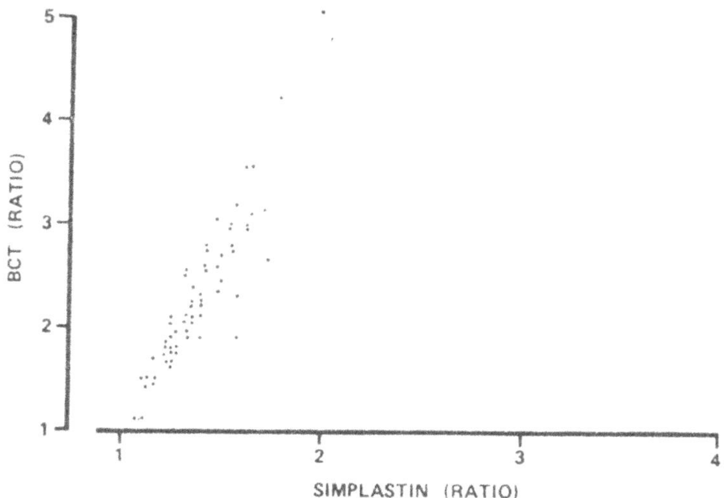

Fig. 1. Simplasin ratio

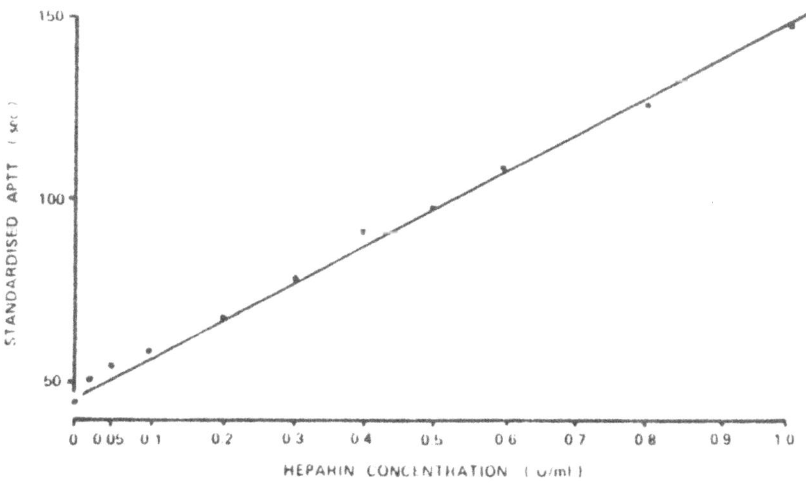

Fig. 2. The effect of increasing concentrations of heparin, added to 'pooled' normal plasma _in vitro_, on the standardised APTT method

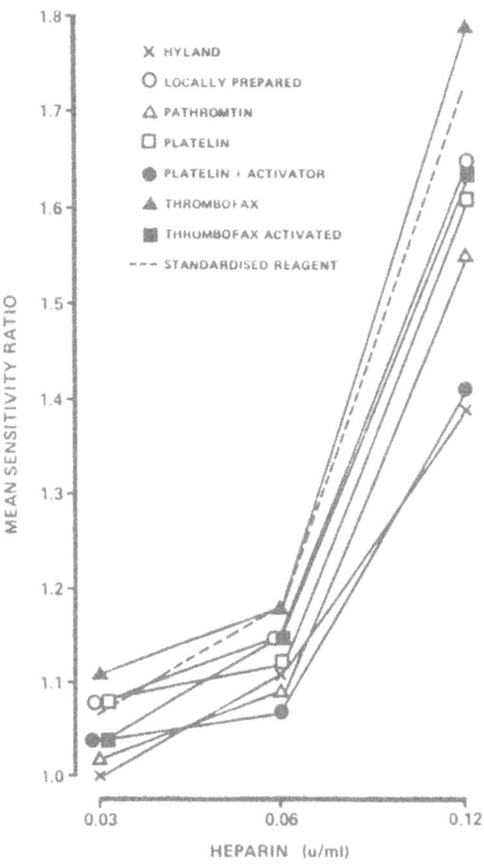

Fig. 3a

assist greatly in the provision of improved safety in laboratory control of anticoagulant administration using the Quick prothrombin time test.

The question of control of heparin dosage is just as complex (Thomson 1981). Heparin concentration or biological effect is measured by clotting times, thrombin times, anti-Xa assay. The APTT is the most widely used in the USA and UK. If it is agreed that heparin dosage control is required and, in view of the high risk of haemorrhage associated with its administration this seems essential, there remains the problem of methodology. As the APTT is the method generally adopted, it is important to consider its reliability. A number of surveys have indicated the insensitivity and unreliability of some commercial procedures. Good sensitivity and linearity of response of a wide range of blood heparin concentrations is possible. Fig. 2 shows the response of the standardised reagent and technique from the National (UK) Reference Laboratory. Figs. 3 a and b show the

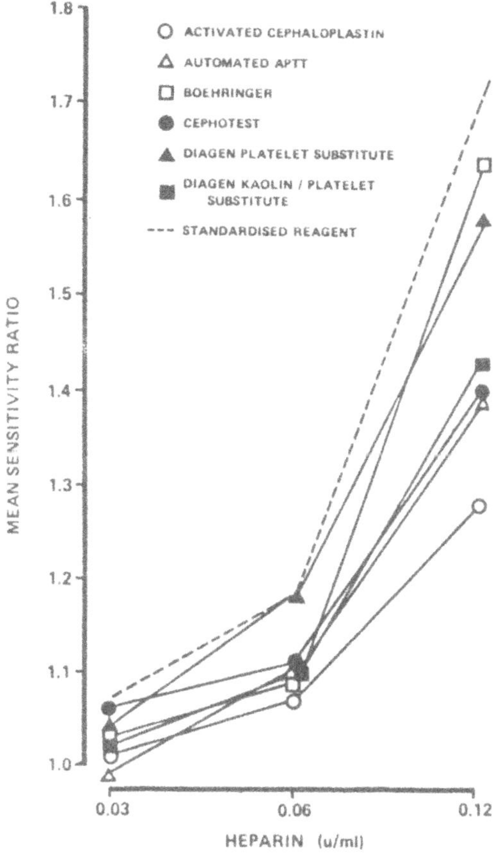

Fig. 3b

response of a variety of APTT reagents to increasing concentrations of heparin. There is a great deal of work to be done to improve the performance of many of the APTT techniques which are currently in wide-spread use.

REFERENCES

Barrit, D.W., and Jones, S.C. (1960) Lancet 1:1309

Coon, W.W., Mackenzie, J.W., and Hodgson, P.E. (1958) Surg. Gynae. Obstet. 106:129

Douglas, A.S., McNicol, G.P. (1976) In: Human Blod Coagulation 2. Ed. Biggs, R. Blackwell, Oxford

Gallus, A.S., Hirsh, J., Tuttle, R.J., Trebilcock, R., O'Brien, S.E., Carroll, J.J., Minder, J.H., and Hudecki, S.M. (1973) New Engl. J. Med. 288:545

Hull, R., Delmore, T., Genton, E., Hirsh, J., Gent, M., Sackett, D.; McLoughlin, D., and Armstrong, R., (1979) New. Engl. J. Med. 301:855

Hume, M., Sevitt, S. and Thomas, D.P. (1971) In: Venous thrombosis and pulmonaru embolism. Harvard University Press, Cambridge Mass.
International Multicentre Trial (1973) Lancet 2:45
Kakkar, V.V., Corrigan, T.P., Spindler, J., Fossard, D.P., Flute, P.T., Crellin, R.Q., Wessler, S., and Yin, E.T. (1972) Lancet 2:10
Lam-Po-Tang, P.R.L.C., and Poller, L. (1975) Thrombos.et Diathes. Haemorrh. 34:419
Medical Research Council (1959) Brit. Med. J. 1:803
Sevitt, S., and Gallagher, N.G. (1959) Lancet 2:918
Sise, H.S., Moloney, W.C., and Guttas, C.G. (1975) Am. Heart J. 53:132
Taberner, D.A., Thomson, Jean M., and Poller, L. (1976) Brit. Med. J. 2:83
Thomson, Jean M. (1981) Am. J. Clin. Path. Suppl. (In press)
Zilliacus, H. (1946) Acta Med. Scand. Suppl. 171

PART 3

VASCULAR COMPLICATIONS OF DIABETES MELLITUS

BLOOD VISCOSITY AND THE COMPLICATIONS OF DIABETES

C.R.M. Prentice and G.D.O. Lowe

University Department of Medicine
Royal Infirmary
86 Castle Street
Glasgow G4 OSF - UK

Increased viscosity in diabetes mellitus was forst noted by Skovborg et al. (1966) and has since been confirmed by several groups including Isogai et al. (1976) and Barnes et al. (1977) although the results are somewhat conflicting. These studies have mostly been carried out in older diabetics in whom the presence of atherosclerosis may cause secondary changes or mask understanding of the underlying haemostatic abnormalities. It is important also to take into account the variable clinical features such as smoking, renal impairment or diabetic retinopathy. We have taken the opportunity to study a homogeneous group of younger insulin treated male diabetics and compared them with an age and smoking matched control group of normal people. The main measurements included haematocrit, plasma fibrinogen (measured by the Clauss technique), plasma viscosity (measured by BS M3 capillary viscometer), and whole blood viscosity at a high (100s-1) and low shear rate (0.94s-1) in a rhombo-spheroid rotational viscometer. The low shear rate studies were measured in a Contraves Model LS 30 viscometer.

We have studied three groups of individuals - diabetics without vascular complications, diabetics with vascular complications proved by the presence of retinopathy, and normal healthy controls (males) matched for age and smoking habits. The results indicated that both groups of diabetics had a higher mean blood viscosity than matched controls (Table 1) at the high shear rate ($p < 0.05$) and at the low shear rate ($p < 0.01$). The diabetics with complications had even higher viscosity readings which were significantly greater than the diabetics without complications. This was due in part to the fact that diabetics with complications had higher haematocrits than both the diabetics without complications and the controls. However blood viscosity corrected to a standard haematocrit of 45% was greater in

Table 1. Blood viscosity and its determinants in diabetics and controls

	Controls	Diabetics - no retinopathy	Diabetics - retinopathy
STUDY I			
Number	38	20	18
Blood viscosity, 100s-1 (cP)	6.75 ± 0.08	7.07 ± 0.14*	7.53 ± 0.17*
Haematocrit (%)	44.8 ± 0.4	44.9 ± 0.7	47.3 ± 0.9 *
Corrected blood viscosity (cP)	6.78 ± 0.05	7.08 ± 0.12*	7.19 ± 0.11*
Fibrinogen (g/L)	2.50 ± 0.09	2.90 ± 0.14*	3.45 ± 0.29*
Plasma viscosity (cP)	1.34 ± 0.01	1.41 ± 0.02*	1.41 ± 0.03*
STUDY 2			
Number	28	14	14
Blood viscosity 0.94s-1 (cP)	18.7 ± 0.6	21.2 ± 0.8*	24.3 ± 1.1
Haematocrit (%)	45.2 ± 0.6	45.7 ± 1.0	48.5 ± 1.0*
Corrected blood viscosity	18.6 ± 0.5	20.7 ± 0.8	21.7 ± 0.8*
Fibrinogen (g/L)	2.58 ± 0.009	2.99 ± 0.17	3.11 ± 0.19*

Results are given as mean ± SEM. cP = centipoise. Corrected blood viscosity corrected to standard haematocrit of 45%. Subscript * indicates significant difference from matched controls.

both groups of diabetics than in controls, the differences being greater at a low shear rate. This was mainly due to the high fibrinogen levels and plasma viscosity values in both groups of diabetics. The fibrinogen levels in the two groups of diabetics were not significantly different. It is interesting that the highest level of haematocrit and blood viscosity were found in the patients with proliferative retinopathy compared to those with only background retinopathy although the numbers studied were too small to be significant.

It appears, from this study, that young male diabetics have increased blood viscosity at both high and low shear rates compared to non diabetics and this is present before the onset of clinically detectable vascular disease. The increased viscosity is only partly due to haematocrit for it persists after correction of haematocrit suggesting that plasma proteins such as fibrinogen are largely responsible for the increased viscosity. The changes are greater at low rather than at high shear rates. This may be of clinical importance for viscosity may be highest in the post capillary venules where early retinal changes are found in diabetics.

The diabetics with retinopathy had significantly higher whole blood viscosity, especially at low shear rates, than those without retinopathy due to their increased haematocrit. This has been observed in only one previous study (Labib et al., 1971). The mechanism of the increased haematocrit is uncertain. In our study it was not due to difference in smoking habits. Hyperglycaemia may possibly cause an increase in haematocrit through an osmotic diuresis leading to loss of plasma volume. However in our study poor control of plasma glucose was not significantly increased in the group with complications. Alternatively, the microangiopathy in diabetic with vascular complications might lead to increased plasma permeability and reduced plasma volume (Langer et al., 1971). The present study does not indicate the role of whole blood viscosity in the pathogenesis of diabetic microangiopathy and further work is required to establish whether reduction in viscosity may prevent or reduce vascular complications .

In a further study we have looked at the level of circulating platelet aggregates as tested by the Wu and Hoak technique in the three same groups, as seen in figure 1. There was a wide scatter in the circulating platelet aggregate results but the group of diabetics with complications had significantly higher values than the other two groups (Lowe et al., 1980). The level of circulating platelet aggregates did not correlate with fibrinogen values, platelet count, glucose level or any of the clinical features of the diabetics including age and duration of diabetes. Previously we had considered that there might be a correlation between fibrinogen levels and circulating platelet aggregates but this was not sustained in the present study. However the presence of circulating platelet aggregates in diabetics with complications might aggravate the degree of microangiopathy in patients who already had some evidence of vascular disease.

The fact that whole blood viscosity and circulating platelet

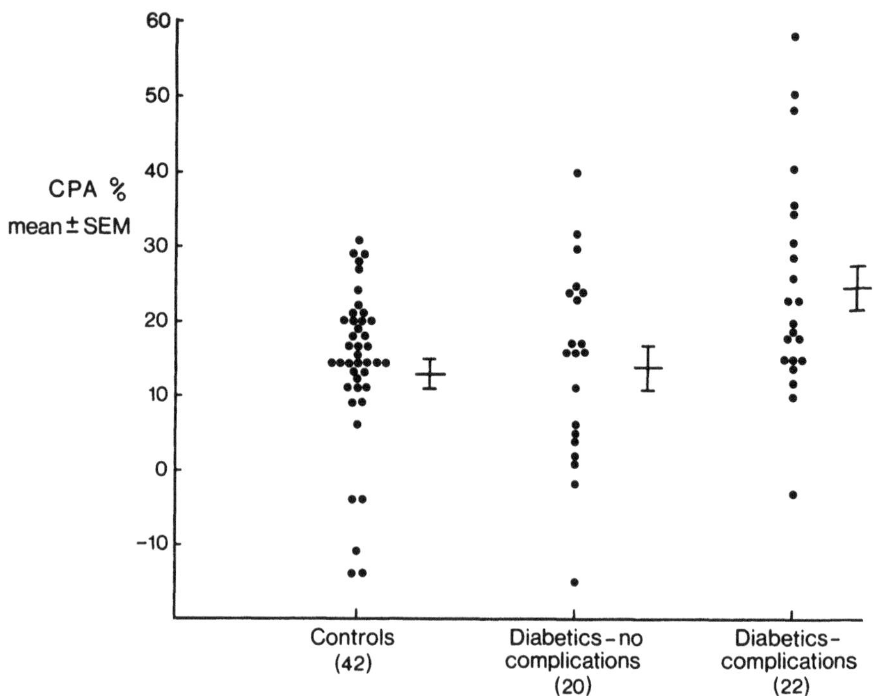

Fig. 1. Circulating platelet aggregates in control and patient groups.

aggregates are greatest in diabetics with vascular complications support the possibility that these abnormalities might contribute to the vascular disease. Wether treatment of these abnormalities either by measures to lower viscosity, such as venesection or haemodilution, or by the use of platelet inhibitory drugs remains to be seen.

REFERENCES

Barnes, A.J., Locke, P., Scudder, P.R., Dormandy, T.L., Dormandy, J.A., Slack, J., 1977, Is hyperviscosity a treatable component of diabetic microcirculatory disease? Lancet 2:789-791.

Isogai, Y., Lida, A., Michizuchi, K., Abe, M., 1976, Haemorheological studies on the pathogenesis of diabetic microangiopathy. Thrombo. Res. 8 (Suppl. II):17-24.

Labib, M.A.M., Higazi, A.M., El-Ebrashby, N., El-Ashmaway, S., Madkour, M.K., Barhooma, G.A., 1971, Studies on diabetic retinal vascular changes with special reference to blood coagulation and viscosity. Bull. Ophthalmol. Soc. Egypt. 64:457-482.

Langer, L., Bergentz, S.E., Bijure, J., Fagerberg, S.E., 1971, The effect of exercise on haematocrit, plasma volume and viscosity in diabetes mellitus. Diabetologia 7:29-33.

Lowe, G.D.O., Signorello, M., Parker, J.L.S., Manderson, W.G., Forbes, C.D., and Prentice, C.R.M., 1980, Platelet aggregates and plasma fibrinogen in diabetes. Microvascular Research 20, 259 (Abstract).

Skovborg, F., Nielsen, A.V., Schlichtkrull, J., Ditzel, J., 1966, Blood viscosity in diabetic patients. Lancet 1:129-131.

FACTORS CONTRIBUTING TO PLATELET HYPERACTIVITY IN DIABETES MELLITUS

E. Dupuy and P.J. Guillausseau

Département d'Hematologie Biologique
Hôpital Lariboisiere
2, Rue Ambroise-Pare
75475 Paris, France

Diabetes mellitus is associated with a high prevalence of atherosclerotic and microvascular disease (31). Platelets may play a part in the development of these vascular complications. Hyperaggregability is frequently reported in diabetes mellitus (1, 2, 7-9, 11, 16, 20, 27). Some factors which could contribute to platelet hyperactivity have been studied.

It has been shown by several authors (1, 2, 8, 9, 11) that in response of low doses of ADP, both primary and second wave responses are increased in diabetes mellitus.

Platelet aggregation has been studied in 163 diabetic subjects compared to 163 control subjects (11).

The clinical characteristics of these patients are summarized in Table 1. This diabetic population is composed of 95 males and 68 females with a mean age of 53 ± 16 years (range 17-82 years). The retinopathy is classified as absent (109 subjects), isolated microaneurysms (24 subjects), microaneurysms with exudates (21 subjects), proliferative retinopathy (9 subjects). A neuropathy is present in 44 subjects and ischemic heart disease in 25 subjects.

The control population is composed of 108 males and 55 females with a mean age of 46.3 ± 8.9 years (range 24-58 years).

In these 163 diabetic subjects, we confirm the hyperaggregability in the presence of two concentrations of ADP (0.6 μM; 1.2 μM). This hyperaggregability is associated with an absence of disaggregation in response to low dose of ADP (0.6 μM). The difference is highly significant (table 2).

Platelet hyperaggregability in diabetes mellitus has been attributed either to plasma factors (7, 16, 20, 33) or to platelet abnormalities (1, 2, 13, 27, 29, 32). Using isolated gel filtered platelets Bensoussan et al. (1) have shown that ADP hyperaggregation

Table 1. Diabetic Subjects

Sex	95 ♂ 68 ♀
Age	53 ± 16.5 years (17-82 years)
% theoretical weight (according to Lorentz)	108 ± 20% (76-194 %)
Mean duration of diabetes	8 ± 8 years (few weeks - 40 years)
Treatment	
insulin	76 subjects
oral antidiabetic drugs	68 subjects
diet	19 subjects

Table 2. Platelet Disaggregation in the Presence of ADP 0.6 μM

	Controls N = 163	Diabetics N = 163
Absence of disaggregation	0	63
	$\chi^2 = 46.6$	$P < 5.10^{-4}$

in diabetics with proliferative retinopathy is related to a platelet factor and no effect of the diabetic plasma on normal platelets has been noticed in this study.

Specific platelet factors which could play a role in the platelet hyperactivity in diabetes have been related in the literature.

Fibrinogen is an essential cofactor for ADP induced aggregation (3). Specific receptor sites have been demonstrated on the platelet membrane after stimulation by ADP or epinephrine, in the presence of calcium, for the fibrinogen binding (18, 23, 28).

H. Lee et al. (19) have studied the fibrinogen binding in 16 diabetics compared to 9 non diabetic subjects. Among the diabetics, 8 patients present severe retinopathy (1 maculopathy, 7 proliferative retinopathy), the other ones have a few microaneurysms.

ADP platelet aggregation is increased in all diabetics compared to controls. There is a correlation between ADP induced aggregation and haemoglobin AL concentration (19).

Fibrinogen binding has been assessed in washed platelets in the presence or the absence of ADP as previously described by H. Lee et al. (18).

The mean percentage platelet bound fibrinogen is higher in diabetics compared to controls. The difference is signigicant in a relationship between ADP platelet hyperactivity and the quality of the metabolic control of the diabetes. The increased fibrinogen binding is not related to platelet aggregation but to the severity of the microvascular complication.

It is suggested that platelets can participate in the early stages of intrinsic coagulation by two different pathways (34). The contact product forming activity (CPFA) defined by the ability of ADP stimulated platelets to activate F XII (35), the collagen induced coagulant activity (CICA) defined by the ability of collagen stimulated platelets to activate F XI in the absence of F XII (34). A two to three times increase of platelet coagulant activities (PCA) in patients with transient ischemic attacks has been described by Walsh et al. (35). Levy-Toledano et al. (21) have shown a significant increase of CPFA as well as CICA in diabetics with vascular complications; in contrast no significant difference is observed between the diabetics without complications and the control group for these contact related coagulant activities. The availability of platelet factor 3 activity (PF3A) is increased in both groups of diabetics.

This activity would be supplied by platelet lipoproteins located in the membrane and the increased PF3A could reflect an altered disposition of membrane components. Increased CPFA may be related to enhanced ADP responsiveness and increased F XII activation on the surface of possible modified diabetic platelet membrane.

It is well established that thromboxane A2 (TXA2) produced by platelets from arachidonic acid promotes cell aggregation (15) whereas prostacyclin (PG12) produced by endothelial cells inhibits ADP platelet aggregation (24). Modifications of this regulatory system may play a role in the development of thrombotic disorders (25). Halushka et al. (13) originally showed an increased production of PGE-like material in diabetic platelets. More recently, Halushka et al. (14) demonstrated an increased synthesis of thromboxane B2 (TXB2), stable metabolite of TXA2 in diabetic platelets. Gerrad et al. (12) have demonstrated an alteration in the balance of prostaglandins and thromboxane synthesis in rats rendered diabetic by injection of streptozocin. Conversion of arachidonic acid to TBX2 is increased in the diabetic rats; it is associated to a decrease in vascular (aortic) production of 6 keto PGF1α. The authors suggest that these changes observed in arachidonic acid metabolism may reflect a significant imbalance in TXA2 and PGI2 in diabetic rats compared to control ones. Such modifications may have a role in the modification in ADP platelet sensitivity and the development of the microvascular complications in diabetes mellitus.

β-Thromboglobulin (BTG) is a specific platelet protein located in the α granules (26), released during platelet aggregation (22). An increase of plasmatic BTG level reflects an in vivo platelet activation. An increase of plasmatic BTG has been described in clinical disorders associated to either platelet activation or thrombotic complications (10, 30). Some authors have reported increased plasmatic BTG level in diabetic patients (4-6); but no correlation has been found between high plasmatic BTG level and simultaneous HbA1 level (9). Preston et al. (29) report a correlation between high level of BTG and circulating platelet aggregates in diabetic microangiopathy.

In conclusion, ADP platelet hyperactivity is well established in diabetes mellitus (1, 2, 8, 9, 11, 27, 32). Therefore, some platelet factors could contribute to this ADP platelet hyperaggregability. An increase of fibrinogen binding on the platelet membrane, an increase of platelet coagulant activities has been noticed in diabetics with severe retinopathy (19, 21). Modifications of the thromboxane production in diabetic platelets (14) and increase of the plasmatic BTG level (4-6, 29) could also have a role in the development of vascular complications.

However if platelets may have a role in the development of vascular complications, modifications of the interaction of platelet-vessel wall play also an important role in the development of thrombotic complications in diabetes.

REFERENCES

1. D. Bensoussan, S. Levy-Toledano, P. Passa, J. Caen, J. Canivet, Platelet hyperaggregation and increased plasma level of von Willebrand factor in diabetics with retinopathy. Diabetologia 11:307-312 (1975).
2. D. Bensoussan, S. Levy-Toladano, P. Passa, Anomalies de l'hémostase primaire au cours de la microangiopathie diabétique. Nouv. Pres. Med. 36:2383-2386 (1976).
3. G. Born, M. Cross, Effects of inorganic ions and plasma proteins on the aggregation of blood platelets by adenosine diphosphate. J. Physiol. (London) 170:397-414 (1964).
4. D. Borsey, J. Dawes, D. Fraser, C. Prowse, R. Elton, B. Clarke, Plasma β-thromboglobulin in diabetes mellitus. Diabetologia 18:353-357 (1980).
5. A. Burrows, S. Chavin, T. Hockaday, Plasma β-thromboglobulin concentrations in diabetes mellitus. Lancet 1:253-237 (1978).
6. J. Campbell, J. Dawes, D. Fraser, D. Pepper, B. Clarke, L. Duncan, J. Cash, Plasma β-thromboglobulin in diabetes mellitus. Diabetes 26:1175-1177 (1977).
7. B. Coller, R. Frank, R. Milton, H. Gralnick, Plasma cofactors of platelet function: correlation with diabetic retinopathy and hemoglobins Ala-c. Ann. Intern. Med. 88:311-316 (1978).
8. J. Colwell, P. Halushka, Platelet function in diabetes mellitus. Brit. J. Haemat. 44:521-526 (1980).
9. J. Davis, P. Phillips, K. Yve, H. Lewis, C. Hartman, Platelet aggregation. Adult onset diabetes mellitus and coronary artery disease. JAMA 239:732-734 (1980).
10. M. Denham, M. Fischer, G. James, M. Hassan, β-thromboglobulin in clinical conditions. Lancet 1:1154-1158 (1977).

11. E. Dupuy, P. Guillausseau, P. Gaudel, G. Kartalis et al., Fonctions plaquettaires et angiopathie diabétique. Nouv. Pres. Med. 8:3123-3125 (1979).
12. J. Gerrard, M. Stuart, G. Rao, M. Steffes, M. Hauer, D. Brown, Alteration in the balance of prostaglandin and thromboxane synthesis in diabetic rats. J. Lab. Clin. Med. 95:950-958 (1980).
13. P. Halushka, D. Lurie, J.A. Colwell, Increased synthesis of prostaglandin-E-like material by platelets from patients with diabetes mellitus. N. Engl. J. Med. 297:1306-1310 (1977).
14. P. Halushka, J.A. Colwell, C. Rogers, C. Loadholt, B. Garner, Increased thromboxane (TXB2) synthesis by platelets from patients with diabetes mellitus (DM): studies with a TX synthetase inhibitor and a TX receptor antagonist. Clin. Res. 27:269 A (1979).
15. M. Hamberg, J. Svensson, B. Samuelsson, Thromboxanes: a new group of biologically active compounds derived from prostaglandin endoperoxides. Proc. Natl. Acad. Sci. 72:2994-2998 (1975).
16. H. Kwaan, J. Colwell, S. Cruz, N. Survenwela, J. Dobbie, Increased platelet aggregation in diabetes mellitus. J. Lab. Clin. Med. 80:236-246 (1972).
17. M. Lagarde, M. Dechavanne, Increase of platelet prostaglandin cycle endoperoxides in thrombosis. Lancet I:88 (1977).
18. H. Lee, A. Nurden, A. Thomaidis, J. Caen, Relationship between fibrinogen binding and the platelet glycoprotein deficiencies in Glanzmann's thrombasthenia type I and type II. Br. J. Haemat. in press.
19. H. Lee, C. Paton, P. Passa, J. Caen, Fibrinogen binding and ADP induced aggregation in platelets from diabetic subjects. (submitted for publication).
20. G. Leone, B. Bizzi, F. Accorra, P. Boni, Functional aspects of platelets in diabetes mellitus. In: Platelet aggregation and drugs. L. Caprino and F. Rossi eds., Academic Press New York, p.49-61 (1974).
21. S. Levy-Toledano, A. Demoszynska, E. Dupuy, P. Gaudel, J. Lubetzki, J. Caen, P. Castaldi, Platelet coagulant activities in diabetic patients. In: Cellular and biochemical aspects in diabetic retinopathy. INSERM symposium n° 7, 69-74 (19787.
22. C. Ludlam, J. Cash, Studies on the liberation of β-thromboglobulin from human platelets in vitro. Br. J. Haematol. 33: 239-249 (1976).
23. G. Marguerie, T. Edgington, E. Plow, Interaction of fibrinogen with its platelet receptor as part of a multistep reaction in ADP-induced platelet aggregation. J. Biol. Chem. 255: 154-161 (1980).
24. S. Moncada, S. Grygelowski, S. Bunting, J. Vane, An enzyme isolated from arteries transforms prostaglandin endoperoxides to an unstable substance that inhibits platelet aggregation. Nature 263:663-666 (1976).

25. S. Moncada, E. Higgs, J. Vane, Human arterial and venous tissues generate prostacyclin, a potent inhibitor of platelet aggregation. Lancet 1:18-22 (1977).
26. S. Moore, D. Pepper, D. Cash, The isolation and characterization of a platelet specific β-globulin (βthromboglobulin) and the detection of anti-urokinase and anti-plasmin released from thrombin-aggregated washed human platelets. Biochem. Biophys. Acta 379:360-369 (1975).
27. J. Mustard, M. Packham, Platelets and diabetes mellitus. New Engl. J. Med. 297:1345-1347 (1977).
28. E. Peerschke, M. Zucker, R. Grant, J. Egan, M. Johnson, Correlation between fibrinogen binding to human platelets and platelet aggregability. Blood 55:841-847 (1980).
29. F. Preston, J. Ward, B. Marcola, N. Porter, W. Timperley, B. O'Malley, Elevated β-thromboglobulin and circulating platelet aggregates in diabetic microangiopathy. Lancet 1: 238-240 (1978).
30. C. Redman, M. Allington, F. Bolton, G. Stirrat, Plasma β-thromboglobulin in pre-eclampsia. Lancet 2:248-251 (1977).
31. H. Root, E. Bland, W. Gordon, Coronary atherosclerosis in diabetes mellitus. A post-mortem study. JAMA 113:27-30 (1939).
32. J. Sagel, J. Colwell, L. Crook, M. Laimins, Increased platelet aggregation in early diabetes mellitus. Ann Intern. Med.82: 733-738 (1975).
33. K. Sarji, H. Schraibman, A. Chambers, R. Nair, J. Colwell, Quantitative studies on von Willebrand factor in normal and diabetic subjects, role of vWF in second-phase platelet aggregation. Microcirculation 2:296-297 (1976).
34. P. Walsh, The effects of collagen and kaolin on the intrinsic coagulant activity of platelets. Brit. J. Haematol. 22: 393-405 (1972).
35. P. Walsh, Platelet coagulant activities and haemostasis. A hypothesis. Blood 43:597-605 (1974).

PLATELET ACTIVITY AND BLOOD LIPID CHANGES IN DIABETES MELLITUS

F. Riolo, G. Davì, S. Novo, A. Pinto, G. Mendola, G. Avellone, M. Russotto, and A. Strano

Institute of Clinical Medicine and Medical Therapy
University of Palermo
Piazza delle Cliniche, 2
90127 Palermo, Italy

An altered platelet function can often be found in diabetes mellitus (2, 3, 4, 10, 13, 16, 17, 23, 24). Several studies have pointed towards an increased sensitivity of platelets to ADP induced aggregation (3, 6, 23) in diabetic patients; this phenomenon can also be found in diabetics without apparent vasculopathy and in subjects with altered glucose tolerance (3, 23).

The increase of the second phase of platelet aggregation found in diabetics is reversible with the use of inhibitors of the prostaglandin-synthetases enzyme such as aspirin (23). It is thus possible that an increased prostaglandin synthesis can be involved in the augmented second phase of platelet aggregation that can be found in patients with diabetes mellitus (8).

In fact, Halushka found that platelets of diabetic subjects are significantly more sensitive to the aggregating effects of arachidonic acid and synthetize a major quantity of a prostaglandin E-like substance in answer to ADP, adrenaline, collagen and arachidonic acid.

Platelets of diabetic patients synthetize a greater quantity of thromboxane A_2 than those of control subjects (9). There is then a positive correlation between glucose plasmatic levels and thromboxane A_2 platelet synthesis in diabetic patients but not in the control subjects. Platelets of diabetic patients are also less sensitive to the antiaggregating action of imidazole, inhibitor of thromboxane-synthetases and of 13-azaprostanoic acid, antagonist of thromboxane-endoperoxides (9).

An increased malondialdehyde release, index of an augmented activity of the enzyme thromboxane-synthetases (5), has been shown in pregnant diabetic women who are hypersensitive to aggregating agents (25). Increased serum levels of PGF_2 and PGE_2 have been found in patients with juvenile diabetes (1).

Nordoy has demonstrated increases of lipidic phosphorus in 4 of the 5 phospholipidic fractions of the platelets obtained from subjects with juvenile or mature diabetes mellitus (20). An increase of the arachidonic acid content of phospholipids and of platelet phospholipase A_2 activity could contribute to the thromboxane increase formed by the platelets of diabetic subjects and such increase could be closely related with the changes of haematic lipids.

We have therefore deemed of interest to carry out a study, on diabetic patients, on the intraplatelet prostaglandin metabolism evalued through the platelet formation of malondialdehyde, platelet release (BTG), platelet turnover (Platelet regeneration time), in relation to the presence or absence of a vascular pathology and both to the coexisting alterations of the lipid metabolism and to the kind of therapy followed in the immediate months before the study.

PATIENTS STUDIED AND METHODS

The study was carried out on 60 diabetic patients, 36 males and 24 females, with an average age of 52.3±12.4 years; 38 showed macroangiopathic complcations (18 ischaemic heart disease, 8 chronic cerebral vasculopathy, 12 atherosclerosis obliterans of the lower limbs at II - III stage). Twenty control subjects of age between 18 and 50 years were included in the study. Blood samples were drawn after overnight fasting; therapy with antiaggregating agents had been suspended at least two weeks prior to the study.

Platelet malondialdehyde formation was evalued on platelet pellets after thrombin stimulation (final concentration 1 U/ml) according to Okuma's method (21).

Plasma levels of betathromboglobulin (BTG) were evalued with radioimmunologic method (Ammersham kit).

In 20 of the diabetic patients (10 with macroangiopathy and 10 without vascular complications) we have also evalued platelet regeneration time according to Stuart (26).

In 30 of the diabetics we have determined, besides MDS formation, also HDL-cholesterolemia on serum with an enzymatic method (after precipitation of the other proteins with PEG) (29). Of these 30 patients 9 were under treatment with sulphonilurea plus phenformin, 12 with insulin and 9 on diet alone.

RESULTS

Figure 1 shows how MDA formation is significantly higher in the diabetic patients and particularly in those who have vascular complications. A similar pattern is also shown for the plasma levels of BTG that are clearly higher ($p<0.01$) both in diabetic patients with macroangiopathic lesions and in those who do not show vascular lesions (Fig. 2).

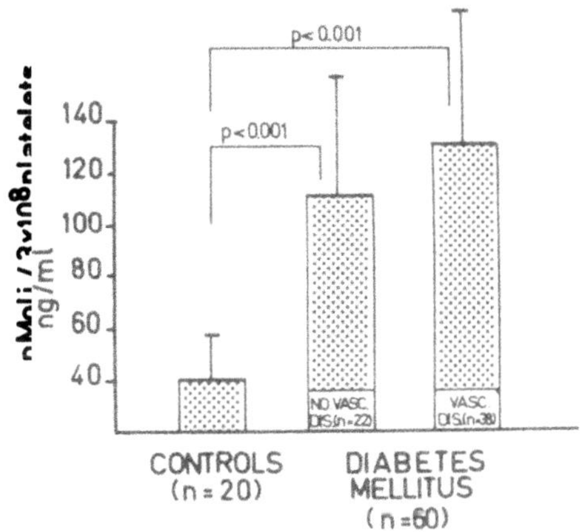

Fig. 1. MDA formation by platelets.

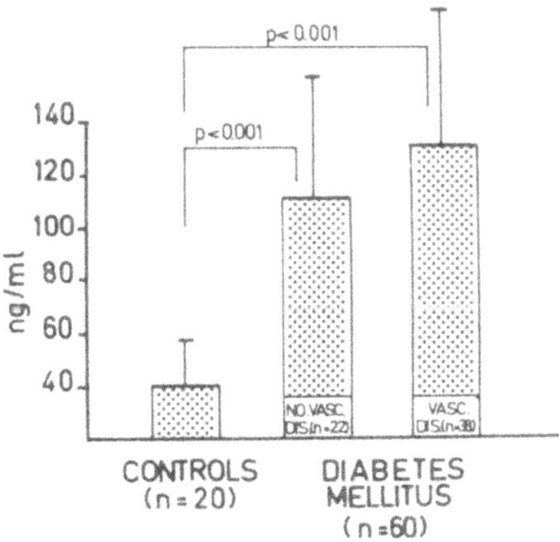

Fig. 2. Betathromboglobulin plasmatic levels.

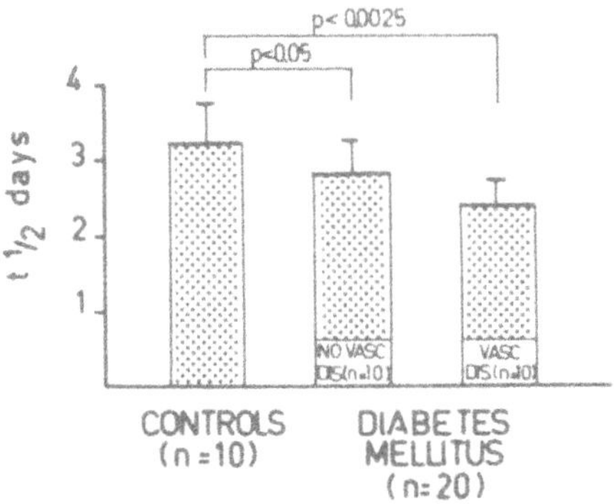

Fig. 3. Platelet regeneration time.

Platelet turnover (Fig. 3) is significantly increased in diabetic patients, particularly in those who present macroangiopathy.

Table I shows the simultaneous behaviour of MDA formation and of HDL-cholesterolemia in the diabetic patients subdivided in relation to the presence of macroangiopathy.

Diabetic patients with vasculopathy present notably reduced HDL-cholesterolemia levels ($p<0.005$) and at the same time a significative increase of MDA formation ($p<0.005$).

Table II shows data concerning MDA formation and HDL-cholesterolemia in relation to the treatment.

Diabetics under sulphonilurea plus phenformin showed significantly increased MDA levels with a reduction of HDL-cholesterolemia levels compared to diabetic patients treated with insulin or on diet alone.

DISCUSSION

The increased malondialdehyde production by platelets, induced by thrombin stimulation, points out the existence of a platelet function activation in patients with diabetes mellitus.

The increased prostaglandin synthesis may not be specific of diabetes but a phenomenon secondary to the presence of a vasculopathy and to the reduced mean life of platelets as we have found. In fact, Garg (7) has found in diabetic patients an increased number of megacariocytes, and these thrombocytes are more sensitive than controls to ADP and adrenaline, and have also an increased release reaction. Furthermore, platelets with a shorter life release more malondialdehyde than controls (14), while platelets of patients with vascular pathology (15) or of smokers (12) synthetize higher quantities of prostaglandin endoperoxides.

Table I

	MDA nMol/$3x10^8$ plts. $\bar{x} \pm$ S.D.	HDL-CT mg/100ml $\bar{x} \pm$ S.D.
Diabetics without vascular diseases (n=12)	0.56±0.21	46.3±8.2
Diabetics with vascular diseases (n=18)	0.83±0.26	34.7±11.64
	$p<0.005$	$p<0.005$

Table II

	MDA nMol/$3x10^8$ plts. $\bar{x}\pm$S.D.	HDL-CT mg/100ml $\bar{x}\pm$S.D.
Diabetics on diet (n=9)	0.62±0.17	39.22±12.31
Diabetics on insulin (n=12)	0.64±0.25	41.8±12.6
Diabetics on sulphonilurea + phenformin (n=9)	0.93±0.29	34.3±10.5
	$p<0.01$ (insulin vs sulphonilurea + phenformin)	

It is possible thus that the platelet changes observed in our diabetic patients are due to a platelet activation from the damaged endothelium and this can be inferred from a higher malondialdehyde production in diabetics with vascular lesions; results similar to ours have been obtained by Neri Serneri (18).

The high BTG levels in diabetics, independently from the presence of vascular complications, suggest that the platelet release is more the result of the metabolic activation than of the vascular damage. This has been confirmed by the results of Preston (22) who after normalization of glycemic values noticed a significant reduction of BTG levels.

Reduced HDL-cholesterol levels together with the increased platelet malondialdehyde formation suggest the presence, in diabetics, of a higher potential capacity to free arachidonic acid from membrane phospholipids as has already been suggested by Nordoy (20).

Patients treated with glibenclamide plus phenformin showed an evident reduction of HDL-cholesterolemia with a clear platelet malondialdehyde increase; a fact that confirms the existence of an interrelation between the two factors.

These data suggest the possibility, in diabetic patients, of a different capacity to free arachidonic acid from membrane phospholipids in relation to the hematic lipoprotein changes as has already been seen in patients with hyperlipoproteinemia type IIa (19, 27, 28).

REFERENCES

1. H.P. Chase, R.L. Williams, S. Dupont, Increased prostaglandin synthesis in chilhood diabetes mellitus. J. Pediatr. 94: 185 (1979).
2. B.S. Coller, R.N. Frank, R.C. Milton, H.R. Gralnick, Plasma cofactors of platelet function: correlation with diabetic retinopathy and haemoglobin A_{1a-c}. Ann. Int. Med. 58:311 (1978).
3. J.A. Colwell, J. Sagel, R. Pennington, M. Meeks, R. Scarpatto, M. Laiminis, Effect of therapy on platelet aggregation in diabetes. Clin. Res. 21:884 (1973).
4. J.A. Colwell, P.V. Halushka, Platelet function in diabetes mellitus. Brit. J. Haemat. 44:521 (1980).
5. U. Diczfalusy, P. Falarderan, S. Hammarstrom, Conversion of prostaglandin endoperoxides to C_1hydroxy acids catalyzed by human platelet thromboxane synthase. Fed. Eu. Biochem. Soc. Let. 82:271 (1977).
6. A.I. Fleischman, M.L. Bierembaum, A. Stier, In vivo platelet function in diabetes mellitus. Thromb. Res. 8:467 (1976).
7. S.K. Garg, H. Lockner, S. Karpatkin, The increased percentage of magathrombocytes in various clinical disorders. Ann. Int. Med. 77:361 (1972).
8. P.V. Halushka, D. Lurie, J.A. Colwell, Increased synthesis of prostaglandin-E-like material by platelet from patients with diabetes mellitus. N. Engl. J. Med. 297:1406 (1977).
9. P.V. Halushka, J.A. Colwell, C. Rogers, C.D. Loudbalt, B. Gartner, Increased thromboxane (TxB_2) synthesis by platelets from patients with diabetes mellitus: studies with a Tx-synthetase inhibitor and Tx-receptor antagonist. Clin. Res. 27:296 (1979).
10. H. Heath, W.D. Bridgen, J.V. Canever, Platelet adhesiveness and aggregation in relation to diabetic retinopathy. Diabetologia 7:308 (1971).
11. A.J. Hellem, Adenosindiphosphate induced platelet adhesiveness in diabetes mellitus with complication. Acta Med. Scand. 190:291 (1971).
12. D.J. Horns, J.M. Gerrard, G.H. Rao, W. Krivit, J.G. White, Smoking and platelet liable aggregation stimulating substances (LASS) synthetizing activity. Thromb. Res.9:661 (1967).

13. E.A. Jaffe, Endothelial cells and biology of factor VIII. New Engl. J. Med. 296:377 (1977).
14. S. Karpatkin, Haeterogenity of human platelets II. Evidence of young and old platelets. Clin. Invest. 48:1083 (1969).
15. M. Lagarde, M. Dechavanne, Increase of platelet prostaglandin cyclic endoperoxides in thrombosis. Lancet 1:88 (1977).
16. E. Lufkin, D.N. Fass, W.M. O'Fallion, E.J.W. Bowie, Increased von Willebrand factor in diabetes mellitus. Metabolism 28: 63 (1979).
17. M. Murray, M.D. Burn, Platelet function in diabetes mellitus. Diabetes 27:342 (1978).
18. G.G. Neri Serneri, G.F. Gensini, R. Abbate, Some aspects of the change of the haemostatic system in diabetes mellitus. In: Atti del Congresso "Giornate Internazionali di Diabetologia". Roma, 17-19 Novembre 1977, p. 133.
19. G.G. Neri Serneri, La sindrome trombofilica nella malattia diabetica. In: Atti 80° Congresso Società Italiana di Medicina Interna, 552, (1979).
20. A. Nordoy, J.M. Rodset, Platelet phospholipids and their function in patients with juvenile diabetes and maturity-onset diabetes. Diabetes 19:698 (1970).
21. M. Okuma, M. Steiner, G.M. Baldin, Studies on lipid peroxides in platelets II. Effects of aggregation agents and platelet antibody. J. Lab. Clin. Med. 77:728 (1971).
22. F.E. Preston, J.D. Ward, B.H. Marcola, N.R. Porter, W.R. Timperley, Elevated betathromboglobulin levels and circulating platelet aggregates in diabetic microangiopathy. Lancet 1: 238 (1978).
23. J. Sagel, J.A. Colwell, L. Crook, M. Laminis, Increased platelet aggregation in early diabetes mellitus. Ann Int. Med. 82:733 (1972).
24. H.N. Seth, Fibrinolytic response to moderate exercise and platelet adhesiveness in diabetes mellitus. Acta Diabet. Lat. 10:306 (1973).
25. M.J. Stuart, H. Erald, J.E. Graeber, D.O. Hakanson, M.K. Barvinchank, Increased synthesis of prostaglandin endoperoxides and platelets hyperfunction in infants of mother with diabetes mellitus. J. Lab. Clin. Med. 94:12 (1979).
26. M.J. Stuart, S. Murphy, F.A. Oski, A simple non radioisotope technic for the determination of platelet life-span. New Engl. J. Med. 292:1310 (1975).
27. M.J. Stuart, J.M. Gerrad, J.G. White, Effect of cholesterol on production of thromnoxane B_2 by platelets in vitro. New Engl. J. Med. 302:6 1980.
28. E. Tremoli, P. Maderna, C.R. Sirtori, Platelet aggregation and malondialdehyde formation in type IIa hypercholesterolemic patients. Haemostasis 8:47 (1979).
29. J. Viikari, Precipitation of plasma lipoproteins by PEG-6000. Scand. J. Clin. Invest. 36:265 (1976).

PLATELET PROSTAGLANDINS AND RELATED COMPOUNDS IN DIABETES MELLITUS

M. Lagarde, P. Berciaud, M. Burtin, M. Soulier, B. Velardo and M. Dechavanne

Inserm U 63, Institut Pasteur, Laboratoire d'Hémobiologie
Faculté Alexis Carrel
69372 Lyon, France

INTRODUCTION

Diabetic patients show a thrombotic tendency with an increase of platelet functions (for a review see reference 1). Prostaglandins and thromboxanes are produced during platelet activation and some of those are potent pro-aggregatory molecules (2, 3). Recently, some investigators have found that diabetic platelet-rich plasmas produce more prostaglandin E-like material than normal platelets when they are aggregated (4). Otherwise, platelets obtained from diabetic subjects are less sensitive to the antiaggregatory effects of imidazole, a thromboxane synthesis inhibitor (5).

In this study, we mainly investigated the part of platelet-poor plasma in platelet reactivity and prostaglandin biosynthesis from exogenous and endogenous arachidonic acid.

METHODS

Patients with various ages (19 to 66 years old) had not taken any drug except for insulin. The average duration of diabetes was about 12 years. Patients were generally free from clinically apparent vascular disease. Among them, twelve showed background retinopathy.

Patient platelets were simultaneously investigated with normal platelets from a donor with the same age and sex.

Blood collection was done on trisodium citrate 3.8% or ACD and platelets isolated from the ACD platelet-rich plasma (PRP) (6). Platelet aggregation was performed according to the method of Born (7). Standard prostaglandins, prostacyclin and thromboxane B2 were generous gifts from Dr. J.E. Pike of Upjohn, Kalamazoo. Endothelial cell microsomes used to inhibit platelet aggregation were obtained from human umbilical cord and their inhibiting activity was completely abolished by 15-hydroperoxy arachidonic acid or tranylcypromine.

Main end-products of exogenous arachidonic acid utilization by platelets were determined with a radiochemical technique (8).

After platelet phospholipid labelling by traces of [^{14}C]-arachidonic acid ($0.4.10^{-6}$M at 50 Ci/mole) Thromboxane B_2, 12-hydroxy-heptadeca-trienoic acid (HHT) and 12-hydroxy-eicosatetraenoic acid (HETE) production under thrombin stimulation, were assayed by the same radiochemical technique (8).

The half-life of thromboxane A_2 in platelet-poor plasma was determined as described by Lagarde et al., (9). Briefly, radiolabelled thromboxane A_2 was generated from human platelets as the enzymatic source andimmediately put in the plasma. Then, aliqots of plasma were decanted in 80 volumes of methanol to obtain mono-o-methyl thromboxane B_2 from thromboxane A_2 (10). Derivatized thromboxane B_2 was radiochemically assayed (8) and a semi-logarithmic regression leads to half-life determination.

RESULTS

Minimal doses of sodium arachidonate or collagen necessary to induce 50% of platelet aggregation were determined. When PRP was used (Table I) these doses were lower, indicating a hyperaggregability to both inducers.

In contrast, only collagen-induced aggregation was increased when isolated platelets were used (Table II).

Table I. Minimal doses of collagen or sodium arachidonate able to induce 50% of platelet aggregation in PRP.

	Collagen (n = 16)	Sodium arachidonate (n = 29)
Control	0.32 µg/ml	0.29 mM
Diabetic	0.21 µg/ml	0.22 mM
Paired test	0.11 ± 0.14 $p < 0.01$	0.07 ± 0.08 $p < 0.001$

Table II. Minimal doses of collagen or sodium arachidonate able to induce 50% of platelet aggregation in isolated platelets.

	Collagen (n = 15)	Sodium arachidonate (n = 28)
Control	0.55 μg/ml	2.05 μM
Diabetic	0.34 μg/ml	1.96 μM
Paired test	0.20 ± 0.33 $p < 0.05$	0.08 ± 0.71 N.S.

Thus, isolated platelets were hyperactive to collagen but not to sodium arachidonate. Moreover, platelet-poor plasma induced a higher response of platelets to arachidonate. Utilization of exogenous arachidonate by platelets isolated from their plasma was not modified since biosynthesis of prostaglandins and related compounds as well as incorporation of arachidonate in phospholipids were unchanged (Table III).

Table III. Utilization of exogenous sodium arachidonate 10 μM by isolated platelets during 4 min. (nmoles of arachidonate incorporated or transformed/10^9 platelets).

	Control	Diabetic	Paired test
Phospholipids (n = 12)	6.1	4.1	2.1 ± 4.3 N.S.
$PGF_2\alpha$ (n = 13)	0.98	1.0	0.02 ± 0.68 N.S.
PGE_2 (n = 13)	0.91	0.93	0.02 ± 0.46 N.S.
TXB_2 (n = 13)	8.1	7.2	0.9 ± 4.5 N.S.
HHT (n = 10)	3.6	4.2	0.6 ± 3.0 N.S.
HETE (n = 9)	10.9	8.2	2.6 ± 3.9 N.S.

Table IV. Biosynthesis of TXB_2, HHT and HETE from endogenous arachidonic acid after stimulation by thrombin 0.1 U/ml. Results are expressed in percentage of initial radioactivity in phospholipids.

	Control	Diabetic	Paired test	
TXB_2 (n = 29)	4.8	5.5	0.6 ± 1.5	$p<0.05$
HHT (n = 28)	0.66	0.57	0.09± 0.90	N.S.
HETE (n = 28)	3.8	4.4	0.6 ± 1.4	$p<0.05$
TXB_2 + HHT + HETE (n = 27)	9.2	10.4	1.2 ± 3.0	$p<0.05$

In contrast, utilization of phospholipidic arachidonate by the same pathways (as judged by thromboxane B_2, HHt and HETE), under thrombin stimulations was higher in diabetic platelets (Table IV).

These data indicate an enhancement of diabetic platelet phospholipase activity whereas prostaglandin synthesis and lipoxygenase activities seem normal. Besides, the half-life of thromboxane A_2 was considerably increased in diabetic platelet-poor plasma as compared to control (Table V).

Lastly, diabetic platelets showed a refractoriness to prostacyclin and prostaglandin E_1 inhibition. Either in the presence of prostacyclin synthesis or prostacyclin, inhibition of collagen-induced platelet aggregation was lower in diabetics than in controls.

Table V. Half-life (min.) of thromboxane A_2 in platelet poor plasma.

Control (n = 9)	Diabetic (n = 12)
7.2 ± 2.9	12.5 ± 5.9
$p<0.05$	

Table VI. Percentage of inhibition of collagen-induced platelet aggregation. PRP was used. Inhibitors were preincubated 1 min.

	Control	Diabetic	Paired test	
Endothelial microsomes (n=26)	55.8	40.8	14.7±36.3	$p<0.05$
PGI_2 (n=28)	53.6	31.3	22.2±31.2	$p<0.001$
PGE_1 (n=6)	70.3	45.5	24.8±21.6	$p<0.05$

Table VII. Percentage of inhibition of collagen-induced platelet aggregation. Isolated platelets were used. Inhibitors were preincubated 1 min.

	Control	Diabetic	Paired test	
Endothelial microsomes (n=15)	63.0	48.7	14.3±16.6	$p<0.01$
PGI_2 (n=19)	61.5	47.1	14.4±22.6	$p<0.02$

These results were observed with PRP (Table VI) as well as with isolated platelets (Table VII).

DISCUSSION

Susceptibility of diabetic platelet aggregation to arachidonate, only in the presence of plasma, suggests the effect of a plasmatic factor to enhance diabetic platelet aggregation. This fact agrees with other recent works which strongly suggest the formation of certain platelet reactive low molecular weight proteins in some diabetic patients (5). Our results do not indicate an increase of the formation of pro-aggregatory molecules provided from arachidonic acid. But, the increase of half-life of thromboxane A_2 by diabetic plasma could partly explain the hyperaggregability of diabetic PRP to arachidonate. Responsiveness of diabetic platelets to collagen (aggregation) or thrombin (prostaglandin synthesis from endogenous arachidonate) was higher and had a platelet origin. These data lead to two hypotheses; 1: diabetic platelets contained more phospholipidic arachidonate or 2: induced phospholipase activity was in patient platelets. On the other hand, patient platelets showed a refractoriness to prostaglandins I_2 and E_1 known to inhibit platelet functions by increasing platelet cyclic AMP (11, 12). Thus a possibility should be that platelet cyclic AMP, which inhibits phospholipase activity (13), is low in diabetic platelets. These last points agree with the second hypothesis mentioned above.

ACKNOWLEDGEMENTS

This work was supported by grant INSERM ASR n° 5. We gratefully acknowledge Drs F. Berthezene and Grange for sending the patients.

REFERENCES

1. M.M. Bern, Platelet functions in diabetes mellitus. Diabetes 27:342-350 (1978).
2. B. Samuelsson, M. Hamberg, C. Malmsten and J. Svensson, The role of prostaglandin endoperoxides and thromboxanes in platelet aggregation. In: Advances in prostaglandin and thromboxane research. Samuelsson, B. and Paoletti, R. (Eds). New York. Raven Press. 1976, 2, 763-766.
3. J.B. Smith, C.M. Ingerman and M.J. Silver, Effects of arachidonic acid and some of its metabolites on platelets. In: Prostaglandins in haematology. Silver, M.J., Smith, J.B. and Kocsis, J.J. (Eds). New York. Spectrum Publications. 1977, 155.
4. P.V. Halushka, D. Lurie and J.A. Colwell, Increased synthesis of prostaglandin E-like material by platelets from patients with diabetes mellitus. New Engl. J. Med. 297:1306-1310 (1977).
5. J.A. Colwell, R.M.G. Nair, P.V. Halushka, C. Rogers, A. Whetsell and J. Sagel, Platelet adhesion and aggregation in diabetes mellitus. Metabolism 28:394-400 (1979).
6. M. Lagarde, P.A. Bryon, M. Guichardant and M. Dechavanne, A simple method for platelet isolation from their plasma. Thrombos. Res. In press.
7. G.V.R. Born, Aggregation of blood platelets by adenosine diphosphate and its reversal. Nature 194:927-929 (1962).
8. M. Lagarde, A. Gharib and M. Dechavanne, A simple radiochemical assay of thromboxane B_2, 12-hydroxy-eicosatetraenoic acid (HETE) and 12-hydroxy-heptadecatrienoic acid (HHT) synthetized by human platelets. Clin. Chim. Acta 79:255-259 (1977).
9. M. Lagarde, B. Velardo, M. Blanc and M. Dechavanne, Fatty acids

bound to serum albumin decrease the half-life of thromboxane A_2. Submitted for publication.

10. M.W. Anderson, D.J. Crutchley, B.E. Tainer and T.E. Eling, Kinetic studies on the conversion of prostaglandin endoperoxide PGH_2 by thromboxane synthetase. Prostaglandins 16: 563-570 (1978).
11. R.R. Gorman, S. Bunting and O.V. Miller, Modulation of human platelet adenylate cyclase by prostacyclin (PGX). Prostaglandins 13:377-388 (1977).
12. R.R. Gorman and O.V. Miller, Modulation of platelet cyclic nucleotide levels by PGE_1 and the prostaglandin endoperoxides PGG_2 and PGH_1. In: Prostaglandins in hematology. Silver, M. J., Smith, J.B. and Kocsis, J.J. (Eds). New York. Spectrum Publications. 1977, 235-246.
13. E.G. Lapetina, C.J. Schmitges, K. Chandrabose and P. Cuatrecasas, Cyclic AMP and prostacyclin inhibit platelet membrane phospholipase. Biochem. Biophys. Res. Commun. 76:828-835 (1977).

PART 4

PLATELET FUNCTION AND VASCULAR DISEASES

RISK FACTORS FOR CORONARY HEART DISEASE AND PLATELET FUNCTIONS

S. Renaud

Inserm, Unit 63
22 avenue du Doyen Lépine
69500 Bron, France

Introduction

Epidemiologic studies have shown that a number of environmental factors or conditions are associated with coronary heart disease. Most of them are predisposing factors also known as risk factors. Other factors appear to have preventive effects. A list of these factors is reported in figure 1. Dietary saturated fats seem to have a key role since in their absence, as in Japanese in Japan, CHD does not occur whatever are the other risk factors (hypertension, diabetes, smoking) present in this population (1). Thus, saturated fats are considered as being the essential factor, while hypertension, diabetes, smoking, obesity, perhaps even oral contraceptives, might be regarded as predisposing factors. Finally, polyunsaturated fats, calcium and magnesium from the hard water (2) and alcohol (3), appear to be preventive factors.

For decades, blood lipids have been considered the main blood mediator between most of these factors and CHD. In recent years, this concept has been challenged since, many of these factors did not affect much or even at all, serum lipids, particularly serum cholesterol. By contrast blood platelets, involved in both thrombosis and atherosclerosis, appear to have their functions markedly changed by most of the factors associated with CHD.

Saturated fats

In order to determine whether saturated fats would affect platelet functions as shown in animals (4,5) and in pilot studies in man (6,7), groups of male farmers (40-45 years) from two regions of France (Var and Moselle) in which the mortality rate from CHD differed markedly as shown in figure 2, were studied, particularly as regards their

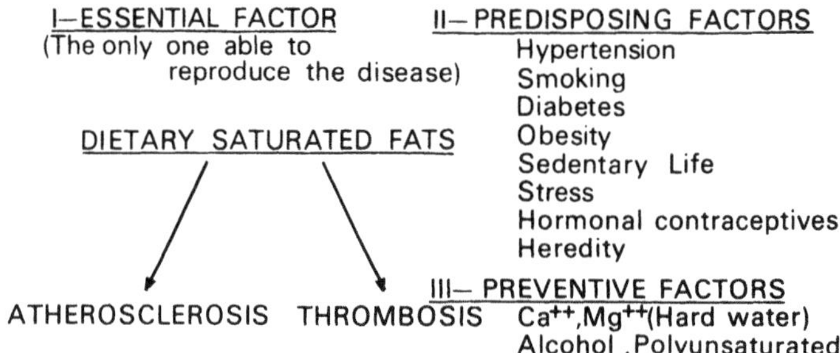

Fig. 1. The risk and preventive factors for coronary heart disease (CHD).

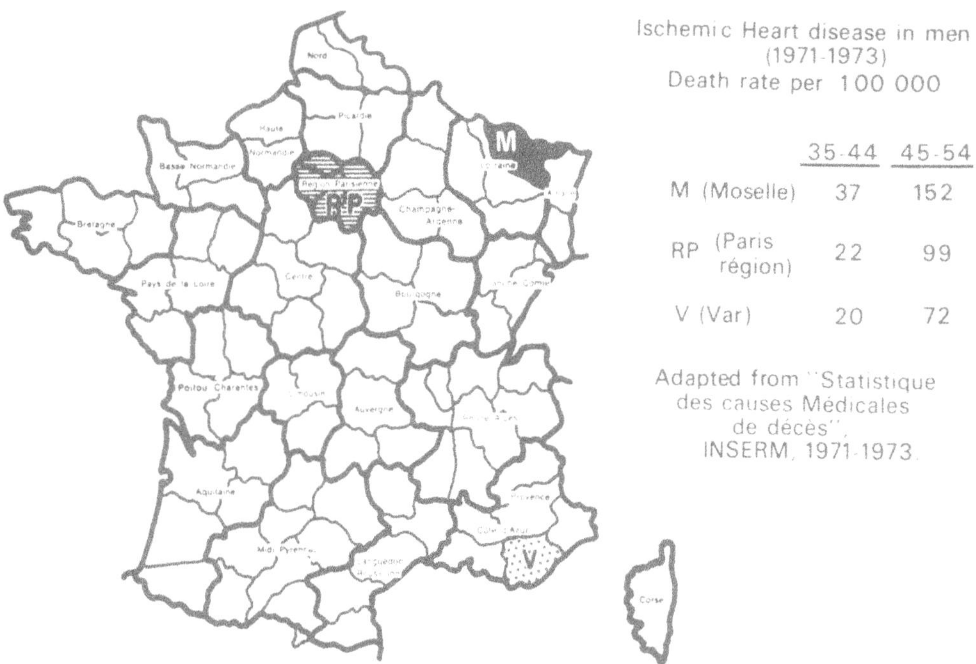

	35-44	45-54
M (Moselle)	37	152
RP (Paris région)	22	99
V (Var)	20	72

Fig. 2. Mortality rate for CHD in Moselle and Var in France (Courtesy of Nutr. Metab. 24 (Suppl 1) 90, 1980).

platelet functions in relation to the intake of saturated fats.

While no difference could be observed in blood between the two regions concerning total cholesterol, HDL-cholesterol or triglycerides, the coagulation was markedly accelerated, as well as the platelet clotting activity (F_3-CT) in farmers from Moselle as shown in figure 3. The response of platelets mostly to thrombin but also to ADP, epinephrine and collagen was more elevated in Moselle farmers.

As shown (figure 4) by the diet chemical analysis, in Moselle there is a significant higher intake of saturated fats (16% of the calories, approximately the level of North America) as compared to Var (12%, approximately the level of Italy).

Diet modification in Moselle farmers

In order to determine whether the abnormal platelet response in Moselle farmers was really due to the diet or whether a genetic factor might be involved, a group of 50 Moselle farmers were persuaded to change their dietary habbits in order to lower their intake of saturated fats to 10% of the calories, and that of polyunsaturated to approximately 12%.

As shown in figure 5, one year after diet modification, the clotting time (PCT) and clotting activity of platelets (F_3-CT) were considerably prolonged and the response to thrombin drastically reduced. These results confirmed that the platelet functions were largely dependent upon the intake of dietary lipids.

Dietary calcium and alcohol

Univariate and multivariate analysis of the results obtained in the 250 French and British farmers studied in 1977-78 indicated (figure 6):

- that the intake of saturated fats was mostly correlated with the clotting activity of the platelets and the response to thrombin
- but also, that the correlations could be significantly improved by including either the alcohol or calcium intake in the analysis.

Both of these factors had a negative sign suggestive of a beneficial effect on the platelet function tests.

Studies in rats fed saturated fats demonstrated that addition of alcohol (6%) to the drinking water was markedly inhibiting the response of platelets to thrombin and ADP aggregation, and prolonged the clotting time (figure 7), despite inducing a significant hypertriglyceridemia.

Similar studies in rats fed saturated fats with an increase in the level of dietary calcium resulted also in a drastic reduction in the platelet reactivity and in the prolongation of the clotting time (figure 8) without changes in the serum cholesterol.

These results indicating that the alcohol and calcium intake have beneficial effects on the platelet hyperactivity induced by saturated fats are consistent with:

- the reported beneficial effect of moderate amounts of alcohol

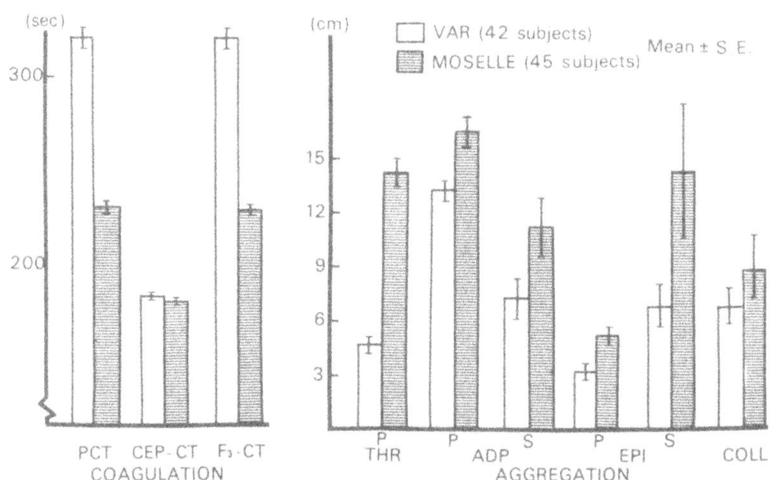

Fig. 3. Compared haematologic results between male farmers (40-45 years) from Var and Moselle in the study performed in the winter of 1977-78.
PCT = Recalcification clotting time of platelet rich plasma (PRP). Evaluates the whole blood clotting activity.
CEP-CT = Cephalin clotting time of platelet poor plasma. Evaluates the clotting activity of the plasmatic clotting factors.
F_3-CT = Recalcification clotting time of washed platelets, resuspended in a standard platelet poor plasma. Evaluates the clotting activity of plateelts (PF_3).
Aggregation: P = primary - S = secondary.
Final concentration of the aggregating agents per ml of PRP.
THR = thrombin, 0.06 NIH Units.
ADP = adenosine diphosphate, 0.92×10^{-6} M
EPI = epinephrine, 1.8×10^{-6} M
COLL = collagen, 126 µg
Highly significant differences ($p<.001$) are observed with the PCT, F_3-CT and thrombin induced aggregation (Courtesy of Nutr. Metab. 24 (Suppl 1):90, 1980).

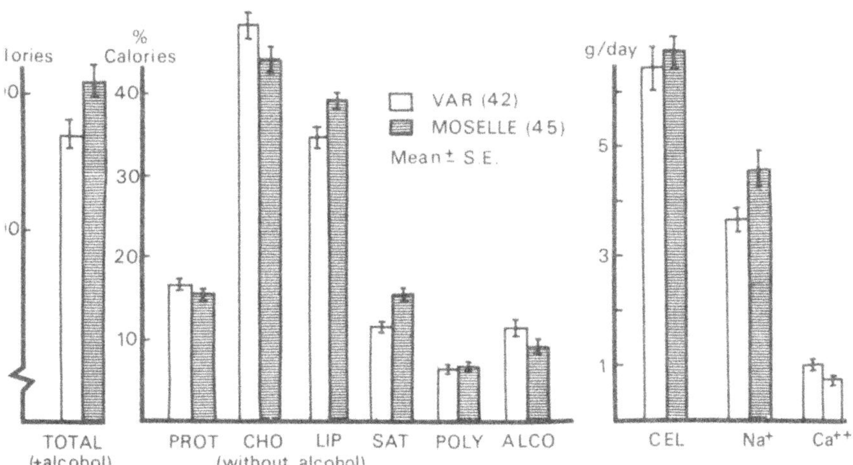

Fig. 4. Compared nutrient intake in the farmers from Var and Moselle studied in figure 3.
PROT = proteins CHO = carbohydrate
LIP = total lipids SAT = saturated fatty acids
POLY = polyunsaturated fatty acids
ALCO = alcohol CEL = cellulose
(Courtesy of Nutr. Metab. as in figures 2 and 3).

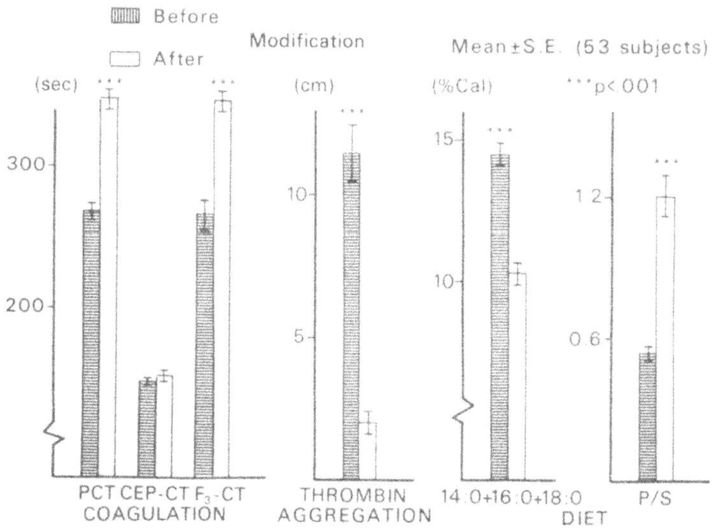

Fig. 5. Coagulation and aggregation to thrombin before, and one year after diet modification in 53 male Moselle farmers. The changes in the intake of saturated fatty acids (14:0+16:0+18:0) and in the P/S ratio are also reported in the figure.

	F3-CT	THR	ADP	EPI	COLL	CHO
SAT (% CAL)	.34	.18	-.16	-.00	.04	.15
SAT-ALCOHOL*	.35	.20	.22	.20	.21	.17
SAT-Ca^{++} *	.38	.23	-.16	.06	.15	.19
18:2 (% CAL)	-.22	-.09	.22	.14	.07	-.30
18:3 (% CAL)	-.31	-.34	.19	.08	-.02	-.13

r = .20, p<.001 ; r = .16, p<.01 ; r = .12, p<.05

* TRIVARIATE ANALYSIS

Fig. 6. Correlations (r) between diet and blood parameters in the 250 male french and british farmers studied in 1877-78. SAT (saturated fats, alcohol, Ca^{++}, 18:2 and 18:3 are diet components determined by chemical analysis of a diet composite collected over a 24 hour-period. F_3-CT, THR ... are the blood parameters as in figure 3. CHO = serum cholesterol.

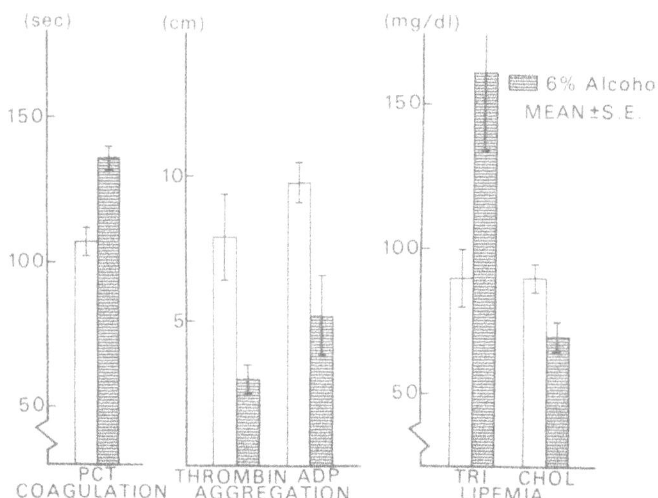

Fig. 7. Influence of 2 months alcohol drinking in rats fed for 6 months a purified diet, containing in weight, 40% of fat. The fat mixture used contained per 100g: corn oil 2, hydrogenated palm oil 20, hydrogenated cocounut oil 18. The main saturated fatty acids of the human diet (14:0+16:0+18:0) represented 75% of the total fatty acids. TRI = triglycerides. CHOL = cholesterol in plasma. Other abbreviations as in Fig.3.

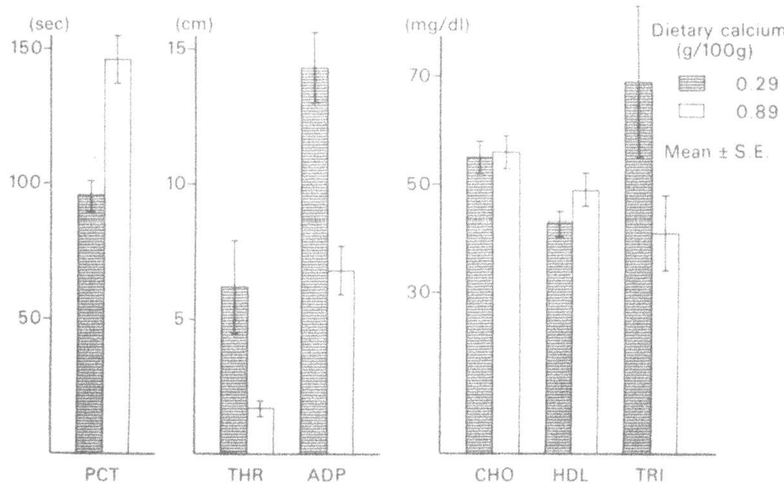

Fig. 8. Influence of dietary calcium on certain blood parameters in rats, fcd for 4 months, purified diet similar to that utilized in the study of figure 7. The only difference was that the slat mixture was decreased to 2 g (per 100 g) in the control group, which supplied, as indicated in the figure 0.29 g of calcium. In the second group, the level of calcium was increased to 0.89 g by addition of calcium carbonate (1 g) and tricalcium phosphate (0.5 g).
CHO = cholesterol HDL = HDL-cholesterol
TRI = triglycerides
Other abbreviations as in figure 3.

on CHD (3)

- the negative association between water hardness and CHD (2), the current available evidence suggesting that the water factor (probably calcium) was not related to blood pressure or serum lipids (8).

Influence of cigarette smoking

There is a well known association between CHD and smoking (11). In order to determine whether cigarette smoking would potentiate the effect of saturated fats on platelet functions, two blood removals were performed in farmers from East and West Scotland.

The first blood removal was performed in fasted subjects, deprived of smoking since the day before, and a second blood removal 10 minutes after having smoked a high nicotine cigarette.

As reported in 1978 (10), it is solely in the Western part of Scotland that the mortality rate from CHD is extremely elevated. Before smoking, the platelet functions tested were already markedly higher in the West part of Scotland (figure 9).

After smoking one cigarette, there was an increase in the reactivity of platelets from 15 to 100% depending on the test, in both regions, which was added to the basic reactivity induced by the saturated fat feeding.

In West Scotland, the elevated intake of saturated fat (16% as compared to 12.6% in the East) appears to be mostly due to a higher consumption of dairy products (butter and cream) (figure 10) in the West.

Physical exercise and platelet functions

A group of 93 Moselle farmers were separated into two groups according to the degree of physical activity determined by the caloric method after withdrawing the basal metabolic rate. This method was shown, in these same farmers, to be strongly correlated with the physical fitness evaluated as the maximum aerobic capacity in the course of exercise ECG (ergometer bicycle).

Results of the platelet functions tested (clotting activity of platelets, response to thrombin, ADP, collagen, epinephrine) indicated that there was no difference between the two groups. In the two groups there was exactly the same intake of saturated fats. By contrast, the level of HDL was significantly higher and that of triglycerides significantly lower in the most active group (figure 11).

Hypertension and platelets

In spontaneously hypertensive rats, we have shown recently (10) that these animals, whatever was the type of diet fed, presented an increase in clotting activity and in the response of platelets to thrombin induced aggregation (figure 12).

By contrast, in human, results obtained so far do not show that

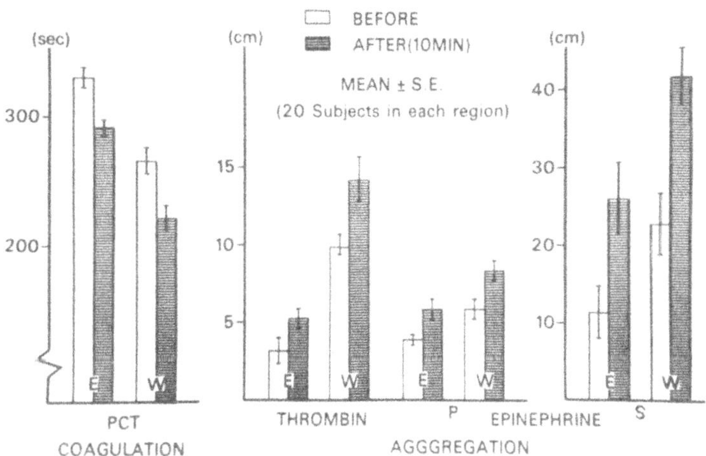

Fig. 9. Haematologic effects of one cigarette, high in nicotine, in farmers from East (E) and West (W) Scotland. Tests were performed on fasted subjects, before and 10 minutes after having smoked a high nicotine cigarette.

	Butter	Cream	Margarine and oil
East	14.5 ± 5.0	3.1 ± 2.7	44.0 ± 6.1
West	40.0 ± 3.5	24.0 ± 9.0	10.1 ± 2.7

Results = Mean ± S.E. in gm/day

Fig. 10. Mean intake of visible fats in the farmers studied in East and West Scotland.

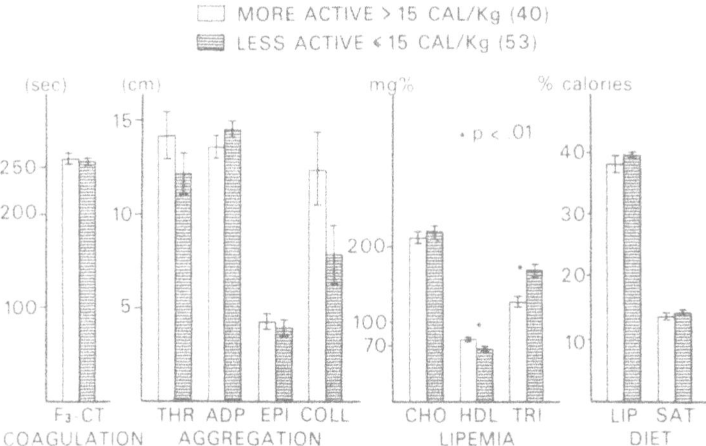

Fig. 11. Physical activity determined by the calorimetric method in 93 Moselle farmers. Abbreviations as in figure 3.

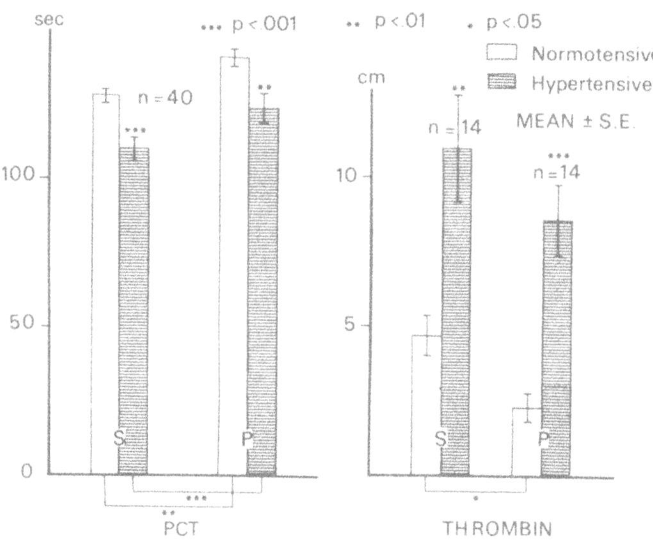

Fig. 12. Influence of spontaneous hypertension in rat, on coagulation and platelet aggregation to thrombin. (Courtesy of Atherosclerosis (101)).
S = saturated P = polyunsaturated diet

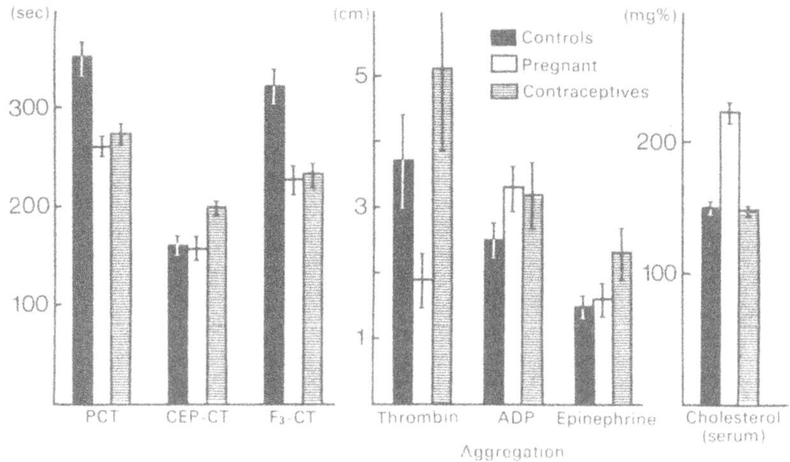

Fig. 13. Influence of pregnancy and oral contraceptives on coagulation andplatelet aggregation in women. Abbreviations as in figure 3.

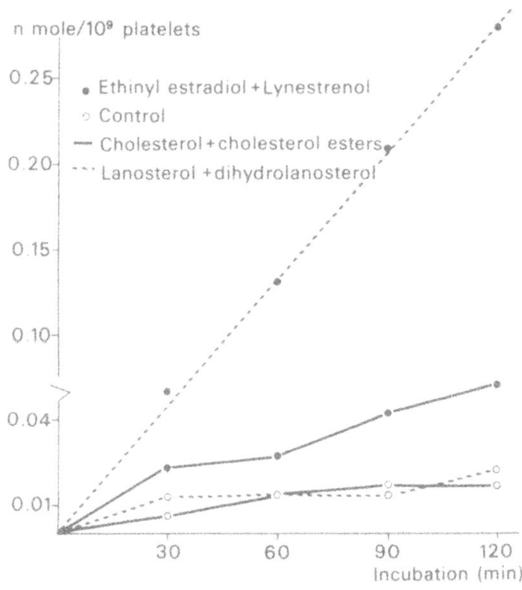

Fig. 14. Kinetics of sodium (^{14}C) acetate incorporation into neutral lipids of rat platelets.
L = lanosterol DL = dihydrolanosterol
CH = cholesterol CE = cholesterol esteres
(Adapted from ref. 17 with the courtesy of Biochim. Biophys. Acta).

hypertension "per se" is associated with an increase in the platelet functions (12).

Diabetes and platelets

Several investigators have shown that platelet functions (particularly aggregation to ADP, collagen and arachidonic acid) were markedly increased in diabetic patients (13) while serum lipids were similar in the diabetic and nondiabetic subjects.

Oral contraceptives and platelets

Oral contraceptives have been associated with thrombotic phenomena, but also with premature CHD (14). Studies we performed more than 10 years ago (15)(figure 13) had indicated that women taking oral contraceptives presented mostly an increase in the clotting activity of their platelets. In female rats, we have shown (16) that the administration of an oral contraceptive was able, in addition to the effect on clotting, to increase the response of platelets to thrombin and ADP induced aggregation. We have recently demonstrated (17, 18) that this hyperactivity of platelets induced by an oral contraceptive was due to an increase in the production of lanosterol, a precursor of cholesterol (figures 14 and 15). Contraceptives are also known to increase triglycerides and lower HDL-cholesterol (19).

Conclusions

As summarized in figure 16, it can be seen that when compared with various blood parameters the effect of environmental factors influencing CHD it is only the platelet functions and HDL-cholesterol which are affected by environmental factors in a way strictly parallel to their known effect on CHD. Consequently, platelet functions might be the main intermediate link between most of the risk (and preventive) factors and CHD, more even than HDL-cholesterol.

Aknowledgments

The main contributors to the studies reported above were, by alphabetical order: Baudier, F., Benoit, C., Ciavatti, M., Covacho, C., Dumont, E., Godsey, F., Mc.Gregor, L., Michel, G., Morazain, R., Ortchanian, E., Thevenon, C. and Symington, I.S.

These studies have been supported by the INSERM (contrats libres CNAMTS and n° 79-5-509-7), the CETIOM in France and by the Tobacco Council of Canada.

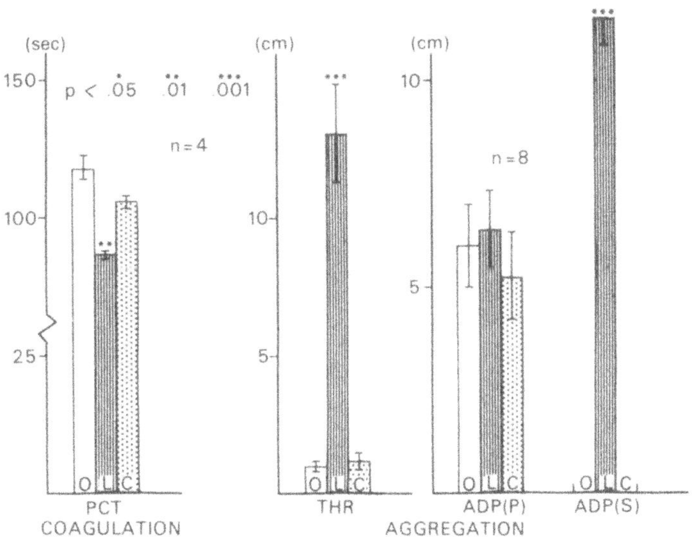

Fig. 15. Compared in vitro effect of lanosterol (L) and cholesterol (C) on coagulation and aggregation on washed platelets of rats.
THR = thrombin ADP = adenosine diphosphate P = primary S = secondary.
Lanosterol and cholesterol were dissolved in alcohol (adapted from ref. 18 with the courtesy of Science).

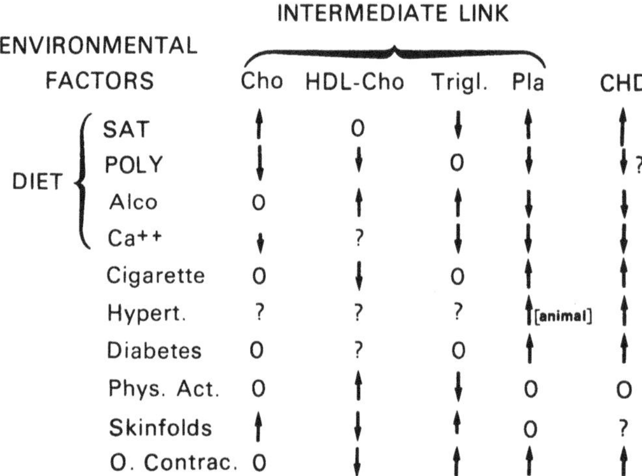

Fig. 16. Influence of the risk an preventive factors on CHD as it can be concluded from the literature. Relationship of these factors to their possible blood mediator.

SAT = saturated fatty acids
POLY = polyunsaturated fatty acids
ALCO = alcohol

Hypert. = hypertension
Phys. Act. = physical activity
O. Contrac. = oral contraceptives

REFERENCES

1. H. Kato, J. Tillotson, M.Z. Nichaman, G. Rhoads and H. Hamilton, Epidemiologic studies of coronary heart disease and stroke in Japanese men living in Japan, Hawai and California. Am. J. Epidem. 97:372 (1973).
2. R. Masironi, Z. Pisa and D. Clayton, Myocardial infarction registry network. Bull. Wld Hlth Org. 57:291 (1979).
3. CH. Hennekens, W. Wilett, B. Rosner, S.D. Cole, S.L. Mayrent, Effects of beer, wine and liquor in coronary deaths. J.A.M.A. 242:1973 (1979).
4. S. Renaud, P. Gautheron, Dietary fats and experimental (cardiac and venous) thrombosis. Haemostasis 2:53 (1973/74).
5. S. Renaud, P. Gautheron, Influence of dietary fats on atherosclerosis, coagulation and platelet phospholipids in rabbits. Atherosclerosis 21:115 (1974).
6. S. Renaud, E. Dumont, F. Godsey, A. Supplisson and C. Thevenon, Platelet functions in relation to dietary fats in farmers from two regions of France. Thromb. Haemostasis 40:518 (1978).
7. J.M. Iacono, R.M. Dougherty, R. Paoletti, C. Galli, A.C.A. Carvalho, A. Ferro-Luzzi, D.G. Therriault, G.J. Nelson, A. Keys, Pilot epidemiological studies in thrombosis. Adv. Exper. Med. Biol. 104:309 (1978).
8. G.W. Comstock, Water hardness and cardiovascular diseases. Am. J. Epidemiol. 110:375 (1979).
9. J.T. Doyle, T.R. Dawley, W.B. Kannel, S.H. Kinch, H.A. Kahn, The relationship of cigarette smoking to coronary heart disease. J.A.M.A. 190:108 (1964).
10. M. Fulton, W. Adams and M.F. Oliver, Regional variations in mortality from ischaemic heart and cerebrovascular disease in Britain. Br. Heart J. 40:563 (1978).
11. L. McGregor, R. Morazain, S. Renaud, Platelet functions and phospholipids fatty acid composition in spontaneously hypertensive rats fed saturated or polyunsaturated fats. Atherosclerosis (In press) (1980).
12. M. Matsumoto, T. Nukada, O. Uyama, S. Yoneda, M. Imaizumi, T. Miyamoto and N. Kayama, Thromboxane generation in patients with essential hypertension or cerebrovascular disease and effect of oral aspirin. Thromb. Haemost. 44:16 (1980).
13. A. Butkus, V.A. Skrinska, O.P. Schumacher, Thromboxane production and platelet aggregation in diabetic subjects with clinical complications. Thromb. Res. 19:211 (1980).
    M. Lagarde, M. Burtin, P. Berciaud, M. Blanc, B. Velardo, M. Dechavanne, Increase of platelet thromboxane A_2 formation and of its plasmatic half-life in diabetes mellitus. Thromb. Res. 19:823 (1980).
14. J.L. Mann, N.H.W. Inman, Oral contraceptives and death from myocardial infarction. Brit. Med. J. 2:245 (1975).
15. F. Lecompte, S. Renaud, Influence of pregnancy and oral contra-

ceptives on platelets in relation to coagulation and aggregation. Thromb. Diath. Haemorrh. 29:510 (1973).
16. L. McGregor, R. Morazain, S. Renaud, Effect of different concentrations of an oral contraceptive and of pregnancy on platelet functions and platelet phospholipid fatty acids composition of rats. In: "Haemostasis and Thrombosis" Academic Press Inc., London 1979, p.565.
17. M. Ciavatti, G. Michel, S. Renaud, Biosynthesis of cholesterol and cholesterol precursors in platelets of female rats treated with oral contraceptives. Biochim. Biophys. Acta 620:297 (1980).
18. M. Ciavatti, E. Dumont, C. Benoit, S. Renaud, Oral contraceptives, lanosterol and platelet hyperactivity in rat. Science 210:642 (1980).
19. U. Larsson-Cohn, L. Wallentin, G. Zador, Plasma lipids and high density lipoproteins during oral contraception with different combinations of ethinyl estradiol and levonorgestrel. Horm. Metab. Res. 11:437 (1979).

ON THE MECHANISM OF PLATELET ACTIVATION DURING HEMOSTASIS AND THROMBOSIS AND ON THE EFFECTS OF PLATELET INHIBITING DRUGS

K. Breddin, N. Bender, and C.M. Kirchmaier

Department of Internal Medicine
J.W. Goethe University
Theodor-Stern-Kai 7
D-Frankfurt a.M., Germany

Platelets are essentially involved in primary hemostasis. During the first seconds after a vascular lesion they are stimulated on the damaged vessel wall as well as inside and outside of the vessel. Many of today's concepts on the mechanism of primary hemostasis and also on the first steps in thrombus formation have been derived from aggregometer studies. But it has to be kept in mind that induced or spontaneous aggregation, as they are usually studied in vitro, only occur if the platelets are partially or totally shape changed, have become more adhesive and tend to aggregate much more than the circulating disc-like platelets.

Since the first investigations on platelet function results of in vitro tests have tempted investigators to draw direct conclusions on the mechanism of hemostasis and thrombosis in vivo. For platelet aggregation this started with the investigations of Caarder (1961) who postulated a retention stimulating factor R in erythrocytes which later was identified as adenosine diphosphate (ADP). The investigations of Born (1962) and O'Brien (1962) led to the routine techniques to measure induced platelet aggregation. ADP from then on was in the discussion as a possibly important inducer of hemostasis and thrombosis. Later a number of other aggregation-inducers became known. Collagen and adrenaline have been widely used and Holmsen (1969) described the release reaction which he later differentiated in a first and second phase.

These investigations often led to the conclusion that platelet reactions in vivo occur in a very similar way as aggregation in vivo. Based on the results obtained with the aggregometer numerous investigators began to transform the aggregometer model into the laboratory animal. But it is unlikely that this will lead to a better insight into the physiology and pathophysiology of hemostasis or thrombosis. If sufficiently high doses are used the infusion of ADP, collagen, adrenaline or arachidonic acid leads also in laboratory animals to an intravascular platelet aggregation, to the obstruction of pulmonary capillaries or in other experimental setups to vascular occlusions in other organs. It has become a custom to investigate antithrombotic drugs in such models. Such models are probably not more conclusive than investigations with the aggregometer.

The contact of platelets with artificial surfaces or a reduced temperature lead to a transformation of the platelets in anticoagulated blood or PRP within 10-30 minutes. If hemostasis or thrombus formation are studied in small rat mesenteric vessels an extremely rapid transformation of those platelets can be observed which stick to the damaged vessel wall and to each other. The forming aggregates consist for 15-60 minutes of single platelets which do not fuse. Irreversible aggregation as it occurs under the influence of ADP or collagen in vitro can be observed only rarely and rather late after vascular lesions in vivo.

WHAT IS RESPONSIBLE FOR THE RAPID PLATELET STIMULATION IN VIVO

In our laboratory we define stimulated platelets as thrombocytes which have formed pseudopodes and have sphered. This process is accompanied by enhanced platelet adhesiveness and an enhanced aggregability. Stimulated platelets may transform back into the circulating disc like form in vitro and in vivo within minutes. When we investigated morphologic platelet changes directly after blood sampling we noticed that in some samples of citrated or whole blood which have been fixed directly after the venepuncture up to 80% of the platelets were morphologically changed in contrast to the 20% which we usually find transformed directly after blood sampling (Bender et al., 1979). It seems possible that this effect was caused by the admixture of tissue fluid at blood sampling.

When we deliberately punctured the vessel wall in 10 healthy volunteers, tried to aspirate some tissue fluid and then drew the needle back into the vein to obtain venous blood we found a mean of 65% of morphologically shape changed platelets in the blood samples which were fixed directly after blood sampling in glutardialdehyde. Apparently the addition of small amounts of tissue material directly at blood sampling had induced the shape change within seconds. It seemed likely that this was a still unknown effect of thromboplastin. But we have been able to obtain tissue extracts which are free of any thromboplastic activity and which have a very strong platelet stiulating effect even if highly diluted. During recent years this tissue extract has been named emostasis activating factor (HAF) (Kirchmaier et al., 1979). This material can be obtained from practically all organs with the exception of the brain. Platelets can adhere, change their shape and aggregate without, this form of stimulation as can be shown in different ex vivo tests, but it is likely that in vivo the hemostasis activating factor together with v. Willebrand

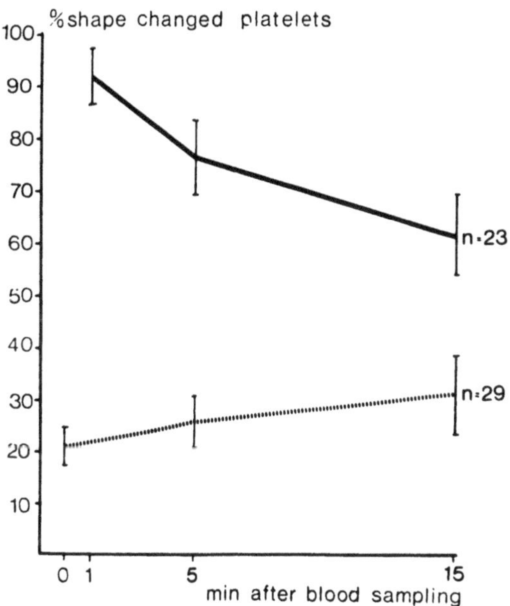

Fig. 1. Normal values of spontaneous platelet stimulation during the first 15 minutes after blood sampling (lower curve). If citrated blood is incubated at 37°C the number of shape changed platelets rises only slowly. The upper curve shows the rapid but reversible platelet stimulation after addition of 40 μg of a tissue extract directly at blood sampling (Kirchmaier et al., 1979).

factor is an important accelerator of platelet stimulation. Platelets regain their disc like form also in vitro within minutes if citrated blood is incubated together with the tissue extracts at 37°C (Fig. 1).

We come to the following hypothesis of the first platelet reactions in primary hemostasis (Fig. 2):

Circulating disc like platelets are rapidly stimulated after contact with lipoproteins which are liberated from damaged cells of the extravascular tissue. This stimulation also depends on the presence of v. Willebrand factor. While it is likely that platelet stimulation by v. Willebrand factor and HAF play a major role in primary hemostasis, it is not yet clear if this mechanism is important for thrombogenesis. A strong platelet stimulating activity was recovered from human atheromatous material, but more investigations are needed to elucidate if this material may propagate arterial thromboses.

We do not yet know the single reactions which lead to thrombus

Induction		Reaction
vascular lesion	⇒	bleeding from damaged vessel
Hemostasis activating factor	⇒	platelet shape change
F. VIII- related antigen	⇒	enhanced adhesiveness
damaged tissue (collagen, basal membranes)	⇒	adhesion and reversible aggregation of stimulated platelets
stimulated, aggregated platelets + thromboplastin	⇒	partial release and activation of thrombin ⇓ coagulation

Reactions in primary Hemostasis

Fig. 2. Hypothesis on the reactions in primary hemostasis.

formation in veins or in atherosclerotic arteries and it is therefore difficult to decide which platelet function should be inhibited by an antithrombotic drug, which inhibits platelet functions. Acetylsalicylic acid (ASA) is a strong inhibitor of induced or spontaneous aggregation and based on the results of aggregometer studies ASA has been investigated as an antithrombotic drug in animal experiments and in clinical studies. 250 mg of acetylsalicylic acid inhibit platelet aggregation for 3-5 days and this effect is caused by the irreversible inhibition of thromboxane A2 formation in the platelets (Hamberg et al., 1974). ASA inhibits cyclooxygenase in platelets and in the vessel wall. Following the concept of an important role of the prostaglandin metabolism for the regulation of blood-vessel wall interactions Moncada and Vane (1979) suggested to use very small doses of ASA in the range of about 100-200 mg/day to test the antithrombotic effect of this drug in future clinical trials. Their hypothesis was that acetylsalicyclic acid inhibits prostacyclin formation in the vessel wall as well as thromboxane A2 formation in the platelets if higher doses of ASA are used and that the antithrombotic effect of ASA might thereby be reduced. This concept is based on the assumption that the antithrombotic effect of ASA is closely correlated with the inhibition of thromboxane A2 formation in the platelets and therefore with the inhibition of platelet aggregation. Several animal studies of different investigators are not compatible with this concept (Busse, Haarmann, Seuter, Zimmerman, 1980). They found that ASA in doses of 1-5 mg/kg which are sufficient to inhibit cyclooxygenase in the platelets had a slight antithrombotic effect but higher doses up to 50 mg/kg were more effective in inhibiting thromboses.

Single doses of ASA between 250 and 500 mg result in a marked and dose dependent prolongation of the Ivy bleeding time. The

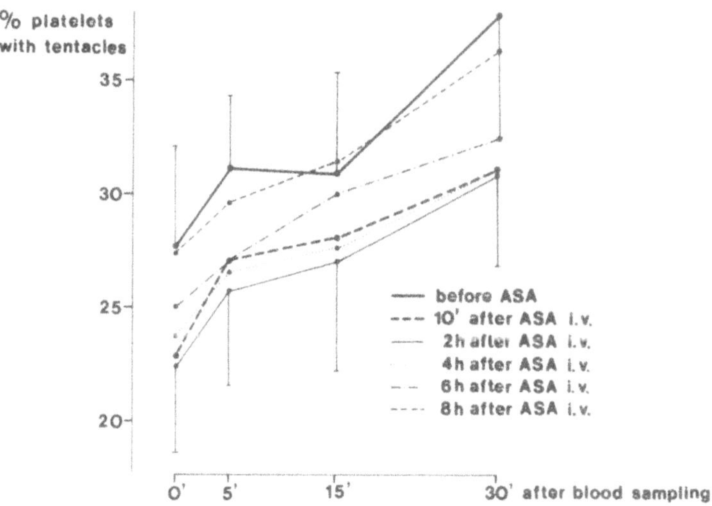

Fig. 3. Effect of 1 g ASA intravenously on platelet stimulation during eight hours. Stimulation was inhibited 10 minutes after injection and remained relatively constant for the next four hours and was slightly reduced after six hours. Eight hours after the injection no stimulation inhibiting effect was present.

prolongation of the bleeding time is marked two hours after ingestion, less pronounced during the following hours but still present after 24 hours. 500 mg are more effective than 250 mg. Pietsch et al. (1979) noticed that after the ingestion or intravenous injection of 500 or 1000 mg ASA the spontaneous platelet shape change after blood sampling was inhibited for 6-8 hours (Kirchmaier et al., 1979) (Fig. 3). In a new test system it is studied, to which extent platelets can be stimulated by hemostasis activating factor containing tissue extracts in venous blood after blood sampling and how fast stimulated platelets are transformed back into the disc form. In this test system 250 mg ASA inhibited platelet stimulation for about 6 hours (Fig. 4). The maximum of this stimulation inhibiting was observed four hours after ingestion. After oral intake of 500 mg ASA the stimulation inhibiting effect was most pronounced after 6 hours (Fig. 5). The initial values were reached after 12-16 hours. 8 hours after ingestion of 1 g ASA the inhibiting effect was most pronounced and lasted also until about 12 hours after the intake (Fig. 6). In this test system dipyridamole was as effective as ASA, but the effect of single doses of 75 or 150 mg lasted for only about 6 hours (Fig. 7). The maximal

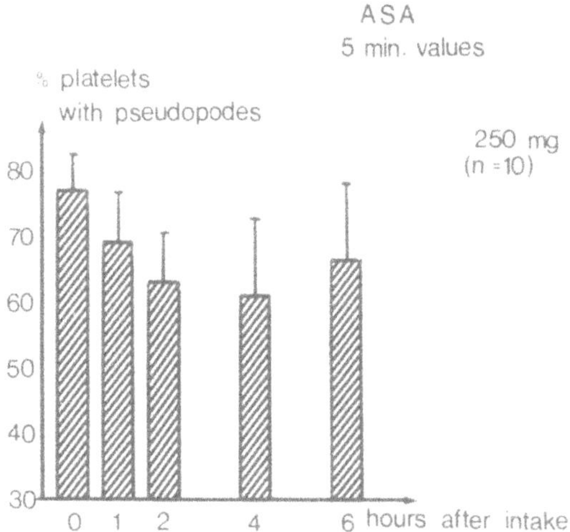

Fig. 4. Effect of oral ingestion of 250 mg ASA on lipoprotein induced platelet stimulation. Results obtained five minutes after blood sampling. Platelet stimulation is inhibited markedly two and four hours after ASA administration. After six hours there is only a slight inhibition.

effect is reached 2-4 hrs after ingestion of the drug. The combination of both drugs did not prolong the duration of the stimulation inhibiting effect of one of the single drugs. We do not yet know if the combination inhibits platelet stimulation as strongly during the first hours after ingestion than one of the single drugs alone.

Clinical trials on the effect of ASA alone or together with dipyridamole have usually been performed in daily doses between 900 and 1500 mg and with a dipyridamole dose of 225 mg/day. If acetylsalicylic acid is administered in doses below 1 g/day platelet stimulation is not continuously inhibited during a 24 hours period 3 x 300 mg are likely to be more effective than 2 x 500 mg for the same reasons. If the inhibition of platelet stimulation is partially or mainly responsible for the antithrombotic action of both drugs, the doses for a continuous inhibition during a 24 hours period would have to be larger than those which are needed to inhibit platelet aggregation.

There are several arguments against the concept that the antithrombotic effect of ASA is caused by the inhibition of cyclooxigenase alone.

1. In most of the clinical trials in which an antithrombotic effect of ASA has been made likely, doses of 9000-1500 mg/day have been administered.

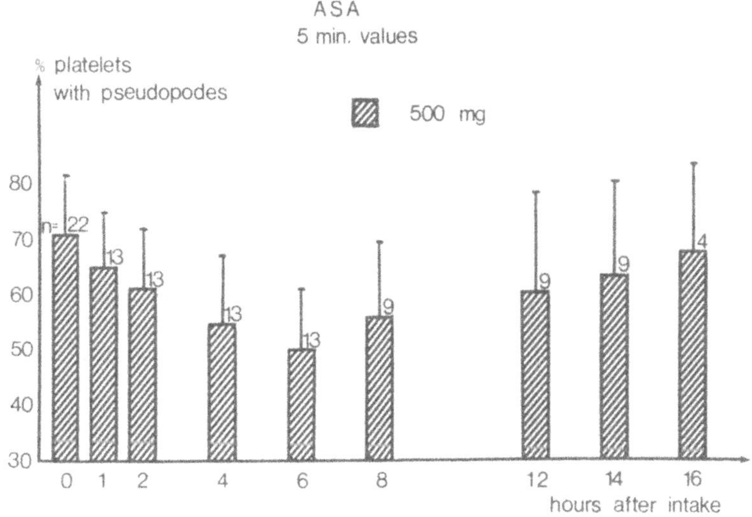

Fig. 5. The effect of 500 mg ASA on platelet stimulation, same technique as in Fig. 4. Stimulation was inhibited markedly from the fourth to the eighth hour, from 12 to 16 hours after the ingestion no or only a minimal inhibition could be detected.

2. Several investigators reported on a dose dependant increase of the antithrombotic effect of ASA in animal models.
3. ASA prolongs the bleeding time and inhibits platelet shape change and HAF induced shape change dose dependent for a much shorter time than platelet aggregation.
4. The total absence of cyclooxygenase in platelets and vessel walls leads to a mild bleeding tendency and not to thromboses as has been shown by Pareti et al. (1980).

Further studies with drugs which either inhibit aggregation or stimulation should verify which effects are important for an antithrombotic effect or if all inhibitory effects contribute to the inhibition of thrombus formation. The different results in two large clinical trials on the effect of ASA in the prevention of death and recurrent infarction after a first myocardial infarction - AMIS (1980) and Paris (1980) - also can possibly be explained by the dose differences between these two studies. In AMIS patients in the ASA group received 2 x500 mg daily, while in the Persantin/Aspirin Reinfarction Study (Paris, 1980) patients in the ASA or in the ASA + Persantin group received 3 x 300 mg daily. If the effect of ASA on platelet stimulation is a main contributing factor of the action of this drug, 3 x 300 mg will result in an inhibition of stimulation for about 16-20 of 24 hours while 2 x 500 mg are effective for only 12-14 hours per

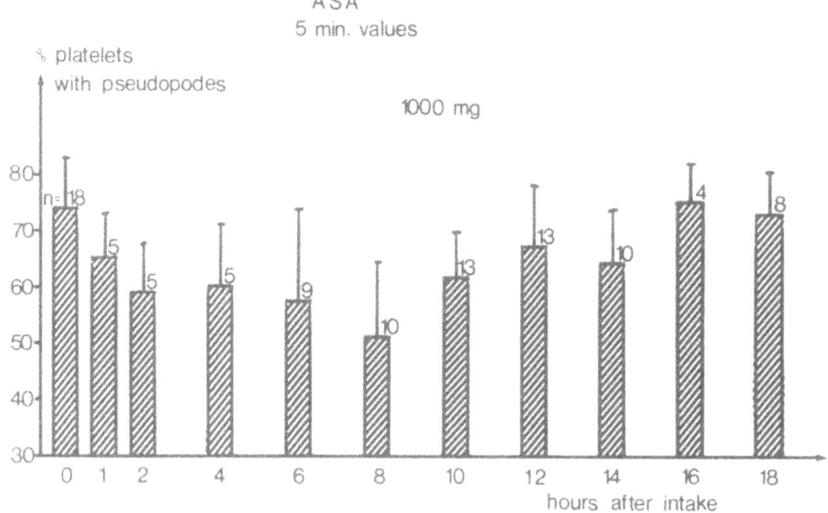

Fig. 6. Lipoprotein-induced platelet stimulation after ingestion of 1 g ASA. A marked inhibition is found from the second to the eighth hour. Before that time and thereafter only a slight or no inhibition is detected. There is not much difference between the results after ingestion of 0.5 and 1.0 g ASA.

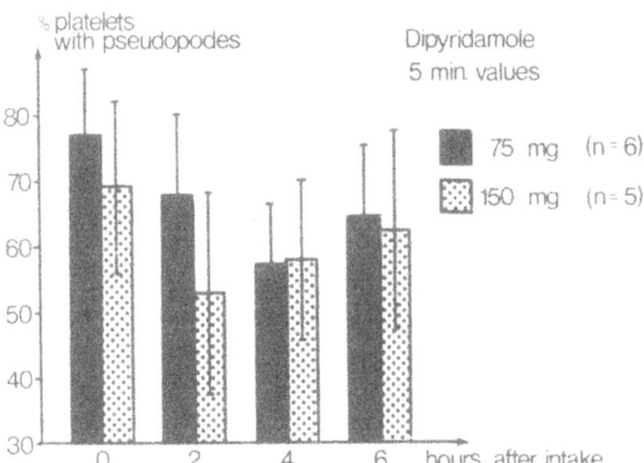

Fig. 7. Tissue extract induced platelet stimulation was inhibited by ingestion of 75 or 150 mg dipyridamole after two and four hours, while after six hours the inhibiting effect was already decreasing.

day. From this point of view ASA should be administered in a form which leads to prolonged resorption and combinations of ASA + dipyridamole also might be more effective if the resorption of both drugs is retarded to result in a continuous inhibition of platelet stimulation.

Ditazole, which does not inhibit platelet aggregation in the doses which are clinically administered has a mild but continuous inhibiting effect on platelet simulation and it also inhibits more effectively laser induced thrombus in our rat mesenteric model. We do not yet know for sure which platelet function should be mainly affected by an antithrombotic drug. For the better evaluation of antiplatelet drugs more sensitive tests to measure primary adhesion and platelet activation will have to be developed and should be standardized.

REFERENCES

Aspirin Myocardial Infarction Study Research Group, 1980, A randomised, controlled trial of aspirin in persons recovered from myocardial infarction. J. Am. Med. Ass.243:661-669.

Bender, N., Kirchmaier, C.M., Bartsch, B., Lindenborn, B., Breddin, K., 1979, Stimulation of blood platelets by extracts of subcutaneous tissue. Trombos. Res.14:341-351.

Born, G.V.R., 1962, Quantitative investigations into the aggregation of blood platelets. J. Physiol. 67-68.

Busse, W.D., Seuter, F., Erfahrungen mit Azetylsalizylsäure, Dipyridamol und Sulfinpyrazon in verschiedenen Tiermodellen. In: K. Breddin, D. Gross (Eds): Thrombosemodelle am Tier. Die Rolle der Prostaglandine für Thrombogenese und Schmerzpathogenese. F.K. Schattauer, Stuttg., New York (im Druck).

Gaarder, A., Jonsen, J., Laland, S., Hellem, A., Owren, P.A., 1961, Adenosine diphosphate in red cells as a factor in the adhesiveness of human blood platelets. Nature 192:531-532.

Haarmann, W., Erfahrungen mit Azetylsalizylsäure, Dipyridamol und Sulfinpyrazon in verschiedenen Tiermodellen. In: K. Breddin, D. Gross, (Eds): Thrombosemodelle am Tier. Die Rolle der Prostaglandine für Thrombogenese und Schmerzpathogenese. F.K. Schattauer, Stuttg., New York (im Druck).

Hamberg, M.J., Svensson, B., Samuelson, B., 1974, Mechanism of the antiaggregating effect of aspirin in human platelets. Lancet i:223-224.

Holmsen, H., Day, H.J., 1971, Adenine nucleotide behaviour during the release reaction induced by ADP and epinephrine. Circulation 44, Suppl. 2 II-81.

Kirchmaier, C.M., Bender, N., Wilhelm, B., Sayegh, A.Al, Breddin, K., 1979, A haemostasis activating factor (HAF) in subcutaneous tissue extracts: effects on morphologic platelet changes, platelet retention and platelet aggregation. Trombos. Res. 16:81-91.

Moncada, S., Vane, J.R., 1979, Arachidonic acid metabolites and the interactions between platelets and blood vessel walls. New Engl. J. Med. 300:1142-1147.

O'Brien, J.R., 1962, Platelet aggregation II. Some results from a new method of the study. J. Clin. Path. 15:452-455.

Pareti, F.I., Smith, J.B., D'Angelo, A., Mari, D., Capitano, A., Mannucci, P.M., 1980, Congenital deficiency of platelet thromboxane and vascular wall prostacyclin in a patient with aspirin-like syndrome. In: E. Deutsch, K. Lechner (Eds): Fibrinolyse, thrombose, haemostase. F.K. Schattauer Stuttg., New York, 619-622.

Persantin-Aspirin Study Research Group, 1980, Persantine and aspirin in coronary heart disease. Circulation 62:449-461.

Pietsch, U., Lippmann, M., Scharrer, I., Breddin, K., 1977, Neue Befunde Wirkung von Azetylsalizylsäure. Die Hemmwirkung auf den Formwandel der Thrombozyten und ihre Bedeutung für die Dosierung als Antithrombotikum. In: K. Alexander, M. Cachovan (Eds): Diabetische Angiopathien: G. Witzstrock Baden-Baden, Köln, New York, 384-351.

Seuter, F., 1976, Inhibition of platelet aggregation by acetylsalicylic acid and other inhibitors. Haemostasis 5: 85-95.

Zimmermann, R., Wirksamkeit antithrombotischer Substanzen an Modellen arterieller und venöser Thrombose am Kaninchen. In: K. Breddin, D. Gross (Eds): Thrombosemodelle am Tier. Die Rolle der Prostaglandine für Thrombogenese und Schmerzpathogenese. F.K. Schattauer Stuttg., New York (im Druck).

METHODS FOR THE DETECTION OF ACTIVATED PLATELETS

F.I. Pareti, A. D'Angelo, and P.M. Mannucci

Centro Angelo Bianchi Bonomi per la Cura delle Malattie Emorragiche
Istituto di Clinica Medica III
Università degli Studi di Milano - Italy

There is substantial evidence that blood platelets may play an important role in the development and progression of premature atherosclerotic disease and its complications. (Mustard and Packham 1975, Ross and Glomset 1976 and Harker et al. 1976). It has been demonstrated that platelet function, as measured by a variety of different *in vitro* methods, is often increased in patients with atherosclerosis and related conditions predisposing to or associated with premature atherosclerosis. However, it is still not known whether the abnormalities of platelet function are primary, that is are induced by changes in the blood associated with the atherosclerosis risk factors or are consequences of the vascular injury, that initiates platelet adherence, followed by the release from platelets of substances that can cause vascular injury and promote the growth of smooth muscle cells and fibroblasts (Mustard and Packham 1975, Harker et al. 1976). The latter hypothesis, assuming that the primary feature in arterial disease is probably damage of the vessel wall rather than hyperreactivity of blood platelets is the commonly favored one. Continuous activation of platelets and local production of thrombin can lead to the presence of either hyperreactive platelets or, if the stimulus is stronger, to the presence of platelets that have released their granules emptied, or "exhausted" platelets can circulate and may be detectable. The presence of the released products in the circulation can serve as an indicator of the existence of vascular disease which has led to platelet activation. On the other hand, intravascular platelet aggregation can lead to an increased rate of removal of platelets from the circulating blood and, through compensatory stimulation of release of platelets from the bone marrow, to increased platelet turnover and shift towards a younger circulating population. Since young platelets have been shown to be functionally more active than older platelets (Karpatkin 1969).

The increased platelet function may well be an epiphenomenon secondary to increased platelet turnover. In patients with atherosclerosis, it should therefore be possible to find both "exhausted" and "hyperreactive" platelets.

When paltelets are exposed in vivo to appropriate stimuli, they adhere, aggregate and release the contents of their storage granules. Moreover they supply "procoagulants" which accelerate thrombin formation, consolidating the aggregates with fibrin. Each of these functional activities has been investigated by many authors, all of whom assume thrombus formation to indicate loss of control of the haemostatic process.

PLATELET ADHERENCE

A number of different methods for the measurement of platelet adherence have been proposed (Wright 1941, Hellem 1960, Salzman 1963, Hirsch et al. 1968, Breddin 1968, Cazenave 1973, Baumgartner and Muggli 1976, Mant 1977). It is clear that the best method on theoretical grounds is one that reproduces as accurately as possible the in vivo conditions, that is one that uses subendothelial tissue as the adhesion surface, whole blood as the source of platelets and appropriate shear rates.

However such a method cannot be used routinely and is not easily reproducible.

Platelet retention on glass beads (Hellem 1971) is a very simple method which has therefore been thoroughly investigated in many laboratories. Although earlier studies suggested that increased adherence to glass might be associated with various thromboembolic conditions (Steele et al. 1971, Heath 1971, Hellem 1971, Achenson et al. 1972, Mason and Summerlin 1972, Steele et al. 1973, O'Brien et al 1974), it is now clear that this test is both nonspecific for thrombosis and insensitive (Hirsch 1977).

PLATELET AGGREGATION

At least three different mechanisms are involved in the process of platelet aggregation:

1) synthesis of prostaglandin endoperoxides and of thromboxane A_2;

2) release of ADP from dense bodies;

3) a third mechanism, independent of TxA_2 production and ADP release which is active in the presence of high concentrations of thrombin and collagen (Smith et al. 1976).

The most widely used in vitro test for the measurement of platelet aggregation involves the use of an aggregometer to measure changes in light transmission or light scattering through citrated platelet-rich plasma that is maintained at 37^{0}C and is stirred at about 100 rpm (Born 1962). Spontaneous platelet aggregation (SPA) is not usually observed in platelet-rich plasma from normal subjects (without addition of aggregating agents). Ten Cate (1977) reported spontaneous platelet aggregation in about 40% of patients with transient ischaemic attacks (TIA) and cerebral infarction. SPA has also been seen in patients with diabetes mellitus (Breddin et al. 1976), angina pectoris, myocardial infarction, peripheral arterial diseases (Wu and Hoak 1976) and in some patients with thrombocystosis. due to myeloproliferative disorders (Preston 1974, Vreeken-Van Aken 1971). Similar results were also obtained by screen filtration pressure methods (Fleischman et al. 1975; Hornstra-Ten Hoor 1975). Platelet aggregation after addition of aggregating agents such as adrenaline, ADP, collagen and thrombin, can be used to detect hyperreactive platelets, which require lower concentrations of inducers than are required to aggregate platelets from "normal" subjects.

Enhanced platelet aggregation with ADP (Kwaan et al. 1972) adrenaline and collagen (Sagel et al. 1975) in diabetics with and without apparent vascular complications (Breddin et al. 1976, Colwell et al. 1977), has been reported. An increase in the sensitivity of platelet aggregation by ADP has also been reported for patients with angina pectoris (Frishman et al. 1974), whereas survivors of myocardial infarction seem to show platelet aggregation enhanced after collagen addition (Salky-Dugdale 1973). A marked increase in the sensitivity to collagen and ADP has been reported for patients with type II hyperlipoproteinaemia (Carvalho et al. 1974, Shattil et al. 1975). These observations do not prove that there is a relationship between enhanced platelet aggregation measured in vitro and the development of vascular or thrombotic complications in these disorders. Moreover, the predictive value of this test remains to be assessed. Finally, special notice should be taken of the many variables that influence the results, including the pH of the plasma, the technique for blood collection and the interval and temperature after collection, the mode of harvesting, the type and rate of stirring and the preparation and strength of the reagents added (Day et al. 1976, Kinlough-Rathbone et al. 1977, Warlow et al. 1974, Mielke 1978).

Recently Wu and Hoak (1974) developed a new method which they claim detects circulating platelet aggregates in vivo by counting the difference between the platelet number in EDTA-blood and blood fixed with formalin. Promising results have been obtained in patients with TIA (Dougherty et al. 1977; Wu and Hoak 1975; Kalendovski et al. 1975), acute myocardial infarction (Gjesdal 1976), acute peripheral insufficiency (Wu and Hoak 1976), recurrent deep vein thrombosis (Wu et al. 1976), migraine and ischaemic retinopathy (Hoak 1977). However Prazich et al. (1977) studying a more limited number of patients with cerebrovascular and cardiovascular diseases, were not able to detect increased platelet aggregates, and inconsistent results have also been obtained by our group for patients with TIA, stroke, angina pectoris and myocardial infarction (D'Angelo et al. 1980 a and b), retinopathy and peripheral arterial diseases (Mari-Moia 1980). Moreover, there is concern about whether the test detects actual circulating aggregates or an increased tendency for certain platelets to form aggregates on exposure to formalin. It is also possible that nonspecific plasma factors in patients with inflammatory disorders might cause rapid clumping of platelets in vitro, while the blood is being taken (Hirsch 1978).

RELEASE REACTION

Once the platelets have been stimulated they release the contents of both the dense bodies and the alpha-granules. In 1975 the Edinburgh group isolated two platelet specific antigens with antiheparin activity. PF_4 and BTG, contained in the alpha-granules (Moore et al. 1975 a and b) and radioimmunoassay for both were developed (Bolton et al. 1976 a and b). It became possible to measure the levels of these two substances in plasma, as an index of the platelet release reaction. Since then high plasma levels of BTG and PF_4 have been reported in a number of patients with deep vein thrombosis (Ludlam et al. 1979), diabetes (Campbell et al. 1977, Burrows et al. 1978, Preston et al. 1978), peripheral arterial disease (Cella et al. 1979, Zahavi et al. 1979) myocardial infarction (Ludlam et al. 1979, Hnadin et al. 1978) and cerebrovascular diseases (Cella et al. 1979). We confirmed this finding in patients with myocardial infarction, angina pectoris (D'Angelo et al. 1980b), stroke TIA (D'Angelo et al. 1980a) and diabetes (Micossi et al. 1980). However, a large overlap with the values for "normal" controls renders it still difficult to differentiate between patients and healthy subjects by means of these tests. Moreover, it is very important that a standardized procedure of blood collection and processing of samples be adopted in order to achieve comparable results. Blood must be collected carefully to avoid release during sampling. We have adopted the modified anticoagulant cocktail suggested by Ludlam and Cash (1976), containing EDTA, theophylline and PGE_1. The blood-anticoagulant mixture must be rapidly cooled in ice and centrifuged within 30 min. Also, even under ideal conditions, there are some doubts that results which are considered to fall into the normal range (less than 40 ng/ml) correspond to the actual levels in the circulation. A major problem is the short half-lives of BTG (100 min) and PF_4 (20 min), which mean that even in normal subjects there is continuous leakage of BTG from the platelets in order to maintain measurable levels in plasma. As stressed by Sixma (1978), a thrombus must grow by 50 ul/hr, or 1 ml/20 hr to give a significant elevation in BTG levels: this may occur in the acute phase of deep vein thrombosis but not in other pathological states in which high levels have been found. The ratio of BTG/PF_4 can be used to detect false high values due to in vitro release. An alternative to measurement of substances released by the platelets into plasma is to determine serotonin, adenine nucleotides, BTG and PF_4 retained within the platelets, i.e. the contents of the dense bodies and alpha-granules.

In vitro experiments have shown that a large proportion of the platelets trapped within a clot may be released following fibrinolysis (Zusel, 1971). Similarly, in vivo, platelets which have undergone aggregate formation or which have been trapped within a thrombus may subsequently be released and return into the circulation. Reimers et al. (1976) have demonstrated that thrombin-degranulated rabbit platelets survive for a normal period of time when transfused into thrombocytopenic animals and that their haemostatic effectiveness is partially maintained. Since these platelets do not restore granules during circulation in the recipient animals (Reimers et al. 1977), the presence in man of circulating "exhausted" (O'Brien 1978) platelets might be detected by finding reduced platelet levels, in relation to the platelet counts, of substances which are extruded during the release reaction.

Such exhausted platelets might still be detectable in the circulation once the released proteins (BTG and PF_4) have been cleared. Moreover serotonin, adeninenucleotides, BTG and PF_4 are present in large quantities within platelet granules: therefore the partial release which might take place in vitro - causing falsely high values of plasma BTG and PF_4, should not significantly alter the pre-existing condition in vivo. Zahavi and Marder (1974) demonstrated the presence of degranulated platelets in patients with platelet antibodies, and since then, "acquired storage pool diseases" have been documented in patients with chronic renal failure, severe cardiac valve disease (Harbury and Galvan, 1977), acute haemolytic anaemia (Russel et al. 1978) and during extracorporeal circulation (Harbury, 1976). Our group has shown that there were low levels of platelet serotonin and adenine - nucleotides in some patients with disseminated intravascular coagulation (Pareti et al. 1976), haemolytic uraemic syndrome, thrombotic thrombocytopenic purpura, systemic lupus erythematosus (Pareti et al. 1980) and after renal transplantation (Capitanio et al. in press). The acquired dysfunction is thought to follow the in vivo exposure of platelets to strong inducers of the release reaction, such as damaged endothelium, thrombin and immunocomplexes. The detection of exhausted platelets in conditions in which the platelet-activating stimuli are less effective is more difficult and requires much more sophisticated in vitro methods, such as platelet serotonin uptake and serotonin storage after addition of imipramine, a drug known to inhibit serotonin uptake at the plasma membrane (Pletscher et al. 1967). In these cases, it is possible that several platelet populations with various degrees of degranulation circulate together. Under such circumstances measurement of serotonin and of serotonin uptake by the platelets may give normal results, due to continuous reuptake by the non-degranulated platelets of amine leaking from the defective cells, which might mask the defect.

However, unlike serotonin, adenine nucleotides are not taken up by the platelets and transferred into storage granules. In survivors of stroke and myocardial infarction - but not in patients with TIA and angina pectoris, we have shown low levels of platelet ADP in the presence of normal serotonin levels and of even increased levels of platelet BTG (D'Angelo et al.1980). O'Brien et al. (1978) suggested that "exhausted" platelets might circulate in several prethrombotic conditions. This seems to be confirmed by our results and may at least partially explain the reason why tests based on platelet adhesion and aggregation give normal or even subnormal values in some patients with vasculopathies and thromboembolic complications (Davies 1973, Zahavi 1977).

PALTELET COAGULANT ACTIVITIES

Platelet coagulant activities are associated with the initiation and early stages of the pathway of blood coagulation. Tests for contact-product-forming activity, collagen-induced coagulant activity and PF_3 mediated factor Xa formation have been developed by Walsh et al. (1972 a and b, 1974, 1976 a and b).

Recently the presence of a weak activator of factor X has also been postulated (Semeraro and Vermylen 1977). High levels of all platelet coagulant activities were found in patients with deep vein thromboses after hip arthroplasty (Walsh et al. 1976a). High PF_3 activity has been reported for patients submitted to coronary angiography (Renaud et al. 1974) and patients with hyperbetalipoproteinemia (Nordøj and Rødset 1977). The exact nature of these various activities are still in doubt and there is no consensus on all the activities. Moreover the methods are cumbersome and not easily reproducible. Other authors have not been able to confirm the results obtained by Walsh (Van Zutphen, 1980).

CONCLUSIONS

Despite the large number of methods that have been developed for detecting the presence of hyperreactive platelets,no reliable test is available to date for identifying "activated platelets" in individual patients. This may well be either because of the poor sensitivity and specificity of the current tests or the time interval between the occurrence of the event triggering platelet activation and performance of the test. These drawbacks do not mean that these tests are of no value, because they may reveal unsuspected contributions of platelets in various pathological conditions. Moreover, combination of several tests might lead to better results: it is therefore advisable that the most sensitive and simple methods will be standardized and used in prospective studies involving large series of well selected patients.

REFERENCES

Acheson, J., Danta, G., Hutchinson, E.C. (1972) Platelet adhesiveness in patients with cerebral vascular disease. Atherosclerosis 15:123

Baumgartner, H.R., Muggli, R. (1976) Adhesion and aggregation: morphological demonstration and quantitation in vivo and in vitro. In: Gordon, J.L. (ed.): Platelets in Biology and Pathology, p. 23 - Elsevier/North - Holland Biomedical Press.

Bolton, A.E., Ludlam, C.A., Moore, S. et al. (1976a) Three approaches to the radioimmunoassay of human beta-thromboglobulin. Brit. J. Haemat. 33:233

Bolton, A.E., Ludlam, C.A., Pepper, D.S. et al. (1976b) A radio-immunoassay for platelet factor 4. Thrombos. Res. 8:51

Born, G.V.R. (1962) Aggregation of blood platelets by adenosine diphosphate and its reversal. Nature 194:927

Breddin, K. (1968) Die Thrombozytenfunktion bei hämorrhagischen Diathesen, Thrombosen and Gefässkrankheiten. Thrombos. Diathes. Haemorrh. (Stuttg.) (Suppl.) 27

Breddin, K., Grun, H., Krzywanek, H.J., Schremmer, W.P. (1976) On the measurement of spontaneous platelet aggregation. The platelet aggregation test III. Methods and first clinical results. Thrombos and Haemostas. 35:669

Burrows, A.W., Chavin, S.I., Hockady, T.D.R. (1978) Plasma-thromboglobulin concentrations in diabetes mellitus. Lancet 1:235

Campbell, I.W., Dawes, J., Fraser, D.M., et al. (1977) Plasma beta-thromboglobulin in diabetes mellitus. Diabetes 26:1175

Capitanio, A., Mannucci, P.M., Pontivelli, C., Pareti, F.I. Detection of circulating released paltelets after venal transplantation. Transplantation (In press)

Carvalho, A.C.A., Colman, R.W., Lees, R.S. (1974) Platelet function in hyperlipoproteinemia. N. Engl. J. Med. 290:434

Cazenave, J.P., Packham, M.A., Mustard, J.F. (1973) Adherence of platelets to a collagen-coated surface: development of a quantitative method. J. Lab. Clin. Med. 82:978

Cella, G., Zahavi, J.n De Hass, H.A. et al. (1979) Beta-thromboglobulin paltelet production time and platelet function in vascular disease. Br. J. Haematol. 43:127

Colwell, J.A., Sagel, J., Crook, L., et al. (1977) Correlations of platelet aggregation, plasma factor activity and megathrombocytes in diabetic subjects with and without vascular disease. Metabolism 26:279

D'Angelo, A., Franchi, F., Vanasia, S., and Mannucci, P.M. (1980a) Haemostatic variables in ischemic cerebrovascular disease. Differences and analogies between stroke and transient ischemic attacks. VIth International Congress on Thrombosis of the Mediterranean League against thromboembolic diseases, Monte Carlo 1980, Abstract, 57

Day, J., Holmsen, H., and Zucker, M.B. (1976) Report of the working party on platelets. Thromb. Haemostas. 36:236

Davies, J.W. (1973) Defective platelet disaggregation associated with occlusive arterial disease. Angiology 24:391

Dougherty, J.H. Jr., Levy, D., Weksler, B.B. (1977) Platelet activation in acute cerebral ischaemia. Serial measurements of platelet function inc cerebrovascular disease. Lancet 1:821

Fleischman, A.I., Bierenbaum, M.L., Stier, A., Sullivan, A. (1975) In vivo platelet function in acute myocardial infarction, acute cerebrovascular accidents and following surgery. Thrombos. Res. 6:205

Frishman, W.H., Weksler, B., CH., Killip, T. (1974) Reversal of normal platelet aggregability and change in exercise tolerance in patients with angina pectoris following oral propanolol. Circulation 50:887

Gjesdal, K (1976) Platelet function and plasma free fatty acids during acute myocardial infarction and severe angina pectoris. Scand. J. Haemat. 17:205

Handin, R.I., Mc Donough, M. Lesch, M. (1978) Elevation of platelet factor 4 in acute myocardial infarction; measurement by radioimmunoassay. J. Lab. Clin. Med. 91:340

Harbury, C.B., Galvan, C.A. (1977) An acquired platelet storage pool deficency in patients with severe valvular heart disease. Thrombos. Haemostas. 38:95

Harbury, C.B., Galvan, C.A. (1977) A bleeding diathesis associated with a platelet sotrage pool deficiency acquired during cardiopulmonary bypass surgery. Thrombos. Haemostas. 38:237

Harker, L.A., Ross, R., Glomset J. (1976) Role of the platelet in atherogenesis. Ann. N. Y. Acad. Sci. 275:321

Heat, H. (1971) Platelet adhesiveness and aggregation in relation to diabetic retinopathy. Diabetologica 7:308

Hellem, A.J. (1960) The adhesiveness of human blood platelets in vitro. University Press, Oslo

Hellem, A.J. (1971) Adenosince diphosphate - induced platelet adhesiveness in diabetes mellitus with complications. Acta Med. Scand. 190:291

Hirsh, J., Glynn, M.F., Mustard, J.F. (1968) The effect of platelet age on platelet adherence to collagen. J. Clin. Invest. 47:466

Hirsh, J. (1977) Hypercoagulability. Sem. Hemat. 14:409

Hirsh, J. (1978) Role of platelets in thrombosis: Rationale for use of antiplatelet drugs. In: Mechanism of Haemostasis and Thrombosis (C.H. Mielke, Jr. and R. Rodvien eds.) 251. Stratton medical books, New York

Hoak, J.C. (1977) Spontaneous platelet aggregation in vivo. Thrombos. Haemostas. 38:174

Hornstra, G., Ten Hoor, F. (1975) The filtragometer: A new device for measuring platelet aggregation in venous blood of man. Thrombos. Diathes. Haemorrh. (Stuttg.) 34:531

Kalendovsky, Z., Austin, J., Steele, P. (1975) Increased platelet aggregability in youngpatients with stroke: diagnosis and therapy. Arch. Neuro. (Chic.) 32:13

Karpatkin, S. (1969) Heterogeneity of human platelets. II. Functional evidence suggestive of young and old platelets. J. Clin. Invest. 48:1083

Kinlough-Rathbone, R.L., Packham, M.A., Reimers, H.J., Cazenave, J.P., Mustard, J.F. (1977) Mechanism of platelet shape change, aggregation and release induced by collagen, thrombin or A 23, 187. J. Lab. Clin. Med. 90:707

Kwaan, H.C., Colwell, J.A., Cruz, S., et al. (1972) Increased platelet aggregation in diabetes mellitus. J. Lab. Clin. Med. 80:236

Ludlam; C.A., Bolton, A.E., Moore, S., and Cash, J.D. (1975) Lancet 2:259

Ludlam; C.A., Cash, J.D. (1976) Studies on the liberation of beta-thromboglobulin from human platelets in vitro. Brit. J. Haemat. 33:239

Ludlam, C.A., O'Brien JR., Bolton, A.E., et al. (1979) A comparison between the plasma concentration of immunologically assayed platelet factor 4 and beta-thromboglobulin and the heparin thrombin clotting time. Thromb. Res. 15:523

Mant, M.J. (1977) Platelet adherence to Collagen: a simple, reproducible quantitative method for its measurement. Thrombos. Res. 11:729

Mari, D., and Moja, M. (1980) Metodi di studio della funzione piastrinica. La Ricerca Clin. Lab. 10(suppl. 2) 19

Mason, R.G., Summerlin, D.C. (1972) Alteration of platelet adhesion to glass in vascular disorders and certain other diseases. Am. J. Clin. Path. 57:611

Micossi, P., Mannucci, P.M. Bozzini, S., etal. (1981) Chlorpropamide alcohol flush (CPAF), diabetic venal and retinal lesions in non-insulin dependent diabetics (NIDD), distribution of lesion-related risk factors. 2nd International Conference on the Diabetes Mellitus, Milano 1981 (Abstract)

Mielke, C.H. Jr. (1978) Techniques to measure platelet function. In: Mechanism of Haemostasis and Thrombosis (C.H. Mielke Jr. and R. Rodvien eds.), 21. Stratton medical books, New York

Moore, S., Pepper, D.S., Cash, J.D. (1975, a) The isolation and characterization of platelet factor 4 released from thrombin-aggregated washed human platelets and its dissociation into sub-units and the isolation of membrane-bound anti-heparin activity. Biochim. Biophys. Acta (Amst.) 379:370

Moore, S., Pepper, D.S., Cash, J.D. (1975, b) The isolation and characteriazation of a platelet specific globulin (beta-thromboglobulin) and the detection of antiurokinase and antiplasmin released from thrombin-aggregated washed human platelets. Biochim. Biophys. Acta (Amst.) 379:360

Mustard, J.F., Packham, M.A. (1975) The role of blood and platelets in atherosclerosis and the complications of atherosclerosis. Thrombos. Diathes. Haemorrh. 33:44

Nordøy, A., Rødset, J.M. (1977) Platelet function and platelet phospholipids in patients with hyperbetalipoproteinemia. Acta Med. Scand. 189:385

O'Brien, J.R., Tulevski, V.G., Etherington, M., et al. (1974) Platelet function studies before and after operation and the effect of postoperative thrombosis. Lab. Clin. Med. 83:342

O'Brien, J.R. (1978) "Exhausted" platelets continue to circulate. Lancet 2:1316

Pareti, F.I., Capitanio, A., Mannucci, P.M. (1976) Acquired storage pool disease in platelets during disseminated intravascular coagulation. Blood 48:511

Pareti, F.I., Capitanio, A., Mannucci, P.M., et al. (1980) Acquirea disfunction due to the circulation of "exhausted" platelets. Am. J. Med. 69:235

Pletscher, A., Burkord, W.P., Tranzez, D.P., Gey, K.F. (1967) Two sites of 5-hydroxy triptamine uptake in blood platelets. Life Sci. 6:273

Prazich, J.A., Rapaport, S.I., Samples, J.R., Engler, R. (1977) Platlet aggregate ratios - standardization of technique and test results in patients with myocardial ischemia and patients with cerebrovascular disease. Thrombos. Haemostas. 38:597

Preston, F.E., Emmanuel, I.G., Winfield, D.A., et al. (1974) Essentiam thrombocythaemia and peripheral ganrene. Br. Med. J. 1:548

Preston, F.E., Marcola, B.H., Ward, J.D., et al. (1978) Elevated beta-thromboglobulin levels and circulating platelet aggregates in diabetic microangiopathy. Lancet 1:238

Reimers, H.J., Kinlough-Rathbone, R.L., Cazenave, J.P., Senyi, A.F., Hirsh, J., Packman, M.A., Mustard, J.F. (1976) In vitro and in vivo functions on thrombin treated platelets. Thrombos. Haemostas. 35:151

Reimers, H.J., Packham, M.A., Kinlough-Rathbone, R.L., Mustard, J.F. (1977) Adenine nucleotides in thrombin-degranulated platelets: Effect of prolonged circulation in vivo. J. Lab. Clin. Med. 90:490

Renaud, S., Gautheron, P., Arbogast, R., Dumont, E. (1974) Platelet factor 3 activity and platelet aggregation in patients submitted to coronarography. Scand. J. Haemat. 12:85

Ross, R., Glomset, J.A. (1976 a) The pathogenesis of atherosclerosis, N. Engl. J. Med. 295:369

Ross, R., Glomset, J.A. (1976 b) The pathogenesis of atherosclerosis. N. Engl. J. Med. 295:420

Russel, N.H., Keenan, J.P., and Frais, M.A. (1978) Thrombocytopathy associated with autoimmune haemolytic anaemia. Br. med. J. 1:604

Sagel, J., Colwell, J.A., Crook, L., Laminis, M. (1975) Increased platelet aggregation in early diabetes mellitus. Ann. Intern. Med. 82:733

Salky, N., Dugdale, M. (1973) Platelet abnormalities in ischemic heart disease. Am. J. Cardiol. 32:612

Salzman, E. (1963) Measurement of platelet adhesiveness. J. Lab. Clin. Med. 62:724

Semeraro, N., and Vermylen, J. (1977) Evidence that washed human platelets po-sess factor X activator activity. Brit. J. Haematol. 36:107

Shattil, S.H., Anaya-Galindo, R., Bennet, J., et al. (1975) Platelet hypersensitivity induced by cholesterol incorporation. J. Clin. Invest. 55:636

Sixma, J.J. (1978) Techniques for diagnosing prethrombotic states. A review. Thrombos. Haemostas. 40:252

Smith, J.B., Ingerman, G.M., andSilver, M.J. (1976) Effects In: Prostaglandins in Hematology Silver, M.J., Smith, J.B., and Kocsis, J.J. eds. 277 Spectrum Publications, Inc. New York

Steele, P.P., Weily, H.S., Davies, H. (1971) Platelet function in coronary artery disease. J. Lab. Clin. Med. 78:807

Steele, P.P., Weily, H.S., and Genton, E. (1973) Platelet survival and adhesiveness in recurrent venous thrombosis. N. Engl. J. Med. 288:1148

Ten Cate, J.W., In vitro spontaneous platelet aggregation in cerebrovascular disease. Thrombos. and Haemostas. 38:174 (1977)

Van Zutphen, H., Bevers, E.M., Hemker, H.C., and Zwaal, R.F.A. (1980) Contribution of the platelet factor 5 content to platelet factor 3 activity. Br. J. Haematol. 45:121

Vreeken, J., Van Aken, W.G. (1971) Spontaneous aggregation of blood platelets as a cause of idiopathic thrombosis and recurrent painful toes and fingers. Lancet 2:1394

Waelow, C., Corina, A., Ogston, D., and Douglas, A.S. (1974) The relationship between platelet aggregation and time interval after venepuncture. Thromb. Diath. Haemorrh. 31:133

Walsh, P.N. (1972a) The role of platelets in the contact phase of blood coagulation. Brit. J. Haemat. 22:237

Walsh, P.N., (1972b) The effects of collagen and Kaolin on the intrinsic coagulant activity of platelets. Evidence for an alternative pathway in intrinsic coagulation not requiring factor XII. Brit. J. Haemat. 22:393

Walsh, P.N. (1974) Platelet coagulant activities and haemostasis: a hypothesis. Blood 43:597

Walsh, P.N., Rogers, P.H., Marder, V.J., Gagnatelli, G., Escovitz, E.S., Sherry, S. (1976a) The relationship of platelet coagulant activities to venous thromboembolism following hip surgery. Brit. J. Haemat. 32:431

Walsh, P.N., Pareti, F.I., Corbett, J.J. (1976b) Platelet coagulant activities and serum lipids in transient cerebral ischemia. N. Engl. J. Med. 295:854

Wright, H.P. (1941) The adhesiveness of blood platelets in normal subjects with varying concentrations of anticoagulants, J. Path. 53:255

Wu, K.K., Hoak, J.C. (1974) A new nethod for the quantitative detection of platelet aggregates in patients with arterial insufficiency. Lancet 2:924

Wu, K.K., Hoak, J.C. (1975) Increased platelet aggregates in patients with transient ischaemic attacks. Stroke 6:521

Wu, K.K., Hoak, J.C. (1976) Spontaneous platelet aggregation in arterial insufficiency. Mechanism and implications. Thrombos. and Hemostas. 35:702

Wu, K.K., Barnes, R.W., and Hoak, J.C. (1976) Platelet hyper-aggregability in idiopathic recurrent deep vein thrombosis. Circulation, 53:687

Zahavi, J., Marder, J.V. (1974) Acquired "storage pool disease" of platelets associated with circulating antiplatelet antibodies. Am. J. Med. 56:833

Zahavi, J. (1977) The role of platelets in myocardial infarction, ischaemic heart disease, cerebrovascular disease, thromboembolic disorders and acute idiopathic pericarditis. Thrombos. Haemotas. 38:1073

Zahavi, J., Jones Nag, Betteridge, D.J., et al. (1979) Platelet factor 4, beta-thromboglobulin, malondialdehyde formation and blood lipids in patients with diabetes mellitus. Thromb. Haemostas 42:334
Zuzel, M. (1971) ADP-induced aggregation of blood paltelets released from clots by fibrinolysis in vitro. Second Congress of the International Society on Thrombosis and Haemostasis, Oslo. Norway, Abstract vol. p. 278

PLATELET FUNCTION CHANGES IN ACUTE MYOCARDIAL INFARCTION

G. Davì, M. Traina [*], S. Novo, V. Albano [**], G.L. Piraino[*], M.P. Muzzo, G. Marano, A. Raineri [*], and A. Strano

Institute of Clinical Medicine and Medical Therapy
[*]Institute of Cardiovascular Physiopathology, [**]Institute of Pharmacology "R" - University of Palermo
Piazza delle Cliniche, 2
90127 Palermo, Italy

Whether the thrombotic component of myocardial infarction is primary or secondary in a given patient, platelet function alterations can influence many mechanisms - operating at the microenvironmental level - from which it depends if the thrombotic lesion grows or sends platelet emboli to the smaller myocardial vessels.

A number of platelet function alterations associated with acute myocardial infarction (A.M.I.) have been reported (1, 2, 3, 4, 5, 6, 7, 8, 9).

Some informations on the dynamics of the changes in the first days following A.M.I. are available for Beta-thromboglobulin (10); circulating platelet aggregates (3); platelet aggregability by the estimation of the threshold concentrations of ADP, collagen and adrenalin (2); platelet sensitivity to arachidonic acid (11).

No information is available on the dynamics of circulating thromboxane B_2, of TxB_2 formation by platelets after an aggregating stimulus and platelet sensitivity to prostacyclin changes; it seemed interesting to evaluate these parameters in A.M.I. patients by serial blood samples up to 10 days.

PATIENTS STUDIED AND METHODS

The material includes a group of 10 patients (2 women and 8 men), aged 57-72 (average age 64.4), with acute myocardial infarction (8 transmural and 2 not transmural), defined by the history and development of ECG and serum enzyme changes, according to the W.H.O. criteria.

No patient received any drug that could influence platelet function for at least 10 days before and during the study and those patients who had received such drugs up to the A.M.I. were excluded.

The clinical course of the patients was classified in 2 cases as mild, in 5 as moderate and in 3 as severe.

Blood samples were collected from the antecubital vein using an 18 G needle and with slight or no stasis.

Plasma PF4 levels were measured on platelet poor plasma using a radioimmunoassay (Abbott Laboratories).

Thromboxane B_2 was detected in plasma with a specific radioimmunoassay (12). Thromboxane B_2 formation by platelets after stimulation with thrombin (5 U/ml) was assayed with a radioimmunoassay, as previously described (12).

Spontaneous platelet aggregation was determined according to Wu and Hoak (13). Platelet sensitivity to prostacyclin was performed, according to Mehta and Mehta (14), to evaluate the amount of prostacyclin required to inhibit ADP-induced platelet aggregation by 50%.

Prostacyclin was a kind gift of Dr. J. Salmon (Wellcome Research Laboratories).

RESULTS

Plasmatic PF4 levels are shown in figure 1 as mean $\pm$ SD for all the patients. Higher values than those of the normal controls(4-10 ng/ml) were observed during the whole period of follow-up.

During the first three days following the chest pain there was a decrease, with the lowest values on the third day (13 ng) with a rising of PF4 levels in the following days (10th day: 27 ng).

Plasmatic thromboxane B_2 levels (Fig. 2) were detected in all the days of observation reaching highest levels in the 5-10 day period (1st day: 0.5 pMol/ml; 10th day: 1.24 pMol/ml).

Thromboxane B_2 formation by platelets (Fig. 3) showed a fall during the first three days, beginning to increase thereafter and reaching highest levels in the 7-10 day period.

A gross spontaneous platelet aggregation (Fig. 4) was positive in only one patient till the 6th day; in the 7-10 day period it was positive in three patients. The extent of platelet aggregation in patients with positive gross spontaneous platelet aggregation ranged from 18.5 - 72 %.

Platelet sensitivity to prostacyclin (Fig. 5) was decreased in all the serial samples (1.86 ng of prostacyclin needed for 50% platelet aggregation inhibition on the 1st day, with a slight increase on the following days - 2.5 ng on the 10th day).

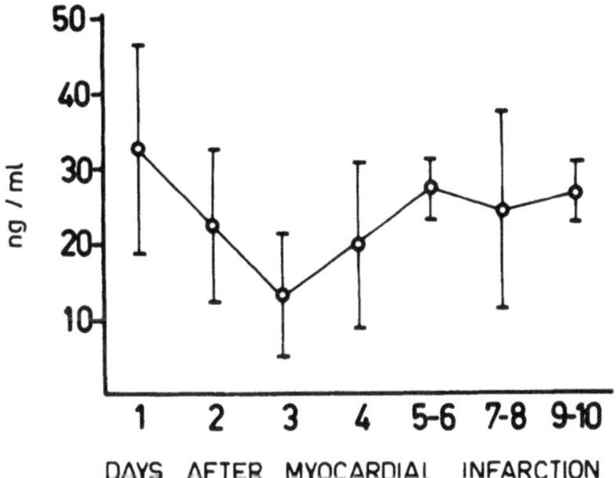

Fig. 1. Plasma platelet factor 4 after acute myocardial infarction; mean ± 1 SD.

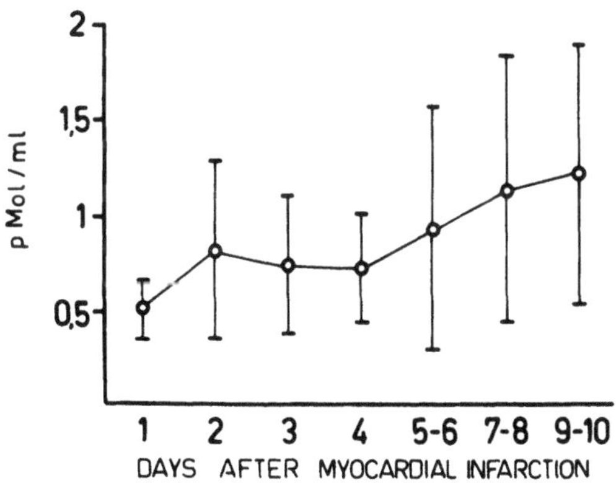

Fig. 2. Plasmatic thromboxane B_2 in the days following acute myocardial infarction; mean ± SD.

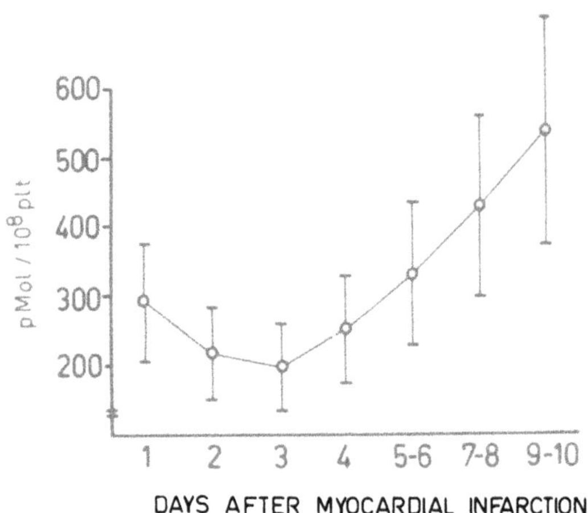

Fig. 3. Thromboxane B_2 formation in PRP (thrombin stimulation, 5 U NHI/ml) after acute myocardial infarction; mean ± 1 SD.

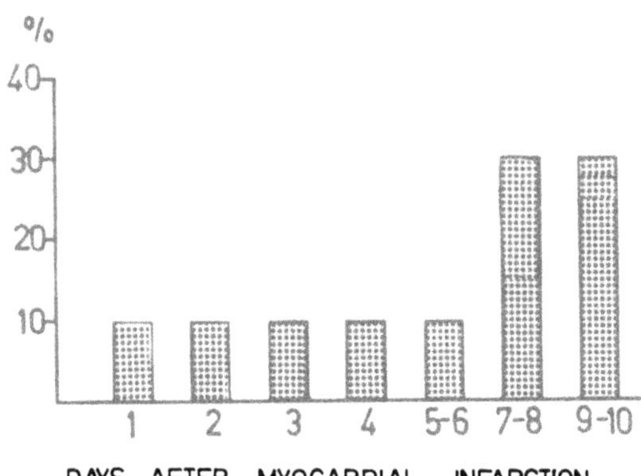

Fig. 4. Gross spontaneous platelet aggregation (%) in the days following acute myocardial infarction; mean ± 1 SD.

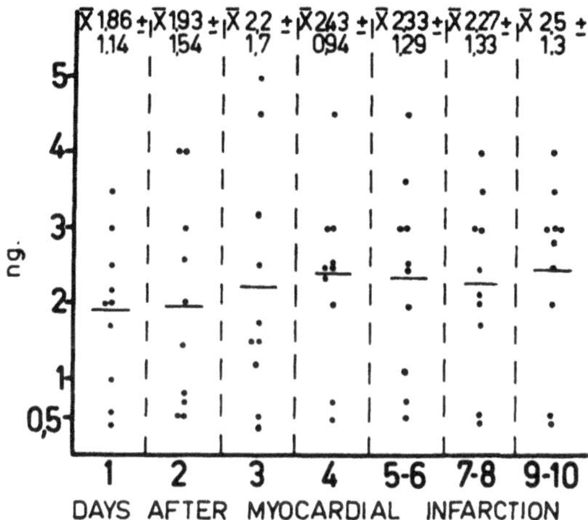

Fig. 5. Prostacyclin needed for 50% platelet aggregation inhibition after acute myocardial infarction; mean ± 1 SD.

DISCUSSION

Handin et al. (6) demonstrated an elevation of platelet factor 4 during the acute phase of myocardial infarction.

In the present study the plasma PF4 level was high on the 1st day followed by an uniform fall during the 2nd and 3rd day and then by an increase after the third day; a similar result was reported by Rasi (10) on the dynamics of the beta-thromboglobulin changes.

Our results showed an increase of spontaneous platelet aggregation in the days 7-10 which can be correlated with the progressive increase in thromboxane B_2 formation by platelets after thrombin stimulus, that was higher than in normal controls in the 7-10 day period. Thromboxane production was decreased on days 2-3 and this may suggest activated and/or exhausted platelets as has been described by O'Brien et al. (15); plasmatic thromboxane, instead, was detected by serial samples up to 10 days.

Mehta and Mehta (3) found that acute transmural myocardial infarction is associated with an increase in circulating platelet microthrombi; the level gradually declined to normal by the 7th hospital day.

In contrast, Gormsen et al. (2) reported uniform changes in ADP and adrenalin induced platelet aggregation; initially a decrease in aggregation was present, changing in a week into increased aggregation. Szczeklik et al. (11) found that platelets became more sensitive to arachidonic acid and also aggregated to a greater extent in response to ADP,4-7 days following myocardial infarction, as compared with 1-2 day values.

The "exhaustion" of platelets, demonstrated by the reduced thromboxane production could explain the "in vitro" decrease of aggregation demonstrated in the first days with a progressive increase in the following days; in fact arachidonic acid and the second phase of ADP induced platelet aggregation are mediated by thromboxane A_2 (17).

In A.M.I. the augmented plasma levels of cathecolamines, FFA (5- 16) and platelet constituents as ADP, PF4, serotonin and TxB_2 could lead to further platelet aggregation "in vivo" that would explain the increased circulating platelet aggregates.

Furthermore, Szczeklik et al. (18) demonstrated that less endogenous TxA_2 is required to trigger platelet aggregation in survival of myocardial infarction.

Another mechanism could also participate in the "in vivo" platelet aggregate formation activity; in the present study the patients with acute myocardial infarction presented, during the whole follow-up period, an evident decreased platelet sensitivity to prostacyclin that provides an additional mechanism involved in "in vivo" increased platelet aggregation that togehter with circulating thromboxane, vasoconstrictive agent, might impair the coronary circulation and thus the platelets could be involved in the extension and expansion of myocardial infarction.

REFERENCES

1. S.C. Sharma, H.N. Setn, Platelet adhesiveness, plasma fibrinogen and fibrinolytic activity in acute myocardial infarction. Brit. Heart J. 40:526 (1978).
2. J. Gormsen, J.B. Knudsen, J.D. Nielsen, O. Amtorp, K. Skagen, Platelet function, coagulation, fibrinolysis, factor XIII and antithrombin III in acute transmural myocardial infarction. In: Proc. of Florence Int. Meet. on Myoc. Inf., May 8-12, 1979, p.233, Excerpta Medica, Amsterdam-Oxford-Princeton (1979).
3. P. Mehta, J. Mehta, Platelet function studies in coronary artery disease. V. Evidence for enhanced platelet microthrombus formation activity in acute myocardial infarction. Am. J. Cardiol. 43:757 (1979).
4. P. Steele, J. Rainwater, R. Vogel, Abnormal platelet survival time in men with myocardial infarction and normal coronary

arteriogram. Am. J. Cardiol. 41:60 (1978).
5. K. Gjesdal, Platelet function and plasma free fatty acids during acute myocardial infarction and severe angina pectoris. Scand. J. Haematol. 17:205 (1976).
6. R.I. Handin, M. McDonough, M. Lesch, Evaluation of platelet factor four in acute myocardial infarction. Measurement by radioimmunoassay. J. Lab. Clin. Med. 91:340 (1978).
7. H.H. Salem, J. Koutts, B.G. Firkin, Circulating platelet aggregates in ischaemic heart disease and their correlation to platelet life span. Thromb. Res. 17:707 (1980).
8. J. Zahavi, The role of platelets in myocardial infarction, ischemic heart disease, cerebrovascular disease, thromboembolic disorders and acute idiopathic pericarditis. Thromb. Haemostas. 38:1073 (1977).
9. M. Packham, Methods for detection of hypersensitive platelets. Thromb. Haemost. 40:175 (1978).
10. V. Rasi, T. Torstila, E. Ikkala, Beta-thromboglobulin in acute myocardial infarction . Acta Med. Scand. (Suppl.) 642:85 (1980).
11. A. Szczeklik, M. Serwonska, W. Lukasiewicz, J. Mruk, J. Musial, Arachidonate versus ADP-induced platelet aggregation in acute myocardial infarction. Thrombos.Haemostas. 42:822 (1979).
12. E. Granström, H. Kindhal, B. Samuelsson, Radioimmunoassay for thromboxane B_2. Analyt. Letters 9;611 (1976).
13. K.K. Wu, J.C. Hoak, Spontaneous platelet aggregation in arterial insufficiency: mechanisms and implications. Thrombos. Haemostas. 35:702 (1976).
14. P. Mehta, J. Mehta, Platelet function studies in coronary heart disease: VIII. Decreased platelet sensitivity to prostacyclin in patients with myocardial ischaemia. Thromb. Res. 18:273 (1980).
15. J.R. O'Brien, M.D. Etherington, R.D. Shuttleworth, Ticlopidine - an antiplatelet drug: effects in human volunteers. Thromb. Res. 13:245 (1978).
16. J. Valles, J. Aznar, M.T. Santos, Platelet fatty acids in acute myocardial infarction. Thromb. Res. 14:231 (1979).
17. E. Marcinkiewicz, L. Grodzinska, R.J. Gryglewski, Platelet aggregation and thromboxane A_2 generation in platelet rich plasma. Pharmacol. Res. Commun. 10:1 (1978).
18. A. Szczeklik, R.J. Gryglewski, J. Musial, L. Grodzinska, M. Serwonska, E. Marcinkiewicz, Thromboxane generation and platelet aggregation in survivals of myocardial infarction. Thromb. Haemostas. 40:66 (1978).

ROLE OF PROSTACYCLIN AND THROMBOXANE A_2 IN ISCHAEMIC HEART DISEASE

G.G. Neri Serneri, G.F. Gensini, G. Masotti, R. Abbate,
A. Morettini, L. Poggesi, and A. Fortini

Istituto di Clinica Medica IV
University of Florence
Florence - Italy

Many investigations have shown that cardiac tissue is able to produce prostaglandins (PGs) of D, E, F series and over all prostacyclin (1-3) both in animals and in humans. Much evidence indicates that the primary site of PGs synthesis is the coronary vasculature and not the cardiac myocytes (3,4).

Thromboxane A (TxA_2) synthesis by normal hearts or by normal coronary vasculature could not be demonstrated (2,5) even if some other vascular beds, such as bovine cerebral microvessels (6) and human fetal vessels (7) seem able to synthetize it. However circulation might be affected by TxA_2 formed during platelet aggregation, which frequently occurs in the coronary vascular bed of patients with IHD (8, 9). In addition to its potent coronary vasoconstrictor activity (10, 11, 12, 13) TxA_2 may affect coronary circulation by its platelet aggregating effect, which may result in the formation of aggregated platelet microthrombi.

Studies on cardiac prostaglandins may gain special importance for patients with IHD because cardiac PGs and specially PGI_2, influence coronary resistance (12, 14, 15) and seem to be involved in the local modulation of vasomotor tone (16, 17). So an impaired prostacyclin production or an increased TxA_2 formation could not only promote platelet aggregation but also may provide an additional stimulus for coronary artery spasm.

In many patients with IHD an increased platelet aggregation has been reported (18, 19) and a significant difference (decreased pla-

---

This investigation has been partially supported by Grant n° 79.010.9083 (Project Atherosclerosis, Consiglio Nazionale delle Ricerche CNR Rome, Italy).

telet aggregation) in platelet aggregation occurs as platelets traverse the diseased coronary vasculature in patients with coronary heart disease (20). Moreover recent studies using ^{111}indium tagged platelets (21, 22) suggest that platelets are sequestered in damaged vessels. So the investigation of the balance between prostacyclin production and thromboxane formation seems to be of special interest in patients with ischaemic heart disease.

THE BIOASSAY OF PROSTACYCLIN IN HUMANS

Prostacyclin production has been demonstrated in isolated organs and in fragments of arterial and venous wall both from humans (23) and various animal species (24, 25). By means of Vane's cascade superfusion technique we bioassayed for the first time the levels of circulating prostacyclin, the production of prostacyclin by the vessel wall and its release into the blood stream in humans (26).

From the pathophysiological point view it is worthwhile to stress that prostacyclin is produced and released by the vessel wall after blood flow changes, such as venous stasis andischaemia (26). Venous stasis of 15 minutes duration induces PGI_2 release (average output 178.4±46.3 ng/min/100 g tissue in young healthy volunteers) immediately after the beginning of venous stasis. Also ischaemia of 3 minutes duration induces a sudden production and release of PGI_2 (average output 333.7±117.1 ng/min/100 g tissue). The release of prostacyclin is phasic and occurs almost exclusively during the first minute of ischaemia. However the prostacyclin production becomes exhausted after 4-6 subsequent short periods of venous stasis or ischaemia. Therefore, in spite of the strong and sudden release induced by venous occlusion and by ischaemia PGI_2 production appears to be limited with time. This fact may be important for some clinical conditions such as angina and/or myocardial infarction with intravascular platelet aggregation and thrombosis.

PLATELET FUNCTION AND THROMBOXANE PRODUCTION IN ISCHAEMIC HEART DISEASE (IHD)

The increased platelet aggregation frequently reported in patients with IHD suggests a possible abnormal platelet function specially of the metabolic pathway of arachidonic acid. Arachidonic acid is a component of the membrane phospholipids of platelets and is released by the enzyme phospholipase. The activation of phospholipase A_2 is not yet completely understood but in general any perturbance of the platelet membrane seems to release arachidonic acid, which is then rapidly metabolized by the enzyme cyclooxygenase in prostaglandin endoperoxide PGG_2. This is converted to PGH_2 which breaks down mainly in thromboxane a , then converted to its stable derivative thromboxane B_2, which is the form usually measured.

In patients affected by IHD (stable angina, unstable angina and patients with a history of myocardial infarction) thromboxane A_2 production has been investigated after platelet aggregation induced by arachidonic acid (1mM). Thormboxane was measured by radiommunoassay (27).

Platelets from patients with IHD produce a significantly larger amount of thromboxane in comparison with controls (Fig. 1). There are many evidences that cAMP can be the intracellular regulator of platelet aggregation (28, 29) probably by modulating the calcium concentration in the vicinity of the contractile proteins (30) and by controlling the availability of arachidonate for prostaglandin synthetase (31). As phospholipase A_2 is activated by calcium released from a dense tubular system (30), a decreased concentration on platelet cAMP could be responsible for the increased activity of the enzymatic system which produces thromboxane A_2. Indeed a feedback mechanism exists which controls platelet aggregability, because prostaglandin endoperoxides and thromboxane A_2 inhibit adenylate cyclase in platelets (32, 33) whereas prostacyclin potently stimulates the adenylate cyclase resulting in an increase of cAMP and an inhibition of platelet aggregation (28, 34, 35).

However the increased conversion of arachidonic acid to thromboxane A_2 observed in patients with IHD is neither related to changes of intraplatelet cAMP level, or to an impaired sensitivity of platelet adenylate cyclase to prostacyclin. The assay of cAMP in platelet rich plasma (radiometric assay 37) showed that cAMP concentration in platelets from patients with a history of myocardial infarction and from patients with angina was not different from that observed in the control group (Tab. I.). Also the formation of cAMP induced by incubation of platelets with 1.5 μM prostacyclin did not differ between patient group and control group, thus indicating the normal responsivity of the platelets from patients with IHD to prostacyclin.

Platelet function is probably influenced also by the action of thrombin (36, 37). In patients with increased platelet aggregation a plasmatic activity can be demonstrated which enhances platelet aggregation (38) related to F. VIII:AGN and activated factor X (39).

In patients with IHD the plasmatic concentration of fibrinopeptide A was investigated by radioimmunoassay (40). The mean value of fibrinopeptide in patients with IHD was significantly ($p<0.001$) higher than the control group (Fig. 2). Although fibrinopeptide A concentration in plasma from patients with history of myocardial infarction (MIP) was higher than in patients with angina, the difference was not significant.

The increased blood concentration of fibrinopeptide A indicates the intravascular formation of thrombin and its activity of fibrinogen. Thus it is likely that the increased production of thromboxane A_2 by platelets from patients with IHD is almost in part the consequence of thrombin action on platelets.

Table 1. Cyclic cAMP levels in paltelet rich plasma.

	controls	MI	EA	SA
cyclic AMP (pMol/10 plt)	7.56±3.96	7.88±3.43	7.32±3.06	6.90±3.07
cyclic cAMP (pMol/10 plt) after PGI 1.5 μM	26.4±15.09	31.45±30.31 n.s.	25.52±16.12 n.s.	24.53±15.22 n.s.

MI = myocardial infarction, EA = effort angina, SA = spontaneous angina.

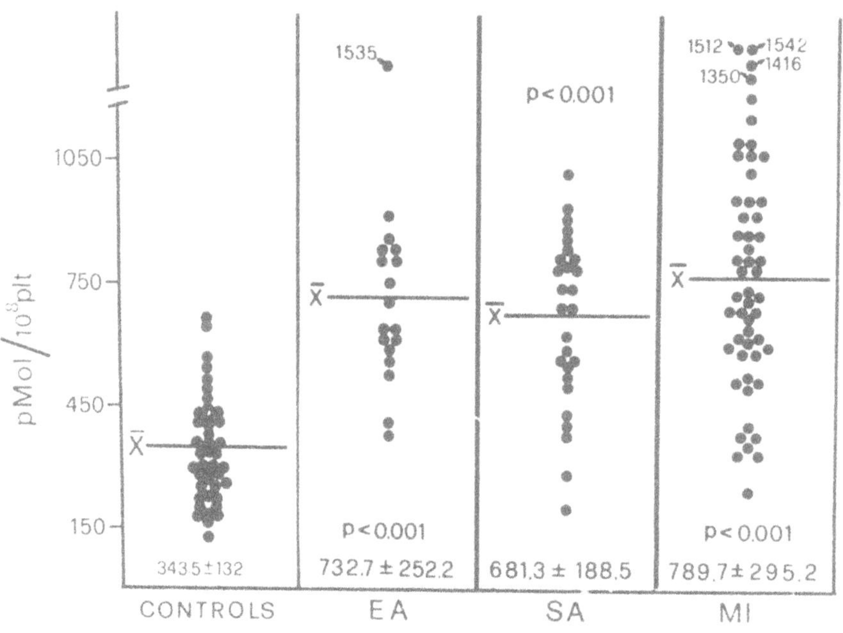

Fig. 1. Thromboxane B production after stimulation with 1 mM arachidonic acid by platelets from patients with ischaemic heart disease and from controls. (EA = effort angina, SA = spontaneous angina, MI = old myocardial infarction).

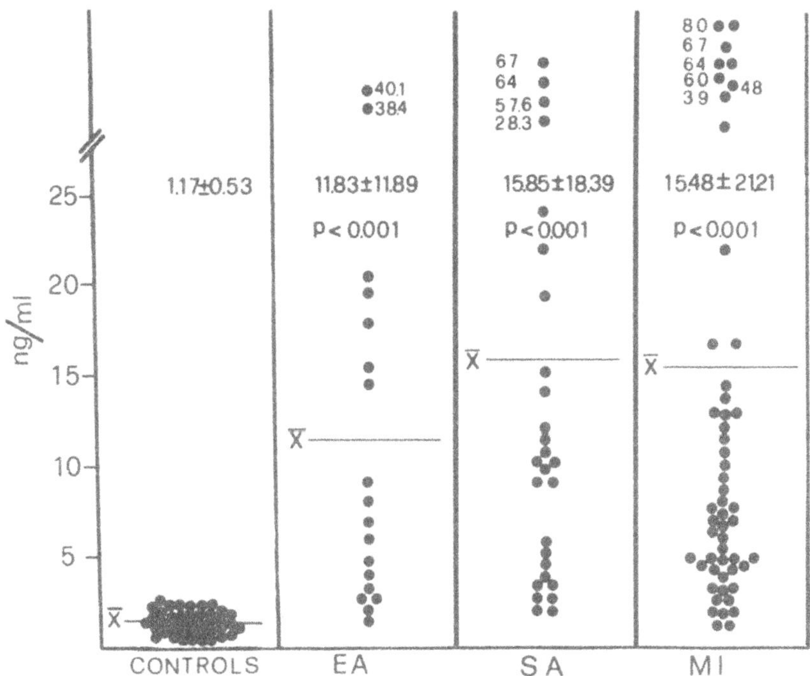

Fig. 2. Fibrinopeptide A levels in plasma from patients with ischaemic heart disease and from controls. (EA = effort angina, SA = spontaneous angina, MI = old myocardial infarction).

THROMBOXANE AND PGI_2 PRODUCTION FOLLOWING ADRENERGIC STIMULATION

Production of prostacyclin and thromboxane in patients with IHD can also be investigated following stimuli able to induce their synthesis and release in plasma. Neri Serneri et al. (41, 42) reported that adrenergic stimulation, obtained by cold stimulation, is able to induce a sudden increase in plasma TxB_2 and in circulating PGI_2. Thus the response of the thromboxane-prostacyclin system to an adrenergic stimulation induced by cold application has been studied in patients with IHD (43). Cold stimulation was performed by immersion of a foot in ice water and by application of ice water on the laterocervical regions for two minutes. In patients with IHD, PGI_2 production was significantly lower than controls, whereas the increase of TxB_2

in plasma was higher in patients than in controls. The increase of TxB_2 in plasma following adrenergic stimulation can be found even after aspirin administration (10 mg/kg). In these conditions platelets are inhibited and produce only amount traces of TxB_2 when stimulated by thrombin. It is worth stressing that whereas TxB_2 formation after adrenergic stimulation is not affected by aspirin administration, the PGI_2 increase is completely inhibited. Thus these findings confirm the significant differences in thromboxane and prostacyclin production observed in unstimulated patients with IHD. Moreover these results may be of importance in relationship to the machanism(s) of coronary vasospasm, because PGI_2 is involved in the control of vascular response to adrenergic stimulation (16, 17, 44) and a diminished production of PGI_2 could facilitate the occurrence of coronary vasospasm frequently induced by adrenergic stimulation (45, 46, 47).

COMMENT

Present results indicate the occurrence in patients with IHD, independently of the different clinical picture, of an impaired prostacyclin production and of an enhanced formation of thromboxane by platelets, associated to a blood clotting activation. The increased formation of thromboxane by platelets and the decreased production of prostacyclin are able to enhance platelet aggregation and thrombus development.

At this stage it is worth stressing the reciprocal relationship between platelets and blood clotting. The increased production of thromboxane by platelets is at least in part due to blood clotting activation leading to an excessive formation of thrombin, as indicated by the increased concentration of fibrinopeptide A in plasma. The concept is very important for the therapeutic management, because the occurrence of a hypercoagulable state suggests that the antiaggregating therapy alone can often be insufficient for the control of platelet hyperaggregability and increased thromboxane production.

The enhanced formation of thromboxane, the reduced production of prostacyclin by the vessel wall after ischaemia and the exhaustion of prostacyclin release after subsequent stimulation could also play a role in the genesis of coronary vasospasm. In dogs with severely reduced coronary blood flow a cyclic standstill of blood flow due to local aggregation of platelets could be observed (48). The low level of circulating prostacyclin, its reduced release by vessel wall after ischaemia and the easy exhaustion after subsequent stimulation in patients with IHD may faciliate the formation of platelet aggregates in coronary vessels undergoing repeated and/or prolonged vasospasm with consequent complete occlusion (49). Moreover, the impaired production of prostacyclin after adrenergic stimulation can by itself be an important factor for vasospasm or for an increase in coronary resistance. In patients with IHD a reflex coronary vasoconstriction in response to a cold stimulus has been demonstrated (50).

The altered equilibrium between thromboxane and prostacyclin and the activation of blood clotting do not seem to be related to different clinical pictures of IHD (stable angina, unstable angina and myocardial infarction), thus suggesting that they could be connected with the alterations in the endothelial wall rather than be a consequence of the coronary disease. In experimental atherosclerosis in rabbits the formation of prostacyclin is very early decreased in damaged endothelium, and a decrease of prostacyclin production by aortic rings (about 40%) can be observed after 1-2 weeks on a hypercholesterolic diet.

The factors and mechanisms responsible for angina and myocardial infarction are far from being known. However our findings indicate that in patients with IHD severe changes in platelet function, in blood clotting and in prostacyclin production exist, and that they can be of importance in coronary vasospasm, angina and myocardial infarction.

ACKNOWLEDGEMENTS

We wish to acknowledge the expert technical assistence of Mrs. Daniela Mazzetti.

REFERENCES

1. P. Needleman, D.L. Kay, P.C. Isakson, et al., Relationship between oxygen tension, coronary vasodilatation and prostaglandins biosynthesis in the isolated rabbit heart. Prostaglandins 9:123-134 (1975).
2. K. Schrör, S. Moncada, F.B. Ubatuba, and J.R. Vane, Transformation of arachidonic acid and prostaglandin endoperoxides by the guinea pig heart. Formation of RCS and prostacyclin. Europ. J. Pharmacol. 47:103-114 (1978).
3. M. Sivakoff, E. Pure, W. Hsueh, and P. Needleman, Prostaglandins and the heart. Fed. Proc. 38:78-82 (1979).
4. A. Wennmalm, Prostaglandin-mediated inhibition of noradrenaline release: VI. On the intra-cardiac source of prostaglandins released from isolated rabbit hearts. Acta Physiol. Scand. 105:254-256 (1979).
5. A.P. Raz, P.C. Isakson, M.S. Minkes, and P. Needleman, Characterization of a novel matabolic pathway of arachidonate in coronary arteries which generates a potent endogenous coronary vasodilator. J. Biol. Chem. 252:1123-1126 (1977).
6. P. Maurer, M.A. Moskowitz, L. Levine, E. Melamed, The synthesis of prostaglandins by bovine cerebral microvessels. Prostagl. Med. 4:153-161 (1980).
7. N.A. Terragno, and A. Terragno, Prostaglandin metabolism in the fetal and maternal vasculature. Fed. Proc. 38:75-77 (1979).

8. H.H. Davis, W.A. Heaton, B.A. Siegel, C.J. Mathias, J.H. Joist, L.A. Sherman, and M.J. Welch, Scintigraphic detection of atherosclerotic lesions and venous thrombi in man by indium^{111} -labelled autologous platelets. Lancet i:1185-1187 (1978).
9. P. Mehta, J. Mehta, C.J. Pepine, et al., Platelet aggregation across the myocardial vascular bed in man: normal versus diseased coronary arteries. Thromb. Res. 14:423-432 (1979).
10. E.F. Ellis, O. Oelz, L.J. Roberts, et al., Coronary arterial smooth muscle contraction by a substance released from platelets: evidence that it is thromboxane A_2. Science 193: 1135-1137 (1976).
11. M. Hamberg, J. Svensson, and B. Samuelsson, Thromboxanes: a new group of biological active compounds derived from prostaglandin endoperoxides. Proc. Natl. Acad. Sci.(Wash.) 72: 2994-2998 (1975).
12. P. Needleman, P.S. Kulkarni, and A. Raz, Coronary tone modulation: formation and actions of prostaglandins, endoperoxides and thromboxanes. Science 195:409-412 (1977).
13. Z.I. Terashi, H. Fukui, K. Nishikawa, et al., Coronary vasospastic action of thromboxane A_2 in isolated, working guinea pig hearts. Europ. J. Pharmacol. 53:49-56 (1978).
14. G. Kaley, The role of prostaglandins in vascular homeostasis. Fed. Proc. 35:2358-2359 (1976).
15. P. Neeldeman, and G. Kaley, Cardiac and coronary prostaglandin synthesis and function. N. Engl. J. Med. 298:1122-1128 (1978).
16. P. Hedqvist, Actions of prostacyclin (PGI_2) on adrenergic neuroeffector transmission in the rabbit kidney. Prostaglandins 17:249-258 (1979).
17. A.G. Herman, T.J. Verbeuren, S. Moncada, and P.M. Van Houtte, Effects of prostacyclin on myogenic activity and adrenergic neurofactor interaction in canine isolated veins. Prostaglandins 16:911-921 (1978).
18. G.G. Neri Serneri, E. Silvestrini, P. Paoletti, and G. Masotti, Studi sulle sindromi trombofiliche. V. L'adesività e l'aggregazione delle piastrine nella malattia ateromasica. Riv. Clin. Med. 68, (suppl. 6), 47 (1978).
19. A. Szczeklik, R.J. Gryglewski, J. Musial, L. Grodzinska, M. Serwonska, and E. Marcinkiewicz, Thromboxane generation and platelet aggregation in survivals of myocardial infarction. Thromb. Haem. 40:66 (1978).
20. P. Mehta, J. Mehta, C.J. Pepine, T.D. Miale, and C. Burger, Platelet aggregation across the myocardial vascular bed in man: normal versus diseased coronary arteries. Thromb. Res. 14:423 (1979).
21. H.H. Davis, B.A. Siegel, J.H. Joist, W.A. Heaton, C.J. Mathias, L.A. Sherman, and M.J. Welch, Scintigraphic detection of atherosclerotic lesions and venous thrombi in mann by indium^{111} -labelled autologous platelets. Lancet i:1185 (1978).

22. M.K. Dewanjee, V. Puster, M.P. Kaye, and M. Josa, Imaging platelet deposition with ^{111}-In-labelled platelets in coronary artery by pass grafts in dogs. Mayo. Clin. Proc. 53:327 (1978).
23. S. Moncada, E.A. Higgs, and J.R. Vane, Human arterial and venous tissue generate prostacyclin (Prostaglandin X), a potent inhibitor of platelet aggregation. Lancet 1:18 (1977).
24. S. Moncada, R. Gryglewski, S. Bunting, and J.R. Vane, An enzyme isolated from arteries transforms prostaglandin endoperoxides to an unstable substance that inhibits platelet aggregation. Nature 263:633 (1976).
25. P. Needleman, S.D. Bronson, A. Wyche, M. Sivakoff, and K.G. Nicolau, Cardiac and renal prostaglandin I_2 - Biosynthesis and biological effects in isolated perfused rabbit tissues. J. Clin. Invest. 61:839 (1978).
26. G.G. Neri Serneri, G. Masotti, L. Poggesi, and G. Galanti, Release of prostacyclin into the blood stream and its exhaustion in humans after local blood changes (ischemia and venous stasis). Thromb. Res. 17:197 (1980).
27. E. Granström, H. Kindahl, and B. Samuelsson, Radioimmunoassay for thromboxane B_2. Analyt. Lett. 9:611 (1976).
28. R.R. Gorman, S.S. Bunting, and O.V. Miller, Modulation of human platelet adenylate cyclase by prostacyclin (PGX). Prostaglandins 13:377 (1977).
29. E.W. Salzman, Platelets, prostaglandins and cyclic nucleotides. In: Platelets: a multidisciplinary approach. 1st ed., p.227, Editors: G. De Gaetano and S. Garattini, Raven Press, New York,(1978).
30. J.G. White, and J.M. Gerrard, Platelet morphology and the ultrastructure of regulatory mechanisms involved in platelet activation. In: Platelets: a multidisciplinary approach. 1st ed. p. 17, Editors: G. De Gaetano and S. Garattini, Raven Press, New York, (1978).
31. M. Minkes, N. Stanford, M.M.Y. Chi, A.R. Roth, P. Needleman, and P.W. Majerus, Cyclic adenosine 3', 5'-monophosphate inhibits the availability of arachidonate to prostaglandin synthetase in human platelet suspensions. J. Clin. Invest. 59:449 (1977).
32. O.V.V. Miller, and R.R. Gorman, Modulation of platelet cyclic nucleotide content by PGE_1 and the prostaglandins endoperoxide PGG_2. J. Clin. Nucl. Res. 2:7 (1976).
33. O.V. Miller, R.A. Johnson, and R.R. Gorman, Inhibition of PGE_1-stimulated cAMP accumulation in human platelets by thromboxane A_2. Prostaglandins 13:599 (1977).
34. R. Korbut, and S. Moncada, Prostacyclin and thromboxane A_2 interaction in vivo. Regulation by aspirin and relationship with anti-thrombotic therapy. Thromb. Res. 13:489 (1978).
35. L.C. Best, T.G. Martin, R.G.G. Russel, and F.E. Preston, Prostacyclin increase cyclic AMP levels and adenylate cyclase activity in platelets. Nature 267:850 (1977).

36. G.N. Brodie, N.L. Baenziger, L.R. Chase, and P.W. Majerus, The effects of thrombin on adenyl cyclase activity and a membrane protein from human platelets. J. Clin. Invest. 51:81 (1972).
37. S. Niewiarowski, and M. Millman, Potentiation of the thrombin induced platelet release reaction by fibrin. Thromb Res. 9:181 (1976).
38. G.G. Neri Serneri, R. Abbate, G.F. Gensini, C. Mugnaini, and A. Lagi, Occurrence of a plasmatic platelet aggregating activity in some patients with increased platelet aggregation. In: Advances in Coagulation, Fibrinolysis, Platelet Aggregation and Atherosclerosis, 1st ed., p. 396, Editor A. Strano, C.E.P.I. Roma (1976).
39. G.G. Neri Serneri, R. Abbate, C. Mugnaini, and G.F. Gensini, Increased platelet aggregation due to a plasma aggregating activity. Identification of the responsible factors. Haemostasis 8 (in press) (1979).
40. V. Hofmann, and P.W. Straub, A radioimmunoassay technique for the rapid measurement of human fibrinopeptide A. Thromb. Res. 11::71 (1977).
41. G.G. Neri Serneri, R. Abbate, G.F. Gensini, L. Poggesi, G. Masotti, S. Favilla, C. Mugnaini, and G. Galanti, Prostacyclin and thromboxane release in plasma after adrenergic stimulation. In: Myocardial Infarction, edited by D.T. Mason, G.G. Neri Serneri, M.F. Oliver, pp. 383-387, Excerpta Medica, Amsterdam (1979).
42. G.G. Neri Serneri, G. Masotti, L. Poggesi, R. Abbate, and M. Mannelli, Prostacyclin and thromboxane A_2 formation in response to adrenergic stimulation in humans. A mechanism for local control of vascular response to sympathetic activation? Card. Res.(1n press) (1981).
43. G.G. Neri Serneri, G. Masotti, L. Poggesi, G. Galanti, A. Morettini, and L. Scarti, Reduced prostacyclin production in patients with different manifestations of ischemic heart disease. Am. J. Cardiol. (1n press) (1981).
44. M.J. Armstrong, G. Thirsk, and J.A. Salmon, Effects of prostacyclin (PGI_2), 6-oxo-$PGF_{1\alpha}$ and PGE_2 on sympathetic nerve function in mesenteric arteries and veins of the rabbit in vitro. Hypertension 1:309-315 (1979).
45. H. Jasue, S. Tanaka, and F. Akiyama, Prinzmetal's variant form of angina as a manifestation of alpha-adrenergic receptor-mediated coronary artery spasm: documantation by coronary arteriography. Am. Heart J. 91:148-155 (1976).
46. D.L. Levene, and M.R. Friedman, Alpha-adrenoceptor-mediated coronary artery spasms. JAMA 236:1018-1022 (1976).
47. D.R. Ricci, A.E. Orlick, P.R. Cipriano, D.F. Guthaner, and D.C. Harrison, Altered adrenergic activity in coronary arterial spasm. Insight into a mechanism based on study of coronary hemodynamics and the electrocardiogram. Am. J. Cardiol. 43:1073-1079 (1979).

48. J.D. Folts, E.B. Crowell, and G.G. Rowe, Platelet aggregation in partially obstructed vessels and its elimination by aspirin. Circulation 54:365 (1976).
49. L.D. Hills, and E. Braunwald, Coronary-artery spasm. N. Engl. J. Med. 299, 695 (1978).
50. G.H. Mudge, R.H. Grossman, R.H. Jr. Mills, M. Lesch, and E. Braunwald, Reflex increase in coronary vascular resistance in patients with ischemic heart disease. N. Engl. J. Med. 295:1333 (1976).

GYKI 14,451, A SYNTHETIC TRIPEPTIDE INHIBITOR OF THROMBIN: "IN VITRO" AND "IN VIVO" STUDIES

E. Tremoli, S. Colli and R. Paoletti

Institute of Pharmacology and Pharmacognosy
University of Milan
Milan, Italy

The search for new compounds active in blood coagulation with different properties to classical anticoagulants, e.g. heparin, has led in the recent years to the development of synthetic low molecular weight peptides, inhibitors of the clotting enzymes (1,2). Among these compounds the benzamidine derivatives and the peptidylarginals have been extensively studied *in vitro* and *in vivo* blood coagulation. The effects of a synthetic tripeptide, GYKI 14,451 (Boc-D-Phe-Pro-Arg-H) have been studied in our Laboratory both *in vitro* on platelets and blood coagulation and *in vivo* in the experimental animal.

GYKI 14,451 at concentrations as low as 1 uM is able, *in vitro*, to prolong significantly the whole blood recalcification time (WBCT), the partial thromboplastin time (PTT) the prothrombin time (PT) and the thrombin time (TT), as shown in Table 1, suggesting that the peptide is a highly effective inhibitor of blood coagulation. In addition GYKI 14,451 at the same concentrations used for clotting tests, completely inhibits thrombin stimulation of platelets (Fig. 1). The inhibition of platelet aggregation was achieved both using platelet rich plasma (PRP) and washed platelets, indicating that the peptide-thrombin interaction is present also in the absence of plasma cofactors. Higher concentrations of the peptide are necessary to inhibit platelet aggregation induced by other aggregating agents, such as collagen (Fig. 2).

To estimate the *in vivo* effects of the peptide, GYKI 14,451 has been administered intravenously and orally to experimental animals. GYKI 14,451 given intravenously to the rat, in the caudal vein, at concentrations of 4 mg/kg is able to prolong significantly plasma thrombin time 15 and 30 min. after the injection (Fig. 3). The prolongation of the plasma thrombin time was present also when the peptide was administered orally (50 mg/kg, by gastric intubation (Table II).

Table I. EFFECT OF GYKI 14,451 "IN VITRO" ON CLOTTING PARAMETERS

GYKI 14,451 μM	WBCT (min.)	GYKI 14,451 μM	PT (sec.)	GYKI 14,451 μM	TT (sec.)
0	10.06±0.80	0	12.8±0.1	0	18.3±0.2
0.6	10.35±0.67	1.25	14.1±0.4	0.3	22.5±0.1
1.25	15.60±1.76	2.5	15.7±0.5	0.6	42 ±0.5
2.5	18.75±2.63	5	17.7±0.1	0.9	72.5±1.2
5	23.8 ±2.59	10	25.6±0.5	1.25	118 ±1.5
10	31.7 ±2.14	20	47.3±1	1.90	146 ±2
20	50			2.5	291 ±1.5
				5	5 min.

Abbreviations: WBCT = Whole Blod Clotting Time
PTT = Partial Thromboplastin Time
PT = Prothrombin Time
TT = Thrombin Time

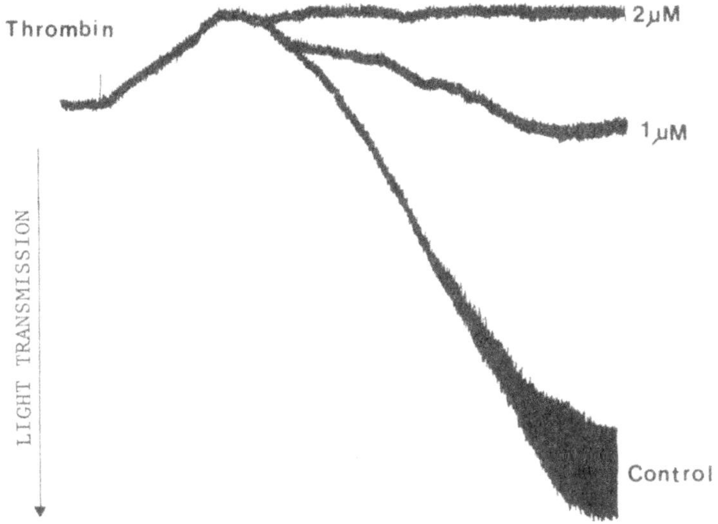

Fig. 1. Thrombin induced aggregation (0.5 U/ml NIH) in washed platelets and inhibition exerted by GYKI 14,451 at two different concentrations.

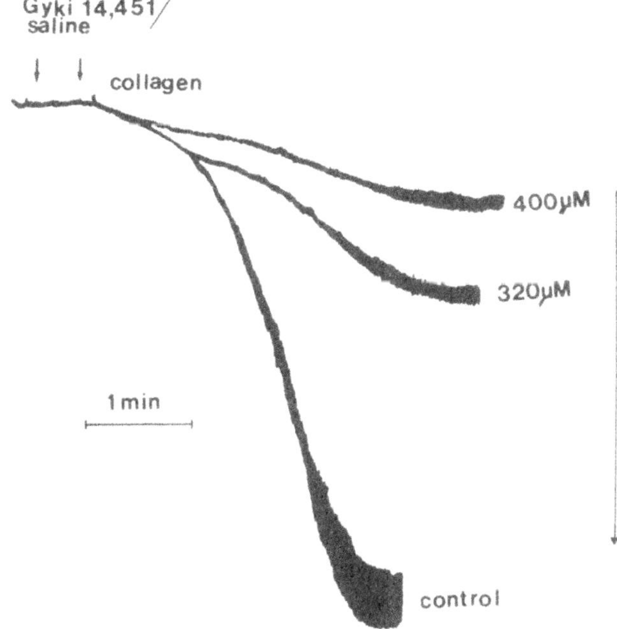

Fig. 2. Collagen induced aggregation (1 ug/ml) in platelet rich plasma (PRP) and inhibition exerted by two different concentrations of GYKI 14,451.

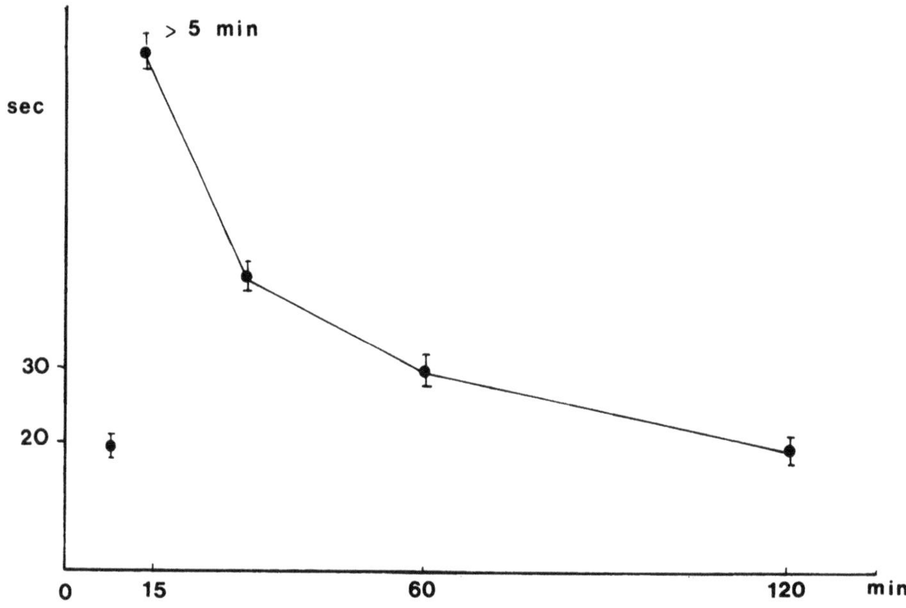

Fig. 3. Effect of GYKI 14.451 (4 mg/kg, i.v.) on plasma thrombin time in the rat. Time after the injection of the peptide is plotted in ascissa.

Table II: EFFECT OF ORAL ADMINISTRATION OF GYKI 14,451 (50 mg/kg) ON THROMBIN TIME (TT) IN THE RAT

GROUP	TIME AFTER THE ADMINISTRATION	TT (sec.)
Controls (6)	--	19.25±0.67
Treated (6)	60 min.	24 ±0.57
Treated (6)	90 min.	38.5 ±0.63
Treated (6)	120 min.	19 ±0.28

In order to verify if the antithrombin activity of GYKI 14,451 observed in in vitro and in vivo studies, would result in an antithrombotic effect, experimental venous thrombosis was induced in the rat, by vena cava ligature.

Spregue-Dawley (Charles River, CD) rats of the average body weight ranging between 250-275 g. were anaesthetized intraperitoneally with sodium pentobarbital (35 mg/kg). GYKI 14,451 or saline were administered either intravenously in the caudal vein (4 mg/kg) or orally (50 mg/kg) by gastric tube. After 15' min. from the injection the abdomen of the animals was opened and venous thrombosis induced by vena cava ligature (3). After three hours from the surgical procedure the abdomen of the animals was reopened and a red thrombus was carefully removed, dried and weighed. GYKI 14,451, injected intravenously, significantly inhibited the occurrence of thrombi in the treated animals. No effect, in contrast, was shown by oral administration of the peptide on the incidence of thrombi, although the mean weight of the thrombi was reduced (Table III).

The in vitro effects of GYKI 14,451 on thrombin and its activity in the prevention of experimental venous thrombosis in the rat, makes the studies on this peptide of interest in view of its potential use in the control and prevention of thromboembolic diseases in human therapy. The lack of a reduction of the incidence of thrombi,

Table III: EFFECTS OF GYKI 14,451 ON EXPERIMENTAL VENOUS THROMBOSIS IN THE RAT

GROUPS	ANIMALS (No.)	INCIDENCE OF THROMBOSIS %	THROMBUS WEIGHT (mean ± SEM)
Controls	12	100	3.65±0.58
GYKI 14,451 (4 mg/kg i.v.)	12	16*	2.06±0.50*
Controls	10	90	4.07±0.42
GYKI 14,451 (50 mg/kg orally)	10	88	3.20±0.39

Thrombus weight is expressed in mg.

* $p<0.001$

observed after oral administration, appears to be linked to the pharmacokinetic of the peptide. As previously reported by Markwardt (1), appreciable and constant blood levels of these peptides are necessary for their activity, as the plasma is their site of action.

Our studies indicate that GYKI 14,451 is able to inhibit blood coagulation processes *in vitro* and *in vivo* as well to prevent the formation of thrombi. The evidence that the inhibitory effect of GYKI 14,451 is related also to the inhibition of thrombin induced aggregation and arachidonic acid metabolism in platelets, suggests a possible therapeutic use for this compound as an alternative to both antiplatelet and anticoagulant therapy.

REFERENCES

1. F. Markwardt, Pharmacological control of blood coagulation by synthetic low molecular weight inhibitors of clotting enzymes. *Trends Pharmacol. Sci.* 1(6):153 (1980).
2. F. Markwardt, G. Wagner, J. Stürzebecher and P. Walsmann, Nα-arylsulfonyl-ω-(4-amidinophenyl)-α-aminoalkylcarboxylic acid amines - Novel selective inhibitors of thrombin. *Thrombosis Res.* 17:425 (1980).
3. I. Reyers, L. Mussoni, M.B. Donati and G. De Gaetano, Failure of aspirin at different doses to modify experimental thrombosis in rats. *Thrombosis Res.* 18:669-674 (1980).

PROSTACYCLIN AND ITS ANALOGUES FOR THE THERAPY OF THROMBOEMBOLIC DISORDERS

B.J.R. Whittle and S. Moncada

Department of Prostaglandin Research
Langley Court
Beckenham, Kent BR3 3BS, U.K.

The discovery that blood vessels synthesize and release an unstable arachidonic acid metabolite, prostacyclin, which is a potent vasodilator and inhibitor of platelet aggregation (Moncada, Gryglewski, Bunting and Vane, 1976) has implicated this prostanoid as an important factor in the regulation of vascular tone and haemostasis (Moncada and Vane, 1979). This bicyclic enol-ether is derived from the fatty acid precursor arachidonic acid via the unstable endoperoxide intermediates. These are transformed by the action of an enzyme system, prostacyclin synthetase, which is located predominantly in vascular endothelium. It has become apparent that prostacyclin has many potential clinical applications for the management of thromboembolic disorders (Table 1).

Prostacyclin has proved valuable in preventing platelet aggregation during interaction with the artificial surfaces of extracorporeal circulatory systems. Thus, prostacyclin improves haemocompatibility during charcoal haemoperfusion in dogs (Bunting and colleagues, 1979) and man (Gimson and co-workers, 1980). Studies in dogs and man have also suggested that prostacyclin can be used as an alternative to heparin for haemodialysis (Woods and colleagues, 1978; Turney and co-workers, 1980). In cardio-pulmonary by-pass experiments in dogs using a bubble oxygenator, prostacyclin in combination with heparin preserved both platelet number and function with minimal fibrinogen consumption and deposit on the arteral filters (Longmore and co-workers, 1979). Preservation of platelet number and function by prostacyclin during extracorporeal oxygenation with a membrane has likewise been demonstrated (Coppe, Wonders, Snider and Salzman, 1979).

Prostacyclin has great clinical potential in the treatment of peripheral vascular disease, its local intra-arterial administration leading to alleviation of pain, regression of necrosis and healing of ulcers in cases of advanced arteriosclerosis obliterans in man (Szczeklik and co-workers, 1979).

Prostacyclin might also be useful in other conditions where excessive platelet aggregation is involved. The microthrombi observed in arterioles and capillaries in conditions of thrombotic thrombocytopenic purpura may result from a deficiency in prostacyclin formation as also suggested in a related condition, haemolytic uraemic syndrome (Remuzzi, Misiani and others, 1978; Hensby, Lewis and others, 1979) and these disorders may thus respond to prostacyclin therapy. Preliminary studies on the use of prostacyclin in persistent foetal circulation (Lock, Olley, Coceani and others, 1979) and severe idiopathic pulmonary artery hypertension (Watkins, Peterson and others, 1980) have also recently been reported. Some of the complications of pre-eclampsia (Remuzzi and others, 1980) and the platelet component of the rejection process during transplant surgery (Mundy, Bewick, Moncada and Vane, 1980) may also respond to prostacyclin therapy. However, such applications are at the moment more speculative and further work is needed before a definite therapeutic role for prostacyclin can be assigned for such utilities.

Although the instability of prostacyclin is considered useful in limiting its biological activity when used for extracorporeal circulations, we have investigated the possibility of developing a short-acting chemically-stable analogue with a biological profile similar to that of prostacyclin.

ACTIVITY OF PROSTACYCLIN ANALOGUES

The elucidation of the chemical structure of prostacyclin (Fig. 1) as (5Z)-9-deoxy-6,9α-epoxy-Δ^5-PGF_1 (Johnson and co-workers, 1976) led to the synthesis of structural analogues by several groups. One such compound 13,14 dehydro prostacyclin methyl ester was reported to be a potent and more stable compound (Fried and Barton, 1977). Although no data on the comparison of the potency of the analogue to prostacyclin on platelet aggregation was presented, its ID_{50} value suggests it to be approximately 5 times less active than prostacyclin on human platelets, but no details of its chemical half-life were given. This analogue was a vasodilator in the cat intestinal vascular bed (Praustian and others, 1977), and in a study where its vasoactive properties on the dog coronary circulation were compared to prostacyclin, it was approximately 3 times less active in increasing coronary sinus blood flow (Hyman, Kadowitz and others, 1978).

An other analogue, 6,9-thiaprostacyclin was reported to be an active, more stable, prostacyclin derivative (Nicolaou, Barnette and others, 1977) although this compound showed divergent biological properties from prostacyclin in that it constricted the cat isolated coronary artery. Following intravenous infusion in the anaesthetized cat, 6,9-thiaprostacyclin lowered systemic BP and elevated superior mesenteric artery blood flow (Lefer, Trachte and others, 1979) and

Table 1. Conditions for which prostacyclin or an analogue may be useful

Coronary thrombosis	Endotoxin shock
Strokes	Pulmonary hypertension
Malignant hypertension	Thrombotic thrombocytopenic purpura
Deep vein thrombosis	Haemolytic uraemic syndrome
Transplant preservation	Disseminated intravascular coagulation
Vascular surgery	Pulmonary embolism
Pre-eclampsia	Persistent foetal circulation
Extra-corporeal circuits	Peptic ulcer

in studies in the canine femoral circulation, it was 10 times less active as a vasodilator than prostacyclin (Horri, Kanayama and others, 1979). These latter workers reported its half-life in neutral solution (determined by biological activity) to be 7 h. This analogue was 10-20 times less active than prostacyclin in vivo in causing disaggregation of platelets from cat blood perfused collagen strips and this effect was not long-lasting (Gryglewski and Nicolaou, 1978). Further, as an inhibitor of rabbit platelet aggregation in vitro 6,9, thiaprostacyclin was 25 times less active than prostacyclin, and possessed thromboxane A_2-like constrictor activity on isolated vascular tissue.

In a study on the vasodilator and anti-aggregating activity of a series of ω-side chain modified analogues, no compound of greater potency or selectivity than prostacyclin towards the platelet actions was reported (Scholkens, Bartmann and others, 1979). The unstable derivative, 20-methyl prostacyclin inhibited the in vitro aggregation of platelets from rat (van Dorp, Evert and van der Wolf, 1978) and rabbit (Gandolfi and Gryglewski, 1978) in doses comparable to those of prostacyclin, whereas the 13,14-didehydro derivative of 20-methyl prostacyclin was slightly more active. Both compounds retained potent vasodilator activities. 20-methyl prostacyclin, like prostacyclin itself, was reported to prevent especially-induced bronchoconstriction in asthmatic patients when given by inhalation in doses causing changes in heart rate (Bianco and others, 1978). The biological activity of some further unstable derivatives of prostacyclin (the 5,6 epimer, the 5,6 methylene and the 4,5 iso compounds) have also been reported by Crane and co-workers (1978) and 12-fluoroprostacyclins by Nicolaou and co-workers, (1978) but none of the more-stable compounds showed enhanced activity as platelet anti-aggregating agents.

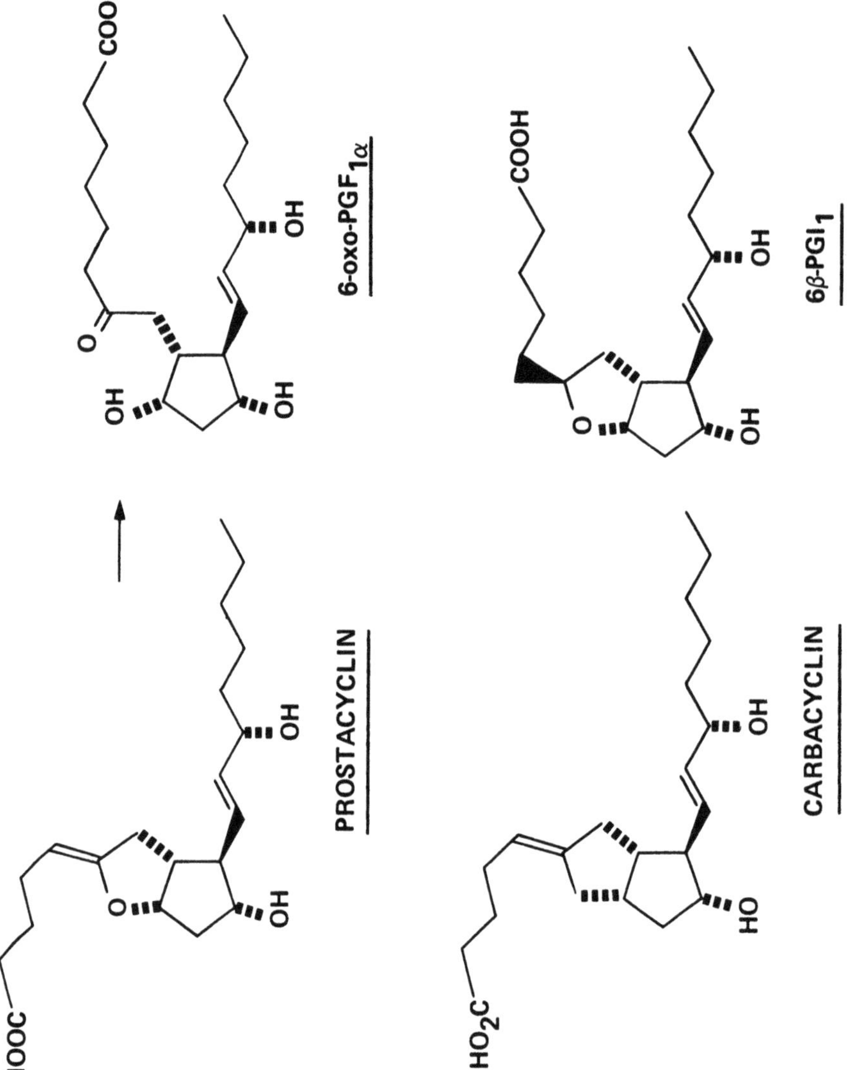

Fig. 1. Chemical structure of prostacyclin and its stable analogues.

ACTIVITY OF STABLE PROSTACYCLIN ANALOGUES

Studies on cardiovascular activity

Anaesthesia was induced in male Wistar rats (250-300 g body weight) and male rabbits (2-2.5 kg) with sodium pentobarbitone (30 mg kg^{-1}, i.v.) and maintained with suppliments (3 mg kg^{-1}). Arterial pressure was recorded from a cannulated femoral artery and heart rate derived by integrating the arterial pulse. Rectal temperature was maintained at 37°C by thermistor-controlled radiant heat. Each compound was injected into a femoral vein in a volume of 0.25 ml and flushed in with 0.25 ml of saline (0.9% w/v). Compounds were administered intra-arterially via catheter inserted retrogradely into the left carotid artery.

Studies on platelet aggregation in vivo

Human blood was freshly collected into plastic vessels containing trisodium citrate (3.15%; 0.1 volume with 0.9 volume blood) and centrifuged (200 g for 15 min) at room temperature. The platelet-rich plasma (PRP) was withdrawn into plastic containers and kept at room temperature. Inhibition of platelet aggregation by prostanoids was determined in a Born-type aggregometer as described previously (Whittle, Moncada and Vane, 1978) by incubating aliquots (0.5 ml) of the PRP for 1 minute at 37°C with or without the inhibitor prior to addition of sufficient adenosine diphosphate (ADP; Sigma Chemical Co.) to just cause maximal aggregation. Dose inhibition curves were constructed for each compound and the ID_{50} (dose causing 50% inhibition) was calculated as the dose required to reduce the control aggregation to 50% of its control amplitude.

Studies on platelet aggregation ex vivo

Studies on the potency of various prostacyclins as inhibitors of platelet aggregation *in vitro* and on cardiovascular parameters *in vivo* provide useful information on their biological profile. However, it has become clear that for any studies on selectivity of action of prostacyclin analogues, these parameters should be assessed simultaneously in the same animal. Therefore, the inhibition of rabbit platelet aggregation *ex vivo* and concurrent cardiovascular changes were determined in both anaesthetised rabbits and dogs (Whittle, Moncada, Whiting and Vane, 1980). To enable a more rapid preparation of samples of PRP so that platelet function could readily and continually be assessed (especially during the administration of labile substances such as prostacyclin) a rapid-spin method for the centrifugation of blood samples was developed. This 'rapid spin' method enabled platelet aggregation to be assessed in platelet rich plasma

(PRP) prepared within 1.5 min of withdrawing the blood sample from the animal (Fig. 2). This technique which allows continual monitoring of platelet aggregation throughout periods of drug infusion, appears particularly useful in the study of labile or rapidly metabolised substances, whose plasma half-life may be far shorter than the time taken to prepare PRP by conventional methods (15-20 min).

Male rabbits (2-2.5 kg body weight) were anaesthetised with sodium pentobarbitone and systemic arterial blood pressure (BP) was recorded from a cannula filled with heparinized saline (5 units/ml) in a femoral artery; no heparin was administered to the animal. Drugs were administered via cannula in the jugular vein. Blood samples (3.0 ml) were slowly collected into a plastic syringe containing tri-sodium citrate (3.18%, 1 vol to 9 vol of blood) from a cannula inserted into the femoral vein, shaken gently and transferred to two Eppendorf plastic tube (1.5 ml) and each was spun separately in a modified Eppendorf centrifuge for 2 sec (maximum centrifuge force, 10,000 g). The PRP from each tube was collected separately and 0.4 ml aliquots were transferred to the aggregometer and incubated at 37°C for 1 min prior to addition of sufficient ADP (15 μM) to produce near-maximal aggregation (Fig. 3). The time-interval between removal of blood samples and the transference of the PRP to the aggregometer was only 1 min (Fig. 2).

Studies on the inhibition of dog platelet aggregation were carried out in comparable fashion using chloralose-pentobarbitone anaesthetized dogs. Blood samples (6 ml) were collected from the left femoral artery into trisodium citrate (0.318% final concentration), PRP prepared by the rapid spin method, and aliquots transferred to an aggregometer. Platelet aggregation was induced by ADP (5 and 20 μM). Blood pressure was recorded from the right femoral artery and drugs administered via the femoral vein.

6β-PGI_1

One of the first chemically-stable analogues to be described was a 5,6-dihydro analogue, 6β-PGI_1 (Johnson et al., 1977, 1979; Whittle, Boughton-Smith, Moncada and Vane, 1978b) whose structure is shown in Fig. 1. This analogue inhibited human platelet aggregation *in vitro* with an ID_{50} 116 ± 20 ng ml^{-1} (Table 2) being some 250 times less active than prostacyclin. As with prostacyclin, its vasodepressor activity was similar when administered by either intravenous or intra-arterial route in both rat and rabbit. The epimer, 6α-PGI_1 was less active on the cardiovascular parameters and platelet aggregation (Table 2).

To study the chemical stability of 6β-PGI_1, aqueous solutions (100-500 μg ml^{-1}) were dissolved in sterile isotonic saline (0.9% w/v; pH 7) and stored at 22°C in stoppered glass vials. At regular intervals the potency of the stored solutions were tested for their ability to inhibit ADP-induced platelet aggregation in human PRP and compared to freshly dissolved compound. There was no loss in biolo-

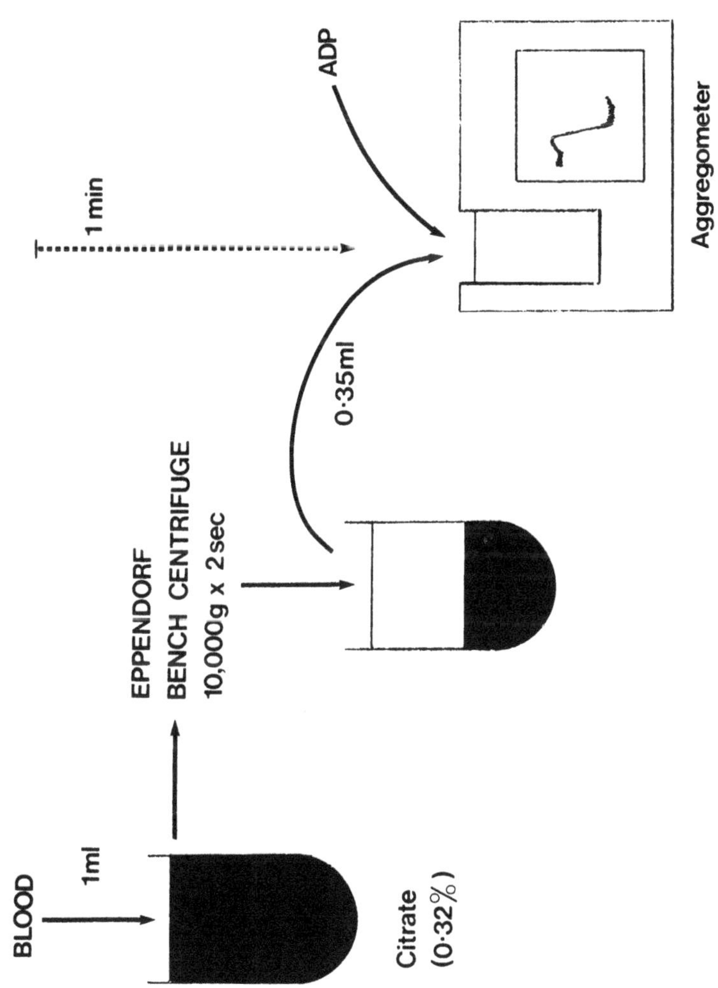

Fig. 2. Rapid-spin preparation of platelet-rich-plasma for *ex vivo* studies on platelet aggregation

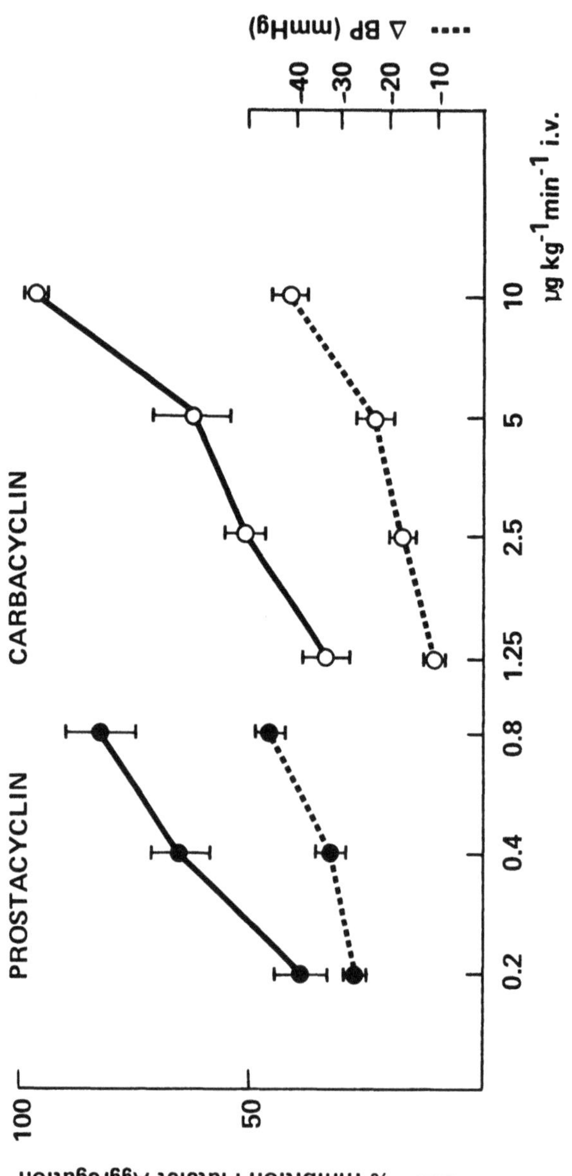

Fig. 3. Effect of prostacyclin or carbacyclin on ADP-induced platelet aggregation *ex vivo* in the anaesthetised rabbit. The aggregometer traces were obtained from samples of PRP prepared by the rapid-spin method.

Table 2. Inhibition of ADP-induced human platelet aggregation by prostanoids following 1 min incubation *in vitro*.

	ID_{50} (ng ml^{-1})	Relative Potency
PGI_2	0.4±0.1	1
PGI_3	0.7±0.2	0.57
6-oxo-$PGF_{1\alpha}$	282±37	0.0014
6-oxo-PGE_1	6±0.7	0.07
PGE_1	21±3	0.02
PGD_2	11±2	0.04
6β-PGI_1	116±20	0.0034
6α-PGI_1	350±30	0.001
Carbacyclin	11±3	0.04

Results shown as ID_{50} values and Relative Potency to prostacyclin are shown as the mean ± S.E. from at least 4 experiments.

gical activity in samples stored for 7 days at room temperature.

Studies were also carried out to investigate actions of 6β-PGI_1 on platelet aggregation *ex vivo* in the rabbit. As is shown in Table 3, 6β-PGI_1 was 80 times less active as prostacyclin as an anti-aggregating agent when infused intravenously and produced greater cardiovascular actions for a comparable degree of platelet inhibition. Thus the biological profile of 6β-PGI_1 different from the parent, prostacyclin.

The biological activity of 5,6-dihydro prostacyclin analogues have also been described by other workers. Both Tonga and colleagues (1977) and Crane and co-workers (1978) have also investigated the anti-aggregatory activity of both the 6α- and 6β- epimers on platelets. In a study on the isolated guinea-pig heart and bovine coronary artery strips, Schror (1979) has observed a divergent profile of activity of both epimers of PGI_1 with prostacyclin. Thus, although these compounds have many of the properties of the parent compound, these 5,6-dihydro analogues cannot be as close mimics of prostacyclin.

Carbacyclin

The synthesis of carbocyclic analogues of prostacyclin have been recently described (Morton, Bundy and Nishizawa; Nicolaou and

Table 3. Effect of intravenous infusion of prostanoids on ADP-induced platelet aggregation *ex vivo* and systemic arterial blood pressure (BP) in the anaesthetised rabbit.

	Infusion $\mu g\ kg^{-1}\ min^{-1}$	Platelet Aggregation % inhibition	Δ BP (mm Hg)
PGI_2	0.25	42±6	-24±3
6β-PGI_1	20	43±13	-33±10
Carbacyclin	2.5	53±8	-15±3
PGE_1	2.5	7±5	-24±7
6-oxo-PGE_1	2.5	56±13	-34±6

Results are the mean ± s.e. mean of (5) experiments using doses of the prostanoids close to their ID_{50} values.

co-workers, 1978). The chemically-stable prostacyclin analogue (5E) 6a-carba-prostaglandin I_2 (carbacyclin, Fig. 1) has proved to be a potent inhibitor of platelet aggregation in human plasma (Table 2). Carbacyclin was active against human platelet aggregation induced by ADP, arachidonic acid and collagen, and also inhibited platelet aggregation in plasma from a variety of species including dog and rabbit (Whittle and co-workers, 1980; Aiken and Shebuski, 1980). As with prostacyclin the antiaggregating action of carbacyclin was enhanced by the phosphodiesterase inhibitor, theophylline (Whittle and co-workers, 1980).

Carbacyclin was a potent inhibitor for *ex vivo* platelet aggregation when infused intravenously in the rabbit (Fig. 4) and dog, being one-tenth as active as prostacyclin (Table 3). Likewise, Aiken and Shebuski (1980) have found this analogue to be effective *in vivo* in reducing thrombus formation in dog coronary arteries. More recent studies with carbacyclin in anaesthetised baboons have indicated inhibition of platelet aggregation *ex vivo* following intravenous or intragastric administration (Adaikan, Karim and Lau, 1980). Other workers have subsequently reported on the anti-aggregating activities of the [(5E) 6a] and the racemic [dl-9α] carbocyclic prostacyclin analogues (Morita, Mori and co-workers, 1980; Ceserani, Grossoni and others, 1980).

In a series of experiments designed to investigate the chemical stability of carbacyclin, acqueous solutions at concentrations of 1-10 $\mu g\ ml^{-1}$ carbacyclin dissolved in sterile isotonic saline (0.9% w/v; pH 7) were stored at 22°C in stoppered glass vials. At regular intervals the potency of the stored carbacyclin solutions were tested for their ability to inhibit ADP-induced platelet aggregation in human PRP and compared to freshly dissolved compound. No loss in biological activity could be detected in samples stored for 30 days at room temperature.

The anti-aggregating action of carbacyclin was, short-lived once the infusion was terminated. As with prostacyclin, its inhibitory action on platelet aggregation ex vivo in the dog and rabbit was no longer significant 10 min after infusion (Fig. 3). Thus, although carbacyclin is chemically stable at physiological temperatures and pH, its similar duration of activity to prostacyclin suggests that in the rabbit and dog, both prostacyclin and carbacyclin are rapidly metabolised. Our studies in the rat indicate that carbacyclin is not inactivated during passage through the pulmonary circulation since the analogue had comparable vasodepressor activity when administered by intravenous or intra-arterial injection (Fig. 5). Like prostacyclin, carbacyclin may not be a substrate for the pulmonary-transport system required for metabolism by 15-PGDH enzyme in intact lung (Hawkins and others, 1978), yet may be metabolised readily in other organs such as the kidney or in vascular tissue (Sun and others, 1979).

The inhibition of platelet aggregation reached plateau levels within 5 mins of starting the intravenous infusion of carbacyclin and was maintained throughout the period of administration in both anaesthetised rabbit and dog. In experiments where near-maximal anti-aggregating doses of carbacyclin were infused for 3 h, the degree of inhibition remained constant, showing no evidence for desensitisation or tachyphylaxis of the platelets to this stable prostacyclin analogue in vivo. Previous studies with PGD_2 in vitro showed that after a 2 h incubation period platelet adenylate cyclase could become refractory to subsequent stimulation with PGD_2 (Cooper, Shafer and co-workers, 1979).

Although PGE_1 has been shown to preserve platelets during in vitro stimulation in a cardiopulmonary bypass circuit (Addenizio and others, 1979), our studies with PGE_1 in vivo have shown a marked fall in BP in doses having little effect on platelet aggregation ex vivo (Table 3). This suggests that PGE_1 would have significantly less clinical value than prostacyclin as an anti-platelet drug. More recently, interest has arisen in a novel stable prostanoid, 6-oxo-PGE_1, a potential metabolite of prostacyclin, which was reported to be a potent vasodilator and inhibitor of platelet aggregation (Quilley, Wong and McGiff, 1979). Our studies on human platelet aggregation in vitro and on rabbit platelet aggregation ex vivo have shown it to be some 10-20 times less active than prostacyclin (Table 2 and 3). This agrees with a recent in vivo study on thrombus formation in dog coronary arteries where 6-oxo-PGE_1 was at least 10 times less active than prostacyclin (Miller and others, 1980). In our studies, this product produced a greater hypotensive response than prostacyclin at doses causing a comparable degree of platelet aggregation, thus exhibiting a different profile of biological activity to either prostacyclin or PGE_1.

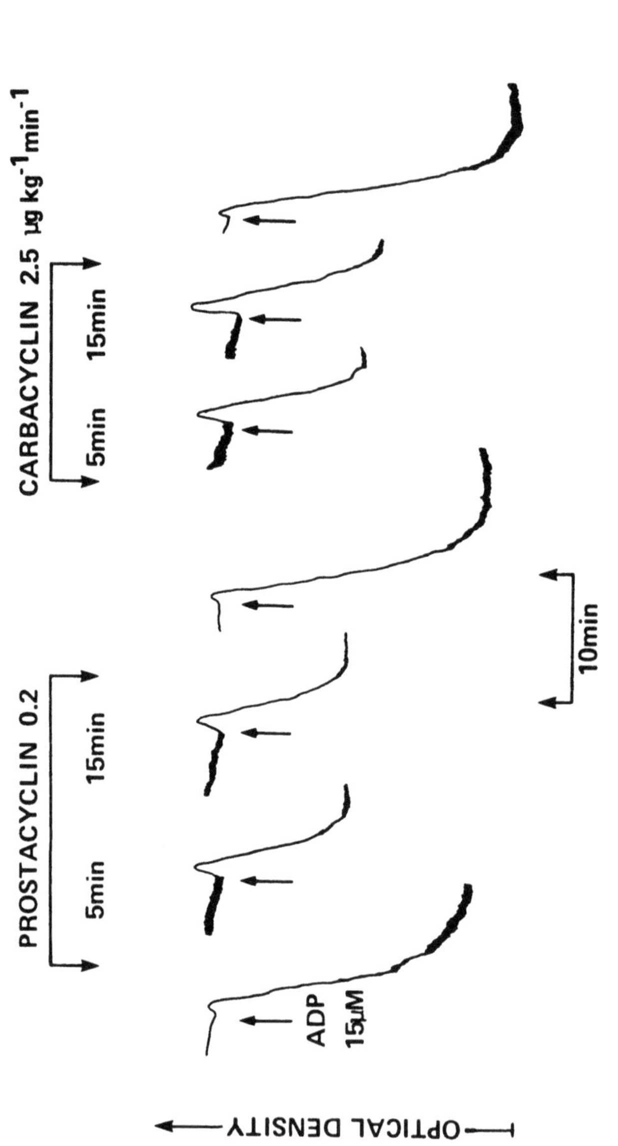

Fig. 4. Inhibition of ADP-induced platelet aggregation ex vivo and fall in systemic arterial blood pressure (BP) by intravenous infusion of prostacyclin or carbacyclin in anaesthetised rabbits. Results, expressed as % inhibition of platelet aggregation compared to the initial controls, and the change in BP, are shown as the mean ± s.e. mean of 4 experiments for each value.

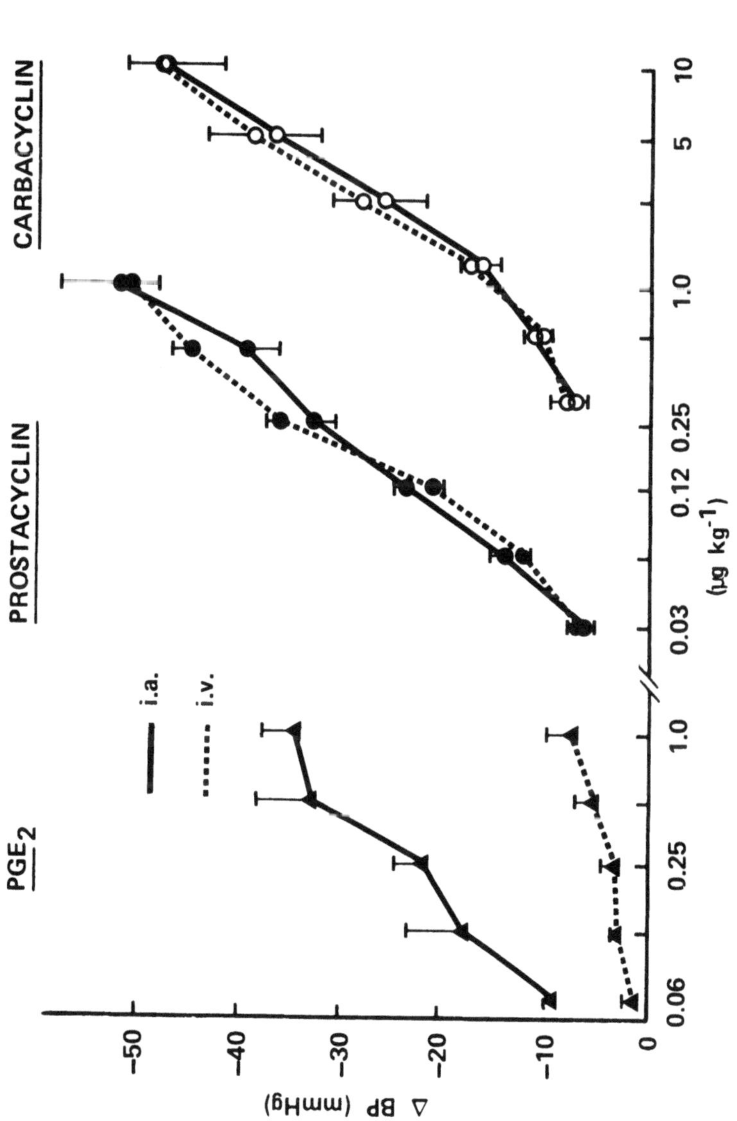

Fig. 5. Effect of prostacyclin, carbacyclin and PGE_2 on systemic arterial blood pressure (BP) in the anaesthetised rat following intravenous or intra-arterial bolus injection. Results shown as the mean ± s.e. mean, are from 4 experiments.

As found with prostacyclin (Whittle, Boughton-Smith and others, 1978b), carbacyclin was an inhibitor of gastric acid secretion in the rat, and also prevented the formation of gastric erosions and intestinal lesions induced by indomethacin (Whittle, Steel and Boughton-Smith, 1980). Previously, the 5,6-dihydro analogue 6β-PGI_1 was shown to inhibit gastric ulceration and gastric output in the rat (Whittle and others, 1978a) and dog (Kauffman, Whittle and others, 1979). Furthermore, a novel series of 16-phenoxy prostacyclin analogues, which were devoid of platelet anti-aggregating actions, were found to be extremely potent anti-ulcer and anti-secretory agents in both rat (Whittle and Boughton-Smith, 1979) and dog (Kauffman, Whittle and others, 1980). Thus, such actions may support a clinical utility for prostacyclin analogues in the therapy of peptic ulceration.

The development of chemically-synthetized prostacyclin analogues have demonstrated the strict requirement of the prostacyclin functional groups for the molecule to possess biological activity. The 5,6-dihydro analogue, 6β-PGI_1 is only a week platelet anti-aggregating agent, although it did retain relatively more of the cardiovascular activity. Indeed, it appears that the binding sites on platelets for prostacyclin and its analogues are more stringent in their structural requirements than those on the vasculature. Carbacyclin appears to be a close mimic of prostacyclin with respect to its haemodynamic and platelet actions and is chemically-stable. Such analogues can serve as reference standards and help to elucidate biological actions and roles under conditions of temperature and pH which would limit the activity of prostacyclin itself.

Both 6β-PGI_1 and carbacyclin are chemically-stable but metabolically-unstable analogues whose biological half-life *in vivo* are close to that of prostacyclin. The development of potent stable prostacyclin analogues with biological profiles very close to the parent compound thus represents the first stage in drug design. The next step is the development of analogues with selective biological actions. However, the desirable degree of selectivity between such parameters as platelet inhibition and cardiovascular activity is as yet unknown, since both activities are clearly of importance in many of the proposed clinical utilities. The rational design of newer analogues will therefore depend on the clinical experience gained with the parent, prostacyclin.

REFERENCES

Adaikan, P.G., Karim, S.M.M. and Lau, L.C., 1980. Prostaglandins and Medicine 5:307-320.
Addonizio, V.P., Macarak, E.J., Niewiarowski, S., Colman, R.W., Edmunds, L.H., 1979. Circ. Res. 44:350-357.
Aiken, J.W. and Shebuski, R.J., 1980. Prostaglandins 19:639-643.
Bianco, S., Robuschi, M., Ceserani, R., Gandolfi, C. and Kamburoff, P.L., 1978. Life Sci. 25:259-264.
Bunting, S., Moncada, S., Vane, J.R., Woods, H.F. and Weston, M.J., 1979. In: J.R. Vane and S. Bergstrom, (Eds.) Prostacyclin, Raven Press, New York, pp. 361-366.
Ceserani, R., Grossoni, M., Longiave, D., Mizzotti, B., Pozzi, O., Dembinska-Kiec, A. and Bianco, S., 1980. Prostaglandins and Medicine 5:131-139.
Cooper, B., Schafer, A.I., Puchalsky, D., Handin, R.I., 1979. Prostaglandins 17:561-571.
Coppe, D., Wonders, T., Snider, M. and Salzman E.W., 1979. In: J.R. Vane and S. Bergstrom, (Eds.) Prostacyclin, Raven Press, New York, pp. 371-382.
Crane, B.H., Maish, T.L., Maddox, Y.T., Corey, E.J., Szekley, I. and Ramwell, P.W., 1978. J. Pharmacol Expt. Ther. 206: 132-138.
van Dorp, D.A., van Evert, W.C., van der Wolf, L., 1978. Prostaglandins 16:953-955.
Fried, J. and Barton, J., 1977. Proc. Natl. Acad. Sci. 74:2199-2203.
Gandolfi, C.A. and Gryglewski, R.J., 1978. Pharmacol. Res. Commun. 10:885-896.
Gimson, A.E.S., Langley, P.G., Hughes, R.D., Canalesa, J., Mellon, D.J., Williams, R., Woods, H.F. and Weston, M.J., 1980. Lancet i:173-175.
Gorman, R.R., Bunting, S. and Miller, O.V., 1978. Prostaglandins 13:389-397.
Gryglewski, R.J. and Nicolaou, K.C., 1978. Experientia 34:1336-1338.
Hawkins, H.J., Smith, J.B., Nicolaou, K.C. and Eling, T.C., 1978. Prostaglandins 16:871-884.
Hensby, C.N., Lewis, P.J., Hilgard, P., Mufti, G.J. and Webster, J., 1979. Lancet ii: 748.
Horii, D., Kanayama, T., Mori, M., Shibosaki, M. and Ikegami, S., 1978. Eur. J. Pharmacol. 51:313-316.
Hyman, A.L., Kadowitz, P.J., Lands, W.E., Crawford, C.G., Fried, J. and Barton, J., 1978. Proc. Natl. Acad. Sci. 75:3522-3526.
Johnson, R.A., Morton, D.R., Kinner, J.H., Gorman, R.R., McGuire, J.C., Sun; F.F., Whittaker, N., Bunting, S., Salmon, J.A., Moncada, S. and Vane, J.R., 1976. Prostaglandins 12:915-928.

Johnson, R.A., Lincoln, F.H., Thompson, J.L., Nidy, E.G., Mizsak, S.A. and Axen, U., 1977. J. Am. Chem. Soc. 99: 4182-4184.

Johnson, R.A., Lincoln, F.H., Smith, H.W., Ayer, D.E., Nidy, E.G., Thompson, J.L., Axen, U., Aiken, J.W., Gorman, R.R., Nishizawa, E.E. and Honohen, T., 1978. In: J.R. Vane and S. Bergstrom, (Eds.) Prostacyclin, Raven Press, New York, pp. 17-28.

Kauffman, G.L., Whittle, B.J.R., Aures, D., Vane, J.R. and Grossman, M.I., 1979. Gastroenterology, 77:1301-1306.

Kauffman, G.L., Whittle, B.J.R., Aures, D. and Grossman, M.I., 1980. In: B. Samuelsson, P.W. Ramwell and R. Paoletti (Eds.) Advances in prostaglandin and thromboxane research, Vol. 8 Raven Press, New York, pp. 1521-1524.

Lefer, A.M., Trachte, G.J., Smith, J.B., Barnette, W.E. and Nicolaou, K.C., 1979. Life. Sci. 25:259-264.

Lock, J.E., Olley, P.M., Coceani, F., Swyer, P.R. and Rowe, R.D., 1979. Lancet i:1343.

Longmore, D.B., Bennet, G., Gueirrara, D., Smith, M., Bunting, S., Moncada, S., Reed, P. and Read, N.G., 1979. Lancet ii: 1002-1005.

Miller, O.V., Aiken, J.W., Shebuski, R.J. and Gorman, R.R., 1980. Prostaglandins 20:391-400.

Moncada, S. and Vane, J.R., 1979. Pharmac. Reviews 30:293-331.

Moncada, S., Gryglewski, R.J., Bunting, S. and Vane, J.R., L976. Nature 263:663-665.

Morita, A., Mori, M., Hasegawa, K., Kojima, K. and Kobayashi, S., 1980. Life Sci. 27:695-701.

Morton, D.R., Bundy, G.L. and Nishizawz, E.E., 1979. In: J.R. Vane and S. Bergstrom (Eds.) Prostacyclin, Raven Press, New York, pp. 31-38.

Mundy, A.R., Bewick, M., Moncada, S. and Vane, J.R., 1980. Prostaglandins 19:595-603.

Nicolaou, K.C., Barnette, W.E., Gaise, G.P., Magolda, R.L., 1977. J. Am. Chem. Soc. 99:7736-7738.

Nicolaou, K.C., Barnette, W.E., Magolda, R.L., Grieco, P.A., Owens, W., Wang, C.L.J., Smith, J.B., Ogletree, M. and Lefer, A.M., 1978. Prostaglandins 16:789-794.

Nicolaou, K., Sipio, W.J., Magolda, R.L., Seitz, S. and Barnette, W.E., 1978. J.C.S. Chem. Commun. 1067-1068.

Paustian, P.W., Chapnick, B.M., Feigen, L.P., Hyman, A.L. and Kadowitz, P.J., 1977. Prostaglandins 14:1141-1152.

Quilley, C.P., Wong, P.Y.K. and McGiff, J.R., 1979. Eur. J. Pharmac. 57:273-276.

Remuzzi, G., Misiani, R., Marchesi, D., Livio, M., Mecca, G. and de Gaetano, G., 1978. Lancet ii:871-872.

Remuzzi, G., Marchesi, D., Mecca, G., Misiani, R., Rossi, E., Donati, M.B. and de Gaetano, G., 1980. Lancet i:310.

Scholkens, B.A., Bartman, W., Beck, G., Lerch, U., Konz, E. and Weithmann, U., 1974. Prostaglandins and Medicine 3:7-22.

Schror, K., 1979. Naunyn-Schmiedeberg's Archiv. Pharmacol. 306: 213-217.
Sun, F.F., Taylor, B.M., McGuire, J.C., Wong, P.Y.K., Malik, K.U., McGiff, J.C., 1979. In: J.R. Vane and S. Bergstrom (Eds.) Prostacyclin, Raven Press, New York, pp. 119-130.
Szczeklik, A., Stawiski, S., Nizankowski, R., Szczeklik, J., Gluszko, P. and Gryglewski, R.J., 1979, Lancet i:1111-1114.
Tonga, G., Gandolfi, C., Andreoni, A., Fumagalli, A., Passarotti, C., Faustini, F. and Patrono, C., 1977. Pharmacol. Res. Commun. 10:909-916.
Turney, J.H., Williams, L.C., Fewell, M.R., Parsons, V. and Weston, M.J., 1980. Lancet ii:219-222.
Watkins, W.D., Peterson, M.P., Crane, R.K., Shannon, D.C. and Levine, L., 1980. Lancet i:1083.
Whittle, B.J.R. and Boughton-Smith, N.K., 1979. In: J.R. Vane and S. Bergstrom (Eds.) Prostacyclin, Raven Press, New York, pp.159-170.
Whittle, B.J.R., Boughton-Smith, N.K., Moncada, S. and Vane, J.R., 1978a. J. Pharm. Pharmacol. 30:597-598.
Whittle, B.J.R., Boughton-Smith, N.K., Moncada, S. and Vane, J.R., 1978b. Prostaglandins 15:955-967.
Whittle, B.J.R., Moncada, S. and Vane, J.R., 1978. Prostaglandins 16:373-388.
Whittle, B.J.R., Moncada, S., Whiting, F. and Vane J.R., 1980. Prostaglandins 19:605-627.
Whittle, B.J.R., Steel, G. and Boughton-Smith, N.K., 1980. J. Pharm. Pharmacol. 32:603-604.
Woods, H.F., Ash, G., Weston, M.J., Bunting, S., Moncada, S. and Vane, J.R., 1978. Lancet ii:1075-1077.

PROSTACYCLIN IN THE TREATMENT OF ATHEROSCLEROSIS OBLITERANS AND OTHER VASCULAR DISEASES

R.J. Gryglewski and A. Szczeklik

Departments of Pharmacology and Internal Medicine
Copernicus Academy of Medicine
Grzegórzecka 16
31-531 Cracow, Poland

Prostacyclin is the main arachidonic acid metabolite produced by the arterial walls (2,3,7) and released into circulation (1,4). In man, prostacyclin acts as a powerful vasodilator and anti-platelet agent (13). Resistance vessels are most susceptible for prostacyclin vasodilatory action, while capacitance vessels show little, if any change, even during administration of high doses of prostacyclin (18). The profound anti-platelet effects induced by prostacyclin can be devided into anti-aggregatory and disaggregatory (5,12,13). The former are reflected by a marked inhibition of ADP - or collagen -induced platelet aggregation, the latter by dispersion of both circulating platelet aggregates and platelet thrombi formed on the collagen surface.

Prostacyclin unites in one molecule powerful biolobical activities affecting the cardiovascular system. This has made it a highly attractive compound for clinical studies and therapeutical trials. First patients treated with prostacyclin were described in 1979 (15).

Both the number ofpatients and their different diagnoses have since increased rapidly. These were all open clinical trials; several double-blind studies are now under way,. The topic was recently reviewed extensively (6,8,9,10,11). A brief summary, therefore is only presented here.

1. Peripheral vascular disease

The results obtained in 65 patients with advanced arteriosclerosis obliterans or thrombangiitis obliterans were recently evaluated (11). Prostacyclin (The Upjohn Company, and The Wellcome Research Laboratories) was administered intra-arterially or intravenously in an average dose 7ng/kg/min for about 72 hours. The follow-up period varied from 4 to 24 months. This therapy led to substantial improvement, as evidenced by total relief of resting pain and healing of ischemic ulcers. There was no improvement in cases with deep gangrene. In 45 per cent of patients treated a persistent, long-lasting improvement was reached (> 2 months). In 40 per cent improvement lasted not longer that two months, and in 15 per cent the results were virtually negative. The efficacy of prostacyclin therapy in advanced peripheral vascular disease depends on the choice of patients, localization of the vascular lesions and the advancement of the disease (14,15).

2. Angina pectoris

In patients with angina of effort, both short-term infusions during atrial pacing as well as prolonged administration of prostacyclin, had no detectable positive effects on symptoms of myocardial ischemia (10,17). On the other hand, 24-72 hrs infusion of PGI_2 at a rate of 5 ng/kg/min to patients with angina at rest (unstable angina) led to radical decrease of nitroglycerin intake and warning of the anginal attacks (16). These observations suggest that prostacyclin might be of therapeutic interest in attacks of angina pectoris precipitated by reduction of oxygen delivery rather than increased oxygen demand.

3. Pulmonary hypertension

Watkins et al. (20) have studied the effects of prostacyclin infusion in a 8-years old girl with severe chronic idiopathic pulmonary hypertension refractory to conventional therapy. They found that prostacyclin provided the greatest degree of pulmonary vasodilatation as compared to prostaglandin E_1 and isoproterenol. We have found (10, 19) that prostacyclin administered intravenously decreased significantly pulmonary artery pressure, pulmonary artery resistance and total pulmonary resistance in patients with pulmonary hypertension secondary to mitral stenosis. These latter findings suggest that prostacyclin might be of interest in preparing patients with pulmonary hypertension for cardiac surgery.

4. Occlusion of central retinal vein

A therapeutic success was reported recently (21) in two patients who had been treated PGI_2, 24 and 48 hours after occlusion of central retinal vein, but not in the one who received the treatment on the seventh day of the disease.

Headache is the most common side-effect experienced by patients receiving prostacyclin infusions. It usually occurs at a high dose (10 ng/kg/min); if the infusion rate is reduced, headache disappears. Other side-effects, recently reviewed (10), include: articular pain, flushing of the face and elevation of serum blood glucose. These side-effects rarely interfere with the usual administration of prostacyclin for a few days.

REFERENCES

1. R.J. Gryglewski, Prostacyclin as a circulating hormone. Biochem. Pharmacol. 28: 3161 (1979).
2. R.J. Gryglewski, Prostaglandins, platelets, and atherosclerosis. CRC series in Biochemistry 7: 291 (i980).
3. R.J. Gryglewski, S. Bunting, S. Moncada, R.J. Flower, J.R. Vane, Arterial walls are protected against deposition of platelet thrombi by a substance (Prostaglandin X) which they make from prostaglandin endoperoxides. Prostaglandins 12: 685 (1976).
4. R.J. Gryglewski, R. Korbut, A. Ocetkiewicz, Generation of prostacyclin by lungs in vivo and its release into arterial circulation. Nature 273: 765 (1978).
5. R.J. Gryglewski, A. Szczeklik, R. Nizankowski, Antiplatelet action of intravenous prostacyclin in man. Thrombos. Res. 13:152 (1978).
6. R.J. Gryglewski, A. Szczeklik, H. Zygulska-Mach, E. Kostaka-Trabka, Prostacyclin and vascular disease. Symposium A. Einstein Coll. of Med., 28-30 October 1980. Raven Press, New York - in press.
7. S. Moncada, R.J. Gryglewski, S. Bunting, J.R. Vane, A lipid peroxide inhibits the enzyme that generates from prostaglandin endoperoxides the substance (prostaglandin X) which prevents platelets from aggregation. Prostaglandins 12: 715 (1976).
8. A. Szczeklik, Prostacyclin and atherosclerosis. Triangle 19: 61 (1980).
9. A. Szczeklik, Cardiovascular actions of prostacyclin in man. International conference on prostaglandins, New york, April 1980, in press.
10. A. Szczeklik, R.J. Gryglewski, Treatment of vascular disease with prostacyclin. In: Clinical pharmacology of prostacyclin, ed. by P. Lewis and J. O'Grady, in press.
11. A. Szczeklik, R.J. Gryglewski, Prostaglandins as therapeutical agents in cardiovascular disease. Proceedings of the meeting "Prostaglandins and the cardiovascular system", Wilrijk (Belgium) 1-3 December 1980, in press (Raven Press).
12. A. Szczeklik, R.J. Gryglewski, E. Nizankowska, R. Nizankowski, J. Musial, Pulmonary and anti-platelet effects of intravenous and inhaled prostacyclin in man. Prostaglandins 16: 651 (1978).
13. A. Szczeklik, R.J. Gryglewski, R. Nizankowski, J. Musial, R. Pieton, J. Murk, Circulatory and anti-platelet effects of intravenous prostacyclin in healthy men. Pharmacol. Res. Commun. 10: 545 (1978).

14. A. Szczeklik, R.J. Gryglewski, R. Nizankowski, S. Skawinski, P. Gluszko, Prostacyclin therapy of peripheral vascular disease. Thrombos. Res. 19: 191 (1980).
15. A. Szczeklik, R. Nizankowski, S. Skawinski, J. Szczeklik, P. Gluszko, R.J. Gryglewski, Successful therapy of advanced arteriosclerosis obliterans with prostacyclin. Lancet 1: 1111 (1979).
16. A. Szczeklik, J. Szczeklik, R. Nizankowski, P. Gluszco, Prostacyclin for unstable angina. N. Engl. J. Med. 303: 881 (1980).
17. A. Szczeklik, J. Szczeklik, R. Nizankowski, P. Gluszko, Prostacyclin for acute coronary insufficiency. Artery - in press.
18. J. Szczeklik, A. Szczeklik, R. Nizankowski, Haemodynamic changes induced by prostacyclin in man. Br. Heart J. 44: 254 (1980).
19. J. Szczeklik, A. Szczeklik, R. Nizankowski, Prostacyclin for pulmonary hypertension. Lancet 2: 1076 (1980).
20. W.D. Watkins, M.P. Peterson, R.K. Brone, D.C. Shannon, L. Levine, Prostacyclin and prostaglandin E_1 for severe pulmonary artery hypertension. Lancet 1: 1083 (1980).
21. H. Zygulska-Mach, E. Kostka-Trabka, A. Niton, R.J. Gryglewski, Prostacyclin in central retinal vein occlusion. Lancet 2: 1075 (1980).

PART 5

FIBRINOLYSIS AND VASCULAR DISEASES

MOLECULAR MECHANISM OF FIBRINOLYSIS

H.R. Lijnen and D. Collen

Center for Thrombosis and Vascular Research
Department of Medical Research
University of Leuven
Belgium

Mammalian blood contains an enzymatic system capable of dissolving blood clots, which is called the fibrinolytic system. A review of the identification of the different components (Table I) has been given by Astrup (1) and by Fearnley (2). The system comprises a proenzyme plasminogen which can be activated to the active enzyme plasmin by several different types of plasminogen activators. Inhibition may occur at the level of the activators or at the level of plasmin.

In this communication we will discuss the properties of the main components of the fibrinolytic system, the molecular interactions between these components and their importance for the regulation and control of fibrinolysis.

MAIN COMPONENTS OF THE FIBRINOLYTIC SYSTEM

Plasminogen

Human plasminogen is a single chain glycoprotein with a molecular weight of about 90,000, containing 2% carbohydrate. The plasma concentration is about 1.5 to 2 µM. Native plasminogen has NH_2-terminal glutamic acid ("Glu-plasminogen") but is easily converted by limited plasmatic digestion to modified forms with NH_2-terminal lysine, valine or methionine (3, 4) ("Lys-plasminogen"). This conversion occurs by hydrolysis of the Arg 67-Met 68, Lys 76-Lys 77 or Lys 77-Val 78 peptide bonds. The hydrodynamic properties of both types have been summarized and discussed elsewhere (5). Single donor plasmas appear to contain different molecular forms of Glu-plasminogen (6, 7, 8, 9).

Lys-plasminogen forms are converted to plasmin by cleavage of a single Arg 560-Val 561 peptide bond (10). The two chain plasmin

Table 1. Survey of Components of the Fibrinolytic System

Plasminogen	proenzyme form of the fibrinolytic enzyme
Plasmin	active fibrinolytic enzyme
Tissue activator of plasminogen	enzymes present in tissues which convert plasminogen to plasmin; may be identical or similar to blood plasminogen activator and to vascular plasminogen activator
Vascular plasminogen activator	plasminogen activator present in endothelial cells
Blood plasminogen activator	plasminogen activator present in blood, most likely identical to vascular plasminogen activator
Streptokinase	streptococcal protein which activates the fibrinolytic system in human plasma
Urokinase	plasminogen activator isolated from urine or kidney cell cultures; different from tissue activator
Hageman factor Hageman factor cofactor High molecular weight kininogen Prekallikrein	plasma proteins involved in intrinsic plasminogen activation, Hageman factor cofactor and prekallikrein may be identical
Antiactivators	general designation for inhibitors of plasminogen activation
Antiactivator in blood	inhibitor of vascular plasminogen activator in blood; its existence is doubtful
Antiplasmins	general designation for plasmin inhibitors
α_2-Antiplasmin	specific fast-reacting plasmin inhibitor in human plasma

molecule is composed of a heavy chain or A-chain originating from the NH_2-terminal part of plasminogen and a light chain or B-chain constituting the C-terminal part (11). The B-chain was found to contain an active site similar to that of trypsin, composed of His 602, Asp 645 and Ser 740 (12). Activation of Glu-plasminigen to plasmin by urokinase in purified systems occurs about 20 times slower than that of Lys-plasminogen (13), but in either case Lys-plasmin is formed. Activation of Glu-plasminogen in the presence of the physiological inhibitor α_2-antiplasmin however generates inhibited Glu-plasmin (14). The exact mechanism of activation of plasminogen in vivo thus remains unsettled.

The plasminogen molecule contains structures, called lysine-binding sites which interact specifically with certain amino acids such as lysine, 6-amino-hexanoic acid and trans-4-aminomethylcyclohexane-1-carboxylic acid. There is one lysine-binding site with high affinity for 6-aminohexanoic acid (K_D = μM), and about four with low affinity (K_D = 5 mM) (15). They are located in the plasmin A-chain (16, 17). One of the functions of these lysine-binding sites in plasminogen is to mediate its interaction with fibrin (18). As will be discussed further they are also very important for the interaction between plasmin(ogen) and α_2-antiplasmin.

Plasminogen activators and inhibitors of plasminogen activators

As illustrated in Fig. 1 plasminogen activation may occur by three different pathways (19). An intrinsic or humoral pathway in which all the components involved are present in precursor form in the blood: its physiological role in the removal of fibrin remains unclear. An extrinsic pathway in which the activator originates from tissues or from the vessel wall and is released into the blood by certain stimuli or trauma, and an exogenous pathway in which the activating substances streptokinase or urokinase may be infused for therapeutic purposes. Some of these activators are counterbalanced by inhibitors.

All plasminogen activators studied so far exert their action through hydrolysis of the Arg 560-Val 561 peptide bond in plasminogen. We will only deal with the properties of the extrinsic activators.

Plasminogen activators are present in many organs, tissues and secretions. These activators appear to be serine proteases with a M_r of approximately 60,000 composed of one polypeptide chain; by limited plasmic action the one-chain activator is converted into a two-chain activator linked by disulfide bonds (20). Both have the same activity in a clot lysis system but differ in their action on synthetic substrates (20). The plasminogen activator found in blood represents released vascular plasminogen activator and these activators are similar or identical to the tissue activator, but different from urokinase (21, 22-24). Recently a plasminogen activator was purified from human melanoma cell cultures which is identical to the activator obtained from human uterus (25). Cash has speculated that plasminogen activator release may be under neurohumoral control. A plasminogen activator releasing hormone (PARH) would constitute the major pathway for the release of plasminogen activator from the endothelial cells, whereas the catecholamine pathway would only be involved in severely stressful situations (26).

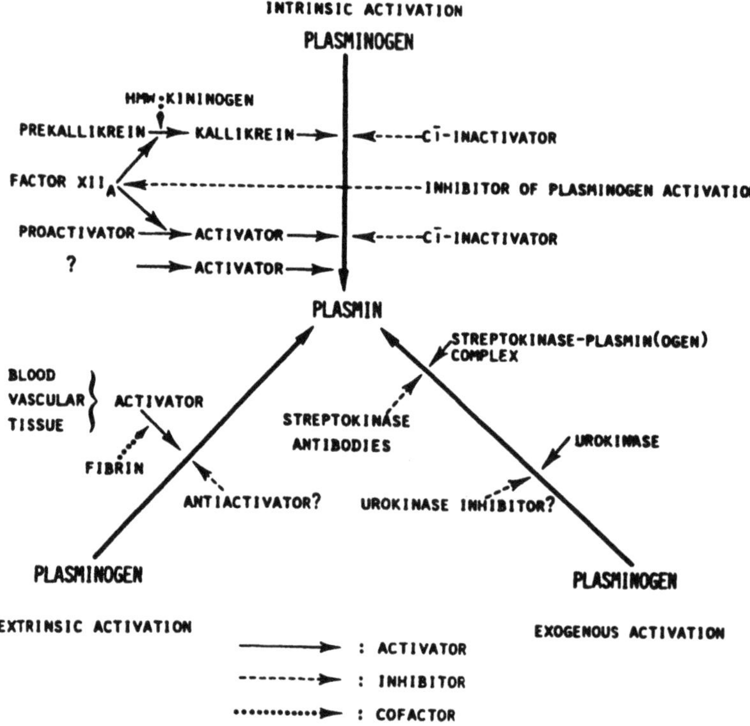

Fig. 1. Schematic representation of activation pathways of plasminogen (⟶) and site of action of inhibitors (--->).

An important property of the blood-vascular-tissue type of plasminogen activator is its high affinity for fibrin which has been used for its isolation (27). Tissue activator is a relatively poor plasminogen activator in pure systems, but fibrin strikingly stimulates the activation (20, 27, 28). From the different half-life of plasminogen activator in vivo and in vitro (29, 30) it can be concluded that a significant amount is cleared in vivo by mechanisms other than neutralization by plasmatic inhibitors. Evidence for the existence of a specific anti-activator in plasma forming a reversible complex with the extrinsic plasminogen activator (31, 32) can at best be regarded as preliminary.

Inhibitors of plasmin

α_2-Antiplasmin

α_2-Antiplasmin is a single chain glycoprotein with M_r 70,000 containing approximately 13% carbohydrate (33, 34). The concentration in pooled normal plasma is approximately 1 μM.

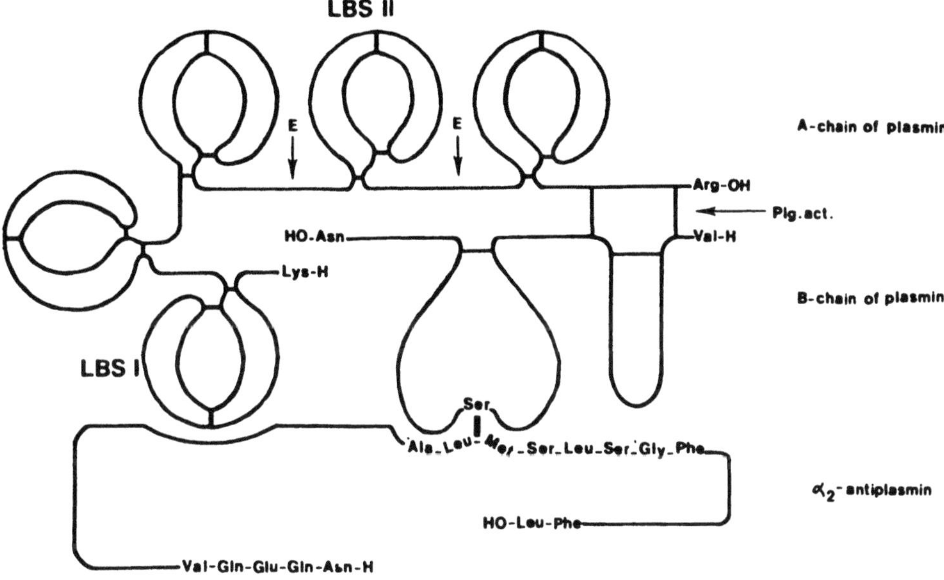

Fig. 2. Schematic representation of the interaction between plasmin and α_2-antiplasmin

Plasmin and α_2-antiplasmin form a stoichiometric 1:1 complex (M_r 150,000) which is devoid of protease or esterase activity (33, 34, 35). Complex formation occurs by strong interaction between the light-(B)-chain of plasmin and the inhibitor. The reaction proceeds in at least two steps: a very fast reversible second order reaction followed by a slower irreversible first order reaction (36, 37) and may be represented by:

$$P + A \underset{k_{-1}}{\overset{k_1}{\rightleftharpoons}} PA \xrightarrow{k_2} PA'$$

The rate of the reaction ($k_1 = 2\text{-}4.10^7\ M^{-1}\ s^{-1}$) is strongly dependent on the availability of free lysine-binding sites and a free active site in the plasmin molecule (36, 38).

The interaction between plasmin and α_2-antiplasmin as proposed by Wiman and Collen (14) is schematically represented in Fig. 2 (19). So far, two cases of congenital α_2-antiplasmin deficiency are reported (39, 40). Both show a bleeding tendency, confirming the physiological importance of the inhibitor.

α_2-Macroglobulin

α_2-Macroglobulin represents the slower reacting plasmin inhibitor of plasma, and its role seems to be to inactivate plasmin formed in excess over the inhibitory capacity of α_2-antiplasmin (41, 42).

REGULATION AND CONTROL OF FIBRINOLYSIS

Turnover studies with labeled components of the coagulation or fibrinolytic system are not continuously active, but designed to be activated in situ when needed for local hemostasis (43). The regulation and control of fibrinolysis occurs at several levels: release of plasminogen activator from the vascular wall, fibrin-associated activation of plasminogen and inhibition of formed plasmin. During the past few years specific interactions at the molecular level have been demonstrated between the different components of the fibrinolytic system which enable us to formulate a molecular model for the regulation of fibrinolysis in vivo.

Plasminogen can specifically bind to fibrin through its lysine-binding sites (18, 44, 45). The tissue activator of plasminogen also binds strongly to fibrin and activates the fibrin-bound plasminogen very efficiently (27, 28). Plasmin molecules bound to fibrin through their lysine-binding sites and involved in fibrin degradation through their active site are protected from rapid inactivation by α_2-antiplasmin (46) (estimated increase in half-life by two orders of magnitude). This explains the directed action of plasmin towards fibrin. Effective clot dissolution in vivo would also seem to require a continuous replacement at the fibrin surface of inactivated plasmin molecules by plasminogen molecules (46). In plasma, α_2-antiplasmin rapidly inhibits plasmin and thereby protects fibrinogen; as soon as plasmin is formed in excess and plasmin-α_2-macroglobulin complex formed, fibrinogen is rapidly degraded (35, 47, 48). These molecular interactions are schematically represented in Fig. 3.

α_2-Antiplasmin not only forms a stable complex with plasmin, but also interacts weakly with the proenzyme plasminogen through the lysine-binding sites (33, 34, 39). Sakata and Aoki (50) reported that α_2-antiplasmin is cross-linked to fibrin when blood is clotted in the presence of factor XIII and calcium ions. They conclude that this would make fibrin clots less susceptible to fibrinolysis by plasmin. Recently we described that histidine-rich glycoprotein (first discovered in 1972 by Haupt and Heimburger (51, 52)) binds to the high-affinity lysine-binding site of plasminogen and thereby prevents binding of plasminogen to fibrin resulting in an antifibrinolytic effect (53). These interactions may play a regulatory role but are not believed to be of primary importance for the mechanism of fibrinolysis.

IN VIVO FINDINGS SUPPORTING THE MOLECULAR MODEL FOR FIBRINOLYSIS

The apparent paradox of an enhanced plasminogen activation by urokinase in the presence of 6-aminohexanoic acid or tranexamic acid in purified systems (27, 53) and the potent antifibrinolytic action of these amino acids in vivo (55, 56) can be explained on the basis of this model. These compounds bind to the lysine-binding sites of plasminogen causing a conformational change: this results in an improved activation by urokinase in vitro, but in vivo they disso-

PHYSIOLOGICAL FIBRINOLYSIS

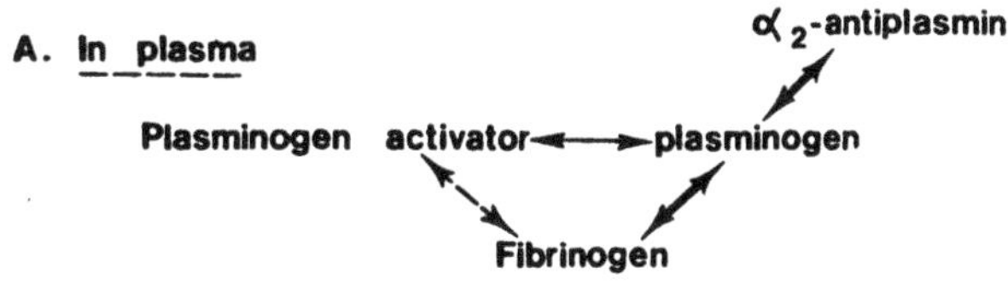

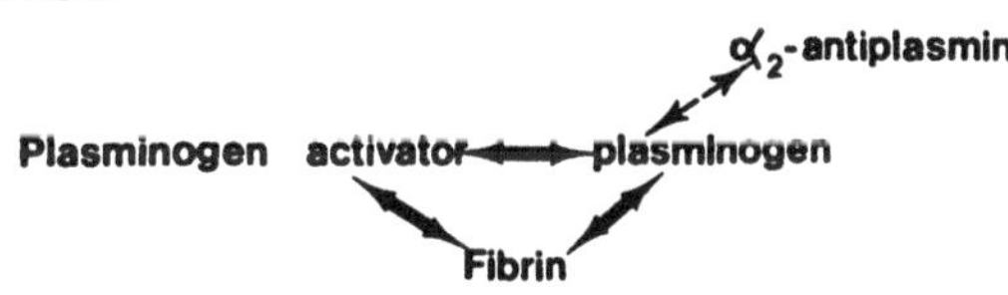

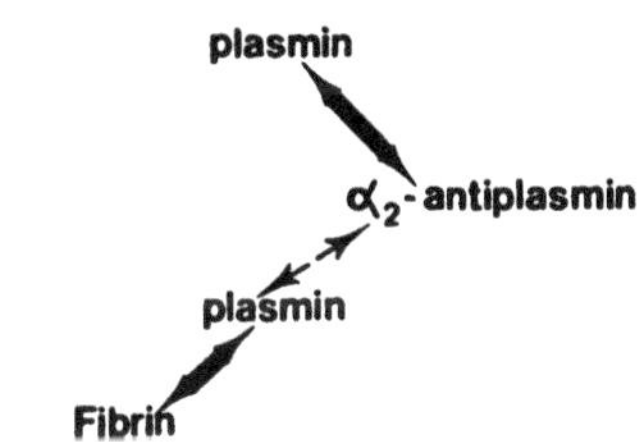

Fig. 3. Schematic representation of the interactions between fibrin(ogen), plasmin(ogen), α_2-antiplasmin and plasminogen activator. The size of the arrows is roughly proportional to the affinity between the different components.

ciate plasminogen from the fibrin surface and thereby prevent activation of fibrin bound plasminogen.

Repeated exhaustive physical exercise in healthy subjects results in the release of large amounts of plasminogen activator into the blood but leads only to minimal plasminogen to plasmin conversion (57). In vivo fibrin formation following infusion of reptilase (58, 59) does not induce an increased level of plasminogen activator in the blood but nevertheless leads to a very marked plasminogen activation. This apparent paradox can also easily be explained on the basis of the above molecular model. In the absence of fibrin, plasminogen activator has a poor efficiency; even high concentrations of activator as released by strenuous physical exercise will not lead to significant plasmin formation. In the presence of fibrin however, plasminogen activator present in blood or released from the vascular wall will efficiently activate fibrin-bound plasminogen (27, 28).

Plasminogen activator is continuously present in the blood of healthy individuals; yet, only very little - if any - plasminogen activation occurs (60). Intravascular coagulation on the other hand is nearly always associated with activation of the fibrinolytic system (61) ("secondary fibrinolysis"), even in the absence of an increased level of circulating plasminogen activator. These observations can be explained by the catalytic role of fibrin which triggers and regulates fibrinolysis.

The two patients described with a deficiency of α_2-antiplasmin presented with a hemorrhagic diathesis (39, 40) while plasma-fibrinogen and fibrinogen degradation products in serum were normal. In the framework of this molecular model for fibrinolysis the bleeding tendency of the patients would be due to premature lysis of hemostatic plugs because due to the absence of α_2-antiplasmin, plasmin molecules generated on the fibrin surface of hemostatic plugs would persist much longer than their normal half-life. The absence of systemic fibrinogen breakdown would then be explained, not by the fact that the other plasma protease inhibitors compensate for the deficient α_2-antiplasmin, but by the lack of systemic plasminogen activation in the absence of fibrin (32).

REFERENCES

1. T. Astrup, Fibrinolysis in the organism. Blood 11:781-806 (1956).
2. G.R. Fearnley, Fibrinolysis. Adv. Drug Res. 7:107-163 (1973).
3. P. Wallén,and B. Wiman, Characterization of human plasminogen. I. On the relationship between different molecular forms of plasminogen demonstrated in plasma and found in purified preparations. Biochim. Biophys. Acta 221:20-30 (1970).
4. P. Wallén,and B. Wiman, Characterization of human plasminogen. II. Separation and partial characterization of different molecular forms of human plasminogen. Biochim. Boiphys. Acta 257:122-134 (1972).
5. B. Wiman, Biochemistry of the plasminogen to plasmin conversion. In: "Fibrinolysis. Current fundamental and clinical aspects" (Gaffney, P.J. and Balkuv-Ulutin, S., eds.). Academic Press, London, p. 47-60 (1978).
6. D. Collen,and L. De Maeyer, Molecular biology of human plasminogen. I. Physiochemical properties and microheterogeneity. Thrombos. Diathes. Haemorrh. 34:396-402 (1975).
7. F.J. Castellino, G.E. Siefring Jr., J.M. Sodetz,and R.K. Brethauer, Amino terminal amino acid sequences and carbohydrate of the two major forms of rabbit plasminogen. Biochem. Biophys. Res. Commun. 53:845-851 (1973).
8. L. Summaria, L. Arzadon, P. Bernabe,and K.C. Robbins, Studies on the isolation of the multiple molecular forms of human plasminogen and plasmin by isoelectric focusing methods. J. Biol. Chem. 247:4691-4702 (1972).

9. W.J. Brockway,and F.J. Castellino, Measurement of the binding of antifibrinolytic amino acids to various plasminogens. Arch. Biochem. Biophys. 151:194-199 (1972).
10. K.C. Robbins, L. Summaria, B. Hsieh,and R.J. Shah, The peptide chains of human plasmin. Mechanism of activation of human plasminogen to plasmin. J. Biol. Chem. 242:2333-2342 (1967).
11. W.R. Groskopf, L. Summaria,and K.C. Robbins, Studies on the active center of human plasmin. Partial amino acid sequence of a peptide containing the active center serine residue. J. Biol. Chem. 244:3590-3597 (1969).
12. L. Sottrup-Jensen, T.E. Petersen,and S. Magnusson, In: "Atlas of protein sequence and structure", Vol. 5, suppl. 3, p. 91 (1978).
13. P. Wallén, and B. Wiman, On the generation of intermediate plasminogen and its significance for activation. In: "Proteases and biological control" (Reich, E., Rifkin, D.B., and Shaw, E., eds.). Cold spring Harbor Laboratory, p. 291-303 (1975).
14. B. Wiman, and D. Collen, On the mechanism of the reaction between human α_2-antiplasmin and plasmin. J. Biol. Chem. 254: 9291-9297 (1979).
15. G. Markus, J.L. De Pasquale, and F.C. Wissler, Quantitative determination of the binding of epsilon-aminocaproic acid to native plasminogen. J. Biol. Chem. 253:727-732 (1978).
16. L. Sottrup-Jensen, H. Claeys, M. Zajdel, T.E. Petersen, and S. Magnusson, The primary structure of human plasminogen: isolation of two lysine-binding fragments and one "mini"-plasminogen (M.W. 38,000) by elastase-catalyzed specific limited proteolysis. In: "Progress in chemical fibrinolysis and thrombolysis, vol. 3" (Davidson, J.F., Rowan, R.M., Samama, M.M., and Desnoyers, P.C., eds.). Raven Press, New York, p. 191-209 (1978).
17. E.E. Rickli, and W.I. Otavsky, A new method of isolation and some properties of heavy chain of human plasmin. Eur. J. Biochem. 9:441-447 (1975).
18. B. Wiman, and P. Wallén, The specific interaction between palsminogen and fibrin. A physiological role of the lysine binding site in plasminogen. Thrombos. Res. 10:213-222 (1977).
19. D. Collen, On the regulation and control of fibrinolysis. Thrombos. Haemostas. 43:77-89 (1980).
20. P. Wallén, M. Rånby, N. Bergsdorf, and P. Kok, Two forms of the tissue plasminogen activator and their enzymatic properties. Prog. Chem. Fibrinolysis Thrombolysis, vol. 5 (in press) (1981).
21. D.C. Rijken, G. Wijngaards, M. Zaal-de Jong, and J. Welbergen, Purification and partial characterization of plasminogen activator from human uterine tissue. Biochim. Biophys. Acta 580:140-153 (1979).
22. E.R. Cole, and F.W. Bachmann, Purification and properties of a plasminogen activator from pig heart. J. Biol. Chem. 252: 3729-3737 (1977).

23. P. Wallén, P. Kok, and M. Rånby, The tissue activator of plasminogen. In: "Regulatory enzymes and their control" (Magnusson, S., Ottesen, M., Foltman, B., Dano, K., and Neurath, H., eds.). Pergamon Press, Oxford, p. 127-135 (1978).
24. E.E. Rickli, and G. Zaugg, Isolation and purification of highly enriched tissue plasminogen activator from pig heart. Thrombos. Diathes. Haemorrh. 23:64-76 (1970).
25. D.C. Rijken, and D. Collen, Purification and characterization of the plasminogen activator from a human melanoma cell culture. Prog. Chem. Fibrinolysis Thrombolysis, 5 (in press) (1981).
26. J.D. Cash, Control mechanism of activator release. In: "Progress in chemical fibrinolysis and thrombolysis, vol. 3" (Davidson, J.F., Rowan, R.M., Samama, M.M., and Desnoyers, P.C., eds.). Raven Press, New York, p. 65-75 (1978).
27. P. Wallén, Activation of plasminogen with urokinase and tissue activator. In: "Thrombosis and urokinase" (Paoletti, R., and Sherry, S., eds.). Academic Press, London, p. 91-102 (1977).
28. S.M. Camiolo, S. Throrsen, and T. Astrup, Fibrinogenolysis and fibrinolysis with tissue plasminogen activator, urokinase, streptokinase-activated human globulin, and plasmin. Proc. Soc. Exper. Biol. Med. 138:277-280 (1971).
29. G. Tytgat, D. Collen, and R.A. De Vreker, Investigations on the fibrinolytic system in liver cirrhosis. Acta Haematol. 40:265-274 (1968).
30. C. Kluft, Quantitation and behaviour of extrinsic or vascular plasminogen activator in blood. Prog. Chem. Fibrinolysis Thrombolysis, 5 (in press) (1981).
31. V. Gurewich, E. Hyde, and B. Lipinski, The resistance of fibrinogen and soluble fibrin monomer in blood to degradation by a potent plasminogen activator from cadaver limbs. Blood 46:555-565 (1975).
32. D. Collen, α_2-Antiplasmin inhibitor deficiency. Lancet I:1039-1040 (1979).
33. M. Moroi, N. Aoki, Isolation and characterization of alpha 2-plasmin inhibitor from human plasma. A novel proteinase inhibitor which inhibits activator-induced clot lysis. J. Biol. Chem. 251:5956-5965 (1976).
34. B. Wiman, and D. Collen, Purification and characterization of human antiplasmin, the fast-acting plasmin inhibitor in plasma. Eur. J. Biochem. 78:19-26 (1977).
35. S. Müllertz, and I., Clemmensen, The primary inhibitor of plasmin in human plasma. Biochem. J. 159:545-553 (1976).
36. U. Christensen, and I. Clemmensen, Kinetic properties of the primary inhibitor of plasmin from human plasma. Biochem. J. 163:389-391 (1977).
37. B. Wiman, and D. Collen, On the kinetics of the reaction between human antiplasmin and plasmin. Eur. J. Biochem. 84:573-578 (1978).

38. B. Wiman, L. Boman, and D. Collen, On the kinetics of the reaction between human antiplasmin and a low-molecular-weight form of plasmin. Eur. J. Biochem. 87:143-146 (1978).
39. K. Koie, K. Ogata, T. Kamiya, J. Takamatsu, and M. Kohakura, α_2-Plasmin inhibitor deficiency (Miyasata disease). Lancet ii:1334-1336 (1978).
40. C. Kluft, E. Vellenga, and E.J.P. Brommer, Homozygous α_2-antiplasmin deficiency. Lancet ii:206 (1979).
41. D. Collen, Identification and some properties of a new fast-reacting plasmin inhibitor in human plasma. Eur. J. Biochem. 69:209-216 (1976).
42. P.C. Harpel, Human alpha 2-macroglobulin. Methods Enzymol. 45:639-652 (1976).
43. D. Collen, G.N. Tytgat, H. Claeys, and R. Piessens, Metabolism and distribution of fibrinogen. I. Fibrinogen turnover in physiological conditions in humans. Brit. J. Haematol. 22: 681-700 (1972).
44. S. Thorsen, Differences in the binding to fibrin of a native plasminogen and plasminogen modified by proteolytic degradation. Influence of omega-amino-carboxylic acids. Biochim. Biophys. Acta 393:55-65 (1975).
45. I. Rákóczi, B. Wiman, and D. Collen, On the biological significance of the specific interaction between fibrin, plasminogen and antiplasmin. Biochim. Biophys. Acta 540:295-300 (1978).
46. B. Wiman, and D. Collen, Molecular mechanism of physiological fibrinolysis. Nature 272:549-550 (1978).
47. S. Müllertz, Different molecular forms of plasminogen and plasmin produced by urokinase in human plasma and their relation to protease inhibitors and lysis of fibrinogen and fibrin. Biochem. J. 143:273-283 (1974).
48. D. Collen, and M. Verstraete, α_2-Antiplasmin consumption and fibrinogen breakdown during thrombolytic therapy. Thrombos. Res. 14:631-639 (1979).
49. B. Wiman, H.R. Lijnen, and D. Collen, On the specific interaction between the lysine-binding sites in plasmin and complementary sites in α_2-antiplasmin and in fibrinogen. Biochim. Biophys. Acta 579:142-154 (1979).
50. Y. Sakata, and N. Aoki, Cross-linking of α_2-plasmin inhibitor to fibrin by fibrin-stabilizing factor. J. Clin. Invest. 65:290-297 (1980).
51. H. Haupt, and N. Heimburger, Humanserumproteine mit hoher Affinität zu Carboxymethylcellulose. I. Isolierung von Lysozym, C_{1q} und zwei busher unbekannten α-Globulinen. Hoppe-Seyler's Z. Physiol. Chem. 353:1125-1132 (1972).
52. N. Heimburger, H. Haupt, T. Kranz, and S. Baudner, Humanserumproteine mit hoher Affinität zu Carboxymethylcellulose. II. Physikalischchemische und immunologische Charakterisierung eines histidinereichen 3,8 S-α_2-Glycoproteins (CM-Protein I). Hoppe-Seyler's Z. Physiol Chem. 353:1133-1140 (1972).

53. H.R. Lijnen, M. Hoylaerts, and D. Collen, Isolation and characterization of a human plasma protein with affinity for the lysine-binding sites in plasminogen. Role in the regulation of fibrinolysis and identification as histidine-rich glycoprotein. J. Biol. Chem. 255:10214-10222 (1980).
54. S. Thorsen, and S. Müllertz, Rate of activation and electrophoretic mobility of unmodified and partially degraded plasminogen. Effects of 6-aminohexanoic acid and related compounds. Scand. J. Clin. Lab. Invest. 34:167 (1974).
55. G.P. McNicol, A.P. Fletcher, N. Alkjaersig, and S. Sherry, Impairment of hemostasis in the urinary tract: the role of urokinase. J. Lab. Clin. Med. 58:34-46 (1961).
56. L. Nilsson, and G. Rybo, Treatment of menorrhagia with an antifibrinolytic agent, tranexamic acid (AMCA). A double-blind investigation. Acta Obstet. Gynec. Scand. 46:572-580 (1967).
57. D. Collen, N. Semeraro, J.P. Tricot, and J. Vermylen, Turnover of fibrinogen, plasminogen and prothrombin during exercise in man. J. Appl. Physiol. 42:865-873 (1977).
58. D. Collen, and J. Vermylen, Metabolism of iodine-labeled plasminogen during streptokinase and reptilase therapy in man. Thrombos. Res. 2:238-250 (1973).
59. D. Collen, and M. Verstraete, Plasmin-antiplasmin complex formation during defibrase infusion in man. Thrombos. Res. 11:417-420 (1977).
60. D. Collen, G. Tytgat, H. Claeys, M. Verstraete, and P. Wallén, Metabolism of plasminogen in healthy subjects: effect of tranexamic acid. J. Clin. Invest. 51:1310-1318 (1972).
61. D. Collen, J. Rouvier, D.F. Chamone, and M. Verstraete, Turnover of radiolabeled plasminogen and prothrombin in cirrhosis of the liver. Eur. J. Clin. Invest. 8:185-188 (1978).

THE BIOLOGICAL ROLE OF FIBRINOLYSIS

J.F. Davidson and Isobel D. Walker

Department of Haematology
Glasgow Royal Infirmary
Glasgow, UK

The fibrinolytic system

Fibrinolysis is a basic defence mechanism of the organism designed to control the deposition of fibrin in the vascular system and elsewhere. This fibrin polymer deposition is regulated by the fibrinolytic system which acts on the insoluble protein and by splitting a limited number of peptide bonds renders it soluble.

Fibrin is of course removed by other enzymes, but the term fibrinolysis is today generally restricted to the "fibrinolysing" action of the plasminogen-plasmin system.

Plasminogen-plasmin

The key component of the fibrinolytic system is the single chain glycoprotein plasminogen which is present in plasma and in most tissues. This polypeptide is the proenzyme from which the highly proteolytic serine protease plasmin is formed by limited proteolysis. Plasmin has broad substrate specificity but it is rendered relatively selective for fibrin by the nature of the molecular biology of the fibrin, plasminogen, plasmin and antiplasmin interactions.

Activators

The conversion of plasminogen to plasmin is brought about by plasminogen activators which are in two categories. Firstly, extrinsic plasminogen activators which are extrinsic to the plasma and secondly, intrinsic plasminogen activators which are intrinsic to the plasma.

The extrinsic activators are either tissue activators, which are firmly fixed in tissues, or endothelial cell activator - vascular activator, which is found in the vascular endothelium and released into the blood. The intrinsic activators are components of the Factor XII activation system and become available by activation of the intrinsic coagulation mechanism. The blood vascular activator is released into the blood continuously and its plasma level shows a marked diurnal variation.

These activators are also regulated by inhibitors, although our knowledge of the anti-activators is less clear than our knowledge of the anti-plasmins. Vascular activator is also regulated by its high affinity for fibrin.

Role of fibrin

Fibrin is central to the whole mechanism of fibrinolysis because the fibrin surface provides a special milieu with optimum conditions for the reaction of the plasminogen-plasmin system. Plasminogen and plasminogen activator bind selectively to fibrin and on the fibrin surface plasmin is formed which immediately interacts with the fibrin. This interaction occupies the active sites of the plasmin and renders them unavailable for interaction and neutralisation by the anti-plasmin in the surrounding plasma. If any plasmin is formed away from the fibrin surface it immediately interacts with the fast anti-plasmin α_2 plasmin inhibitor (α_2PI) and is inhibited. In this way fibrinolysis is made highly specific for fibrin and is contained within the immediate environment of the clot.

Like several parts of the coagulation mechanism it is a surface linked phenomenon. It is only if excessive amounts of plasmin are formed, or if the α_2PI level in the plasma is deficient that the fibrinolytic process can extend out into the general circulation and generalized fibrinolysis ensue.

Fibrinolysis interactions

Fibrinolysis is a complex co-operative reaction at the fibrin surface between activator, plasminogen, plasmin and α_2PI which should it spill over into the surrounding plasma will be met by considerable anti-plasmin activity primarily in the form of α_2PI and secondarily as α_2 macroglobulin (α_2M)(1).

Biological principles of fibrinolysis

The biological principles of the fibrinolytic system are basically similar to those of the coagulation system. An initiating or switch mechanism is required to "start" the system and thereafter serine proteases are generated to achieve the system's biological function. While proteases, however, can generate biological functions they can equally destroy them because proteolysis is an irreversible process and proteases are not endowed with repair functions.

A "stop" mechanism or inhibition mechanism is, therefore, essential to limit proteolysis. This on and off mechanism is controlled by different switches. The on switch is the release or perhaps activation of plasminogen activators. The off switch is the containment of the reaction by the inhibitor α_2PI supplemented if necessary, by α_2M, aided by the constraints of a surface mediated reaction, and the run down of available surface for the fibrinolytic reaction as fibrin is digested.

In addition, the switch on of activation is regulated in a similar fashion with antiactivators. The mechanism of this reaction, unlike the α_2PI mechanism, is poorly understood and is still the subject of some controversy.

The fibrinolytic system in addition to the switch on, switch off mechanisms, has an inbuilt self acceleration process. When plasminogen activator meets plasminogen, if the conditions are right, plasmin is formed: this plasmin, in addition to attacking fibrin, feeds back into the system, and greatly accelerates the conversion of plasminogen to plasmin.

Fibrinolysis activation

Our knowledge of the trigger mechanism is very limited, although we do know that there are several types of plasminogen activators (2). The tissue type of plasminogen activator is firmly fixed in tissues and can be extracted and studied. It is a stable protein which is probably closely related to vascular or endothelial activator, and to the urine activator urokinase.

Activator is also found in human milk, tears, saliva, cerebrospinal fluid and bile. A trigger is therefore available through most body tissues and body fluids which can initiate fibrinolysis. The activation of this trigger appears to be fibrin deposition, ischaemia, hypoxia or a combination of these, but our knowledge of this is very scanty.

The extrinsic activation mechanism of fibrinolysis seems to play an important role in keeping body cavities and channels free from unwanted fibrin. Thus the urinary tract activator urokinase helps to keep the urinary tract free of fibrin. Various duct systems like the lacrimal ducts and bile ducts have plasminogen activator activity which helps to keep them patent. Fibrinolysis also has an important role in the reproductive mechanism. It contributes to maintaining the patency of the reproductive channels and it plays a role in fertilisation. It also is an important component in the mechanism of menstrual bleeding.

The trigger mechanism for activating fibrinolysis in blood is more complicated. Blood contains a certain amount of extrinsic activator in the form of vascular endothelial activator which is synthesized in the endothelial cells of the small veins, stored there and released on demand. The level of this activator in blood shows a marked diurnal variation being lowest in the morning.

Blood also contains two types of intrinsic activators, one which is associated with activation of Factor XII - the intrinsic Factor XII dependant pathway, and the other which is independent of Factor XII - the Factor XII independent pathway. It now seems quite clear that when intrinsic coagulation is activated fibrinolysis is activated at the same time.

Therapeutic possibilities

What are the possibilities for therapeutic manipulation of the fibrinolytic system? The system can be therapeutically activated by infusing either streptokinase or urokinase and a condition of hyper-fibrinolysis induced. This form of therapy has been available for well over 10 years and it has found only limited application in anti-thrombosis therapy. During such fibrinolytic therapy the plasminogen can fall to zero. In such circumstances it may be of benefit to give simultaneously an infusion of plasminogen.

Fibrinolysis can also be augmented by oral anabolic steroid therapy which enhances the production of vascular endothelial activator. This form of therapy, however, has never progressed much beyond the experimental stage.

Very recent developments, however, suggest that certain therapeutic innovations will soon be available to activate fibrinolysis with probably greater potential than streptokinase or urokinase. Furthermore, the day may not be far removed when human plasminogen activator may be available for therapeutic use.

Inhibition of fibrinolysis can be readily achieved yb therapeutic intervention. Plasminogen carries lysine binding sites which react with fibrin and play a key role in the fibrinolysis reaction by attaching plasminogen to fibrin. Lysine or related aminoacids, epsilon aminocaproic acid, or tranexamic acid can occupy these lysine sites and thus prevent the binding of plasminogen to plasmin. This phenomenon explains the marked anti-fibrinolytic properties of these amino acids in vivo.

Fibrinolysis - Experiments of nature

In the past two years there have been reports of congenital abnormalities of the fibrinolytic system which serve to emphasize the importance of its biological role.

Koie et al. (3), Aoki et al. (4) and Kluft et al. (5) have described cases of congenital deficiency of α_2PI. The patients with this deficiency have a severe haemorrhagic diathesis which is most probably due to premature lysis of haemostatic plugs because of the absence of α_2PI and in consequence relatively inhibited local in vivo fibrinolysis. It is particularly interesting also that the administration of a lysine aminoacid, tranexamic acid reduced the frequency and the severity of the haemorrhagic diathesis.

This experiment of nature indicates the very important biological role of α_2PI in haemostasis.

Aoki et al. (6) and Wohl et al. (7) have reported hereditary molecular abnormalities of plasminogen in patients with a history of thrombosis. In Aoki et al. (6) cases the abnormality was a depressed level of plasminogen activity in plasma although the plasma plasminogen antigen level was normal. In Wohl et al. (7) report plasminogen variants named Chicago I and Chicago II are described which have impaired activator binding properties, subnormal functional plasminogen values and subnormal plasmin generation rates.

This further experiment of nature indicates the very important biological role of plasminogen in haemostasis.

Conclusion

The biological role of fibrinolysis is therefore that of a closely controlled fibrin clearing machine which has standing by a potentially massive activating mechanism and in the circulation a massive reserve of inhibitors.

If the machine is triggered into action then its chemical design largely serves to contain it in the immediate environment of its target fibrin.

Should it escape control and its own biological inhibition mechanism prove inadequate then supplementary inhibition can be provided by the lysine amino acids - epsilon aminocaproic acid or tranexamic acid.

Finally while "fibrinolytic therapy" has so far been rather disappointing, new therapeutic innovations are likely to become available in the near future which could have a major impact on antithrombosis therapy.

REFERENCES

1. D. Collen, B. Wiman, The fast acting plasmin inhibitor of human plasma: In: Davidson, J.F., Cepelak, V., Samama, M.M., Desnoyers, P.C. Eds.: Progress in chemical fibrinolysis and thrombolysis, Vol. IV, Edinburgh: Churchill Livingstone, 1979: 11-19.
2. T. Astrup, Fibrinolysis: an overview: In: Davidson, J.F., Rowan, R.M., Samama, M.M., Desnoyers, P.C. Eds.: Progress in chemical fibrinolysis and thrombolysis; Vol. IV, New York: Raven Press, 1978: 1-57.
3. K. Koie, T. Kamiya, K. Ogata, J. Takamatsu, M. Kohakura, α_2 Plasmin - inhibitor deficiency Miyasato disease. Lancet 2 : 1334-1336 (1978).
4. N. Aoki, H. Saito, T. Kamiya, K. Koie, Y. Sakata, M. Kohakura, Congenital deficiency of α_2-Plasmin inhibitor associated with severe haemorrhagic tendency. J. Clin. Invest. 63:877-884. (1979).
5. C. Kluft, E. Vellegua, E.J.P. Brommer, Homozygous α_2-antiplasmin deficiency. Lancet 2 : 206 (1979).
6. N. Aoki, M. Moroi, Y. Sakata, N. Yoshida, M. Matsuda, Abnormal plasminogen. A hereditary molecular abnormality found in a

patient with recurrent thrombosis. J. Clin. Invest. 61: 1186-1195 (1979).
7. R.C. Wohl, L. Summaria, K.C. Robbins, Physiological activation of the human fibrinolytic system. Isolation and characterisation of human plasminogen variants, Chicago I and Chicago II. J. Biol. Chem. 254: 9063-9069 (1979).

FIBRINOLYSIS AND BODY WEIGHT: FIBRINOLYTIC RESPONSE TO VENOUS OCCLUSION IN OBESE CHILDREN

S. Coccheri[*], E. Cacciari[**], G. Fortunato[*], R. Bergamaschi[**], A. Balsamo[**], F. Cipollani[**], and M. Poggi[*]

Department of Angiology and Blood Coagulation[*], and Department of Paediatrics[**], University Medical School and Regional Hospital
Bologna, Italy

Obesity in adults is an important risk factor for cardiovascular diseases. An important role among these factors is played by some alterations in the mechanisms of coagulation. Changes in the fibrinolytic process are significant in obesity, although not always correlated with metabolic disorders involving lipid and glucose regulation (1, 2, 3, 4).

As there are no data, to our knowledge, on the same subject in obese children, we studied some aspects of the hemostatic balance in a group of prepubertal obese subjects clearly defined from the metabolic point of view. The primary goal of the present investigation was to evaluate the fibrinolytic response to venous occlusion in obesity of childhood, a condition certainly devoid of vascular complications but preluding or predisposing to adult obesity and its complications. However, other haemostatic parameters have been measured and an attempt to correlate haemostatic alterations with the metabolic disorders has been preformed.

SUBJECTS AND METHODS

Thirty four prepubertal obese children (18 males, 16 females) with a weight excess between 38% and 89% (mean 51.8% ± 15.6 SD) and chronological age from 5 2/12 and 12 years (mean 9 2/12 years) and 16 prepubertal normal-weight children (13 males, 3 females), their chronological age ranging between 6 2/12 and 13 years (mean 9 7/12 years), were submitted to the following tests:

- One stage clotting determination of factor VIII (F VIII: C) (5)
- Immunologic determination of factor VIII (F VIII: R Ag - Behring Institute)

Table 1. Glycemia and Insulinemia During OGTT and Basal Values of Cortisol, Cholesterol

	chronological age	bone age	weight excess	glycemia (g/1) basal value	peak	increase	area
Obese n 34	9.2±2.4	9.7±2.6	51.8±15.6	0.97±0.08 (^)	1.50±0.25	0.53±0.25	6.07±0.94 (+)
Controls n 16	9.7±2.5	8.3±2.0	-	0.9±0.08	1.36±0.21	0.44±0.19	5.68±0.76

(^) $p < 0.05$ for the difference vs controls

(+) $p < 0.05$ for the correlation with $S.AT_{III}$ ($r = + 0.35$)

(x) $p < 0.05$ for the correlation with $S.AT_{III}$ ($r = + 0.62$)

- Serum AT III (S. AT III) according to Von Kaulla and Von Kaulla (6).
- Immunologic AT III (I. AT III) (Behring Institute)
- Semiquantitative assay of platelet aggregation after rotation (PAT 1) according to Breddin (7)
- Euglobulin lysis time (ELT) (8)
- Same after 5' of venous stasis at the forearm at intermediate pressure between systolic and diastolic (ELTV) (9)
- Plasma α_2 antiplasmin (Chromogenic substrate S 2251)

Metabolic investigations

Oral glucose tolerance test (OGTT): Base value (BV), peak (P), increment rate (IR) and glucose area (A) were recorded.

Insulinaemia during OGTT with recording of the parameters: base value, peak, increment rate, Insulinaemic area (I.A.)
Tolbutamide tolerance test (TTT)
Cholesterol and Triglycerides
Blood cortisol.

RESULTS

1) Metabolic characterization of obese children

The results of this part of the study are partially reported in Table I. Obese children had an average overweight of 51.8% ± 15.6. They showed a higher baseline blood glucose ($p < 0.05$), a somewhat higher glucose peak in OGTT ($p > 0.05$), and higher blood insulin and Triglycerides (mean ± SD) in 34 Obese and 16 Normal Subjects.

insulinemia (μU/ml)						
basal value	peak	increase	area	Cortisol (mg/ml)	Cholesterol (mg/100 ml)	Triglycerides (mg/100 ml)
21.1±11.7	93.1±82.1 (^)	68.7±74.6	302.1±230.6 (^)	159.0±70.9	195.6±36.5 (^)	86.1±29.0
14.5±7.2	45.5±21.4	31.0±20.9	145.1±52.0	167.3±79.0	169.5±26.7 (x)	70.0±34.7

peak values during OGTT; in fact peak insulinaemia ($p < 0.05$) and insulinaemic area ($p < 0.05$) were evidently higher in obese children. They also had a higher average cholesterol level ($p < 0.05$), and a trend to increased triglycerides ($p \approx 0.05$).

No differences were found in regard to other metabolic parameters.

2) Parameters of blood coagulation and fibrinolysis

The results are summarized in Tables 2 and 3. Among the blood coagulation parameters studied (Table 2) no significant difference was found as to F VIII: C and F VIII: R Ag.

AT III as serum antithrombin activity was significantly lower than in controls ($p < 0.01$), though largely within physiologic values.

On the other hand, the immunologic assay of AT III showed that its molecular concentration was slightly but significantly higher in obese compared to control children ($p < 0.05$).

The determination of α_2-antiplasmin showed that the level of the main inhibitor of plasmin is higher in obese compared to control children ($p < 0.001$) (Table 2).

The prevalence of cases with increased platelet aggregation was higher in obese vs. controls. In a larger group whose results will be reported elsewhere the difference in this parameter reached statistical significance.

As seen in Table 3 baseline euglobulin lysis time (ELT) is in the average prolonged in obese children, but differences versus controls are not significant. On the contrary, after 5 min of venous stasis the fibrinolytic response is generally almost absent in obese children, whereas it is evident in controls. The differences between the means of ELTV is highly significant ($p < 0.01$). If we define as non responders those subjects having a ratio ELTV to ELT higher than 0.75, non responders are 76.5% of the obese subjects and 43.7% of control children, the difference approaching significance with the χ^2 test ($\chi^2 = 3.75$; $P = 0.05$). The high proportion of non responders

Table 2. Obese children and controls. Haemostatic investigations.

	VIII AHF %	VIII R Ag %	S.AT III %	IMM.AT III mg%	α_2 APL %	PAT (Breddin) prev. stages 4,5
Obese	133.1±50	116.3±33	120.7±29	29.1±29	159.2±20.4	28.1%
Statistical Analysis	(t) n.s.	(t) n.s.	(t)$p<0.01$	(t)$p<0.05$	(t)$p<0.001$	(χ^2) n.s.
Controls	131.8±52	114.6±28	147.3±27	24.6±3	119±17.4	12.5%

Table 3. Obese children and controls. Euglobulin lysis time (ELT), ELT after venous occlusion (ELTV), average percent difference between ELT and ELTV (Δ%) and prevalence of non responders (having ratio ELTV/ELT > 0.75).

	ELT min.	ELTV min.	Δ % av.	NON RESP. ($\frac{ELTV}{ELT}$ >0.75)
Obese	210±107	203±111	14.9±21	76.5%
Statistical evaluation	(t) n.s.	(t)$p<0.01$	(t)$p\approx0.05$	(χ^2)$p = 0.05$
Controls	168±90	114±68	29.2±28	43.7%

even among controls can be explained by the short duration of venous stasis, which may not be capable of mobilizing the entire fibrinolytic capacity of the vascular walls.

3) Correlations between metabolic and haemostatic indices

The correlations (r) calculated will be shown in more detail in an extended paper. Summarizing, no clotting parameter showed correlation with overwheight. No correlation was found between ELT and any of the metabolic indices.

As seen in Table I, serum AT III correlated inversly with age in the controls ($p < 0.05$). In the obese, such correlation was masked, and substituted by a positive correlation with the glucose area in OGTT ($p < 0.05$).

DISCUSSION

In obese children the capacity of producing growth hormone is lower (10), hyperinsulinism is frequently associated with decreased glucose tolerance (11), testosterone response to hCG stimulation and prolactin production are lower than normal (12, 13).

The present data suggest that a reduced fibrinolytic response to venous occlusion is a very early event in obesity, being present already in overweight children. A high level of α_2 antiplasmin seems also to play a role in the reduced fibrinolytic capacity of the obese child.

No significant changes in F VIII AHF and F VIII R Ag were observed. However, there was an increase in AT III measured immunologically, similarly to the finding of the group of De Gaetano in diabetic children (14). This increase might be the result of an early defense mechanism against low grade activation of blood coagulation. AT III activity in serum was slightly but significantly lower in the obese children, a finding also suggesting low grade activation of clotting and mild consumption of AT III activity in presence of normal or increased AT III production.

The high frequency of altered "spontaneous" platelet aggregation after rotation (PAT) may also be referred to conditions of low grade activation of blood clotting, being the method used especially sensitive to aggregating factors in plasma.

Although none of the haemostatic parameters studied could be correlated with the degree of overweight, obesity seems to alter the normal association of a lowering of AT III activity with progressing age, as observed in the controls.

CONCLUSIONS

It is known that obesity in adult age is a condition predisposing to thrombotic vascular events, to postoperatory DTV and pulmonary embolism, to DTV after oral contraceptives, and possibly to atherosclerosis.A reduced fibrinolytic activity and a reduction of plasminogen activator in the vascular wall in the obese was described by several Authors (1, 2, 3, 4, 5, 16, 17).

Alterations of the hemostatic balance, though moderate, are already evident in obese children. In particular, they are "poor responders" in relation to fibrinolytic capacity, have increased α_2-antiplasmin levels, show no rise in F VIII, but AT III concentration, activity and regulation behave abnormally and platelet aggregation is frequently increased.

From the present results we can infer that in obese children some changes in the hemostatic balance can be observed as a forewarning of a later tendency to vascular thrombotic disease in the adult and mature age. It is still to be established whether the changes found can reverse following effective dietary management or are the expression of a constitutional tendency. Further interesting data may emerge from a comparative study of the hemostatic balance in obese and diabetic children.

REFERENCES

1. L.O. Almèr and L. Janzon, Low vascular fibrinolytic activity in obesity. Thromb. Res. 6:171 (1975).
2. D. Shaw and D. Mac Naughton, Relationship between blood fibrinolytic activity and body fatness. Lancet I:352 (1963).
3. C.P. Warlow, A. Mc Neill, D. Ogston and A.S. Douglas, Platelet adhesiveness, coagulation, and fibrinolytic activity in obesity. J. Clin. Path. 25:484 (1972).
4. C.S. Grace, and R.B. Goldrick, Fibrinolysis and body build. Interrelationships between blood, fibrinolysis, body composition and parameters of lipid and carbohydrate metabolism. J. Atheroscler. Res. 8:705 (1968).
5. K.W.E. Denson, In: Human blood coagulation, haemostasis and thrombosis, by Bigs R., Blackwell, Oxford, 1976, p 682.
6. E. von Kaulla and K.N. von Kaulla, Antithrombin III and diseases. Am. J. Clin. Path. 48:68 (1967).
7. K. Breddin, Undersuchungen über die Agglutinationsbereitschaft der Thrombozyten bei Gefässkrankheiten. In: Emmrich R., und Perlick E., eds: Gefasswand und Blutplasma, Leipzig, 1963, II Symp. Med. Klinik.
8. T. Astrup and J. Rasmussen, Estimation of fibrinolytic activity in blood. In: Proc. VII Int. Congress Haematology, Rome, 1958, p 164.
9. B.R. Robertson, M. Pandolfi and I.M. Nilsson, Fibrinolytic capacity in healthy volunteers as estimated from effect of venous occlusion of arms. Acta Clin. Scand. 138:429 (1972).

10. E. Cacciari, A. Cicognani, P. Pirazzoli, P. Tassoni, F. Zappulla, S. Salardi, F. Bernardi, Relationships among the secretion of ACTH, GH and cortisol during the insulin-induced hypoglycemia test in the normal and obese child. J. Clin. Endocrinol. Metab. 40:802 (1975).
11. E. Cacciari, E. Sarti, A. Cicognani, P. Pirazzoli, P. Tassoni, G. Fabiani, F. Zappulla, F. Bernardi, S. Salardi and L. Mazzanti, Insulin efficiency and release in the obese child before and after loss of weight: a study by means of a mathematical model. In: Cacciari, E., Laron, Z. and Raiti, S., eds: Obesity in childhood, London-New york, 1978, Academic Press, p 19.
12. E. Cacciari, A. Cicognani, P. Pirazzoli, F. Zappulla, P. Tassoni, F. Bernardi, S. Salardi and L. Mazzanti, Effect of obesity on the hypothalamo-pituitary gonadal axis in childhood. Acta Pediatr. Scand. 6:345 (1977).
13. E. Cacciari, E. Fréjaville, A. Balsamo, A. Cigognani, P. Pirazzoli, F. Bernardi and F. Zappulla, Disorder of prolactin secretion in the obese child and adolescent. Arch. Dis. Child (1981) in press.
14. E. Corbella, G. Miragliotta, R. Masperi, S. Villa, A. Bini, G. De Gaetano and G. Chiumello, Platelet aggregation and antithrombin III levels in diabetic children. Haemostasis 8:30 (1979).
15. L.O. Almèr, Effect of obesity on endogenous fibrinolytic activity in diabetes mellitus. J. Med. 6:351 (1975).
16. S. Novo, G. Avellone, F. D'Eredità and A. Pinto: Il tempo di lisi delle euglobuline. Nota I: Comportamento in un gruppo di soggetti giovani sani in relazione al peso corporeo relativo. Boll. Soc. It. Cardiol. 12:2145 (1976).
17. A. Girolami, D. Fioretti and G. Boressi, La fibrinolisi euglobulinica ed il fibrinogeno ematico nell'obesità semplice. Folia Endocrinol. 25:502 (1972).

FIBRINOLYTIC VESSEL WALL ACTIVATOR IN ARTERIAL THROMBOSIS

H. Stormorken

Research Institute for Internal Medicine
Rikshospitalet
Oslo 1, Norway

The general consensus is that the fibrinolytic system is the main defence system against thrombo-embolism on the venous side, as illustrated in Fig. 1. This is reasonable because the venous thrombus is more or less a coagulation thrombus where fibrin is predominant, whereas on the arterial side the platelets are the dominant constituent. However, in a fully developed arterial thrombus there is after all some fibrin, the breakdown of which could lead to instabilization and thus halting further growth. It is even possible that the fibrinolytic system might be of importance in the early phase of thrombus formation, since forming fibrin may induce the platelet release reaction. As the fibrin in this stage is most susceptible to plasmin, and the vessel wall activator is stored very close to the initial events, it is feasible that an attack on the fibrin during formation would be of particular importance as a defence phenomenon. However, there has been very little attempt to devise models to pursue this possibility. So far, the evidence for a role of the fibrinolytic system in the defence against arterial thrombosis stems from observations on different patient-groups, and this evidence is steadily becoming stronger.

However, the fibrinolytic system is rather complicated (Fig. 2) having both an extrinsic and intrinsic way of activation. The final result depends on activators as well as inhibitors in a complicated balance which we have not as yet a satisfactory inventory to evaluate. This is so although many, notably Kluft (1978) have made important contributions. For this reason, most studies have disregarded the intrinsic activator pathway and largely concentrated on studying the release or production of the vessel wall activator. Although it might be that this activator is the most important in the clinical sense, it is a gross oversimplification to disregard the intrinsic part.

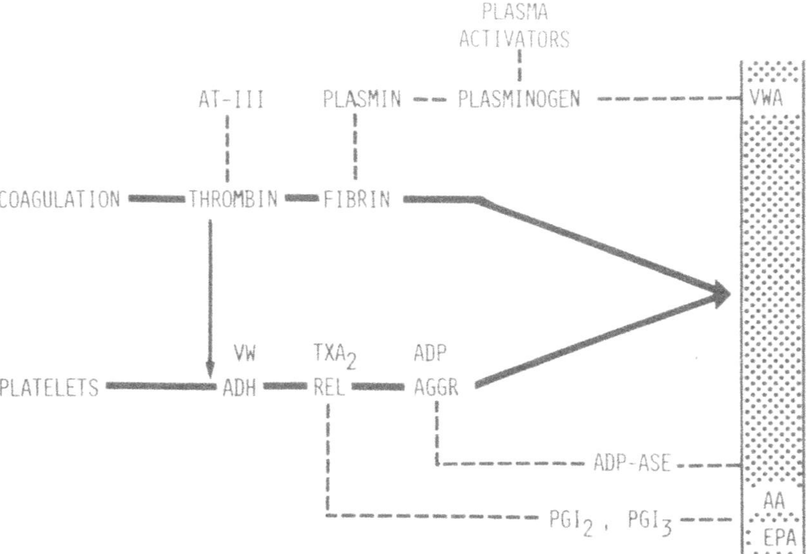

Fig. 1. Defence systems against thrombosis.
VWA - vessel wall activator; vW - von Willebrand factor; ADH - adhesion; TxA_2 - thromboxan A_2; REL - release reaction; ADP - adenosin diphosphate; AGGR aggregation; PGI_2 - prostacyclin; AA - arachidonic acid; EPA - eicosapentaenoic acid.

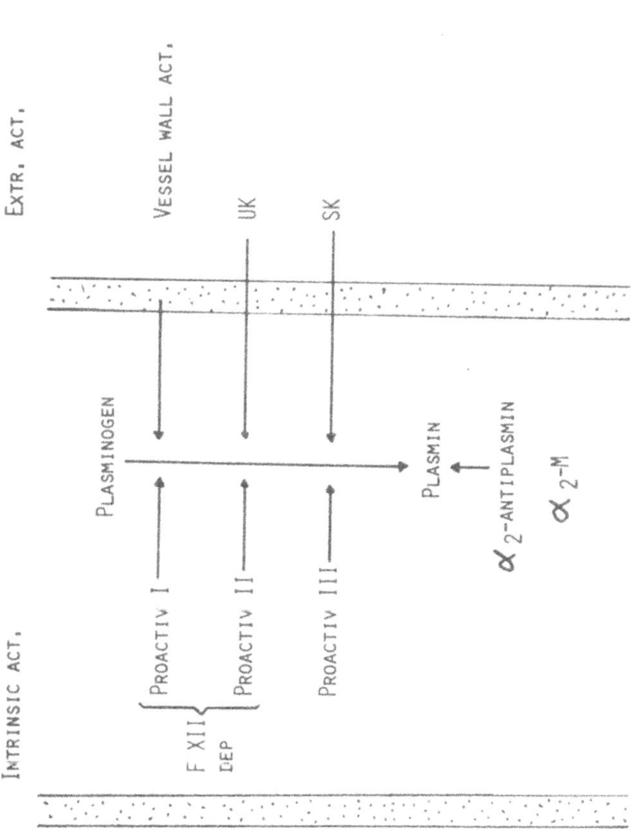

Fig. 2. Fibrinolytic system.
UK - urokinase; SK - streptokinase. (Adapted from Kluft 1978).

But even studying the importance of the extrinsic pathway alone for arterial thrombosis poses methodological problems which may be of importance for the results. Thus the common way of obtaining information is to measure fibrinolytic activity before and after stasis of a vein. Although there is evidence (Almér et al. 1975) that this may be justified , it is not unequivocally proven. Moreover, we have too scanty evidence that the activity in various arterial beds, e.g. cerebral versus coronary, is mirrored equally well by the activity of a special vein. Other uncertainties in the evaluation are inherent in the well known diurnal and day-to-day variation, known and unknown effects of drugs, of exercise and of smoking. The most problematic of these is the day-to-day variation. In 132 patients (Table 1) with recurrent DVT/PE investigated twice for vessel wall activator activity using the 15 min poststasis euglobulin lysis time as parameter, 43 had definite prolonged (>40 min) values on both occasions, whereas 5 were borderline and 16 (12%) had one pathological and one entirely normal result. The release stimulus applied might also be of consequence. Usually stasis, in some studies using a pressure of midway between the diastolic and systolic blood pressure, in others at a fixed level, usually 90 mmHg. In various materials, however, the stasis time varies from 10 through 15 up to 20 minutes. Since it has been shown by the Nilsson-group that maximum release is only attained after 20 minutes, one can easily visualize a different outcome when other times are used. Recently, DDAVP has come into use as a release stimulus, and both intravenous and intrapulmonal application have been attempted. Not sufficiently is known as yet to decide which is the best and most reproducible of these.

After the blood has been drawn, new possibilities for variability occur, such as at which pH the euglobulin is produced, whether dextran sulphate is applied, the ionic strength applied, the use of inhibitors like fluphenamate, and also the time lapse from withdrawal to precipitation. Further, the evaluation might be done either on the fibrin plate or by the euglobulin lysis time, and although there is evidence that this does not make any great difference (Arnesen et al. 1980), not everybody agree in this. The fibrinogen concentration, admittedly of small influence, may however, in large materials have a significant effect. Other uncertainties are derived from variations in the amount of inhibitors precipitated and the possible variation in the degree of activation via the extrinsic or the intrinsic systems. Altogether, even concentrating on the extrinsic activation pathway alone requires a formidable attempt to standardize the circumstances sufficiently for obtaining reliable results.

Irrespective of these difficulties, the majority of the published materials seem to show grossly similar results. Thus, all published papers agree that the extrinsic fibrinolysis system is decreased in diabetes and obesity (for references see Nilsson 1978). Similar conformity exists as to the decrease in hyperlipoproteinemia, which is heavily bound to coronary heart disease. In a recent study (Andersen et al. 1980) 68% of 104 hyperlipemic men showed reduced fibrinolytic activity, particularly applying to type IV in which 95%

Table 1 Methodological Problems

1.	Anatomical geography (Vein - Arteries)
2.	Diurnal, day to day, drugs, smoking, exercise
3.	Release stimulus (Stasis-time - DDAVP-application)
4.	Euglobulin precipitation (pH, Dextransulf., Ionic strength, Flufenamate, etc,)
5	Fibrin plate - Euglobulin Lysis
6.	Fibrinogen concentration
7.	Inhibitors
8.	Extrinsic - Intrinsic activation

had reduced activity. This high figure indicates that the decreased fibrinolysis is secondary to the hyperlipemia. However, in the 55 hyperlipemic persons having been on lipid lowering diet for 3 years and with a marked tendency towards normalization of the lipoprotein pattern, there was very little tendency to normalization of the fibrinolytic activity. this finding therefore speaks for a primary role of fibrinolysis in hiperlipemic persons, but it is obscure indeed why these two abnormalities go together.

There is also new evidence that low extrinsic fibrinolytic activity may participate in the pathogenesis of ischemic cerebral disease and TIA. Thus, Wahlberg et al. (1980) found that in ICD patients the extrinsic activator level was about half of that of a control group. A similar result was found by Mettinger et al. (in press). Additionally, they found no difference between the patients and the control group in antiplasmin, but significantly higher levels of factor VIII : RAg and factor VIII : C than in the controls, which is in line with our findings (Stormorken and Erikssen, 1977) in a prospective study of coronary heart disease. Additionally, they showed that in Group A the angiotensive patients had less than half the level of vessel wall activator than the angionegative patients. (Tables 2 and 3).

Thus, there is increasing evidence that the fibrinolytic system, particularly the extrinsic pathway, may be involved in a series of arterial thrombotic manifestations. But whether this influence is of primary or secondary nature is still unsolved. Only a carefully planned prospective study can answer this question with certainty.

Table 2. Vessel Wall Activator in Recurrent DVT/PE

TOTAL	PATHOLOGIC AT BOTH OCCASIONS	PATHOLOGIC AT FIRST NORMAL AT NEXT	BORDERLINE BOTH	NORMAL
132	43	16	5	68
100%	32%	12%	4%	52%

Table 3. Plasminogen Vessel Activator in ICD-Patients

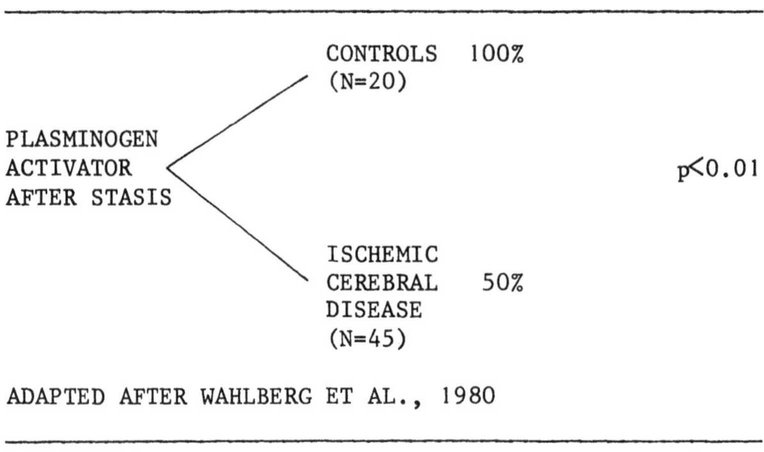

ADAPTED AFTER WAHLBERG ET AL., 1980

Table 4. Plasminogen Vessel Activator anf F.VIII in ICD-Patients

	CONTROLS %	PATIENTS %	P
PLASMINOGEN ACTIVATOR	100	56	<0.01
α2-ANTIPLASMIN	109	108	N.S
F.VIII:RAg	81	110	<0.001
F.VIII:C	77	118	<0.001
	(N=53-80)	(N=58-117)	

ADAPTED FROM METTINGER ET AL. (in press)

REFERENCES

Almér, L.O., Pandolfi, M. and Åberg, M., 1975, The plasminogen activator activity of arteries and veins in diabetes mellitus. Thromb. Res. 6:177-182.

Andersen, P., Arnesen, H. & Hjermann, I., Hyperlipoproteinemia and reduced fibrinolytic activity in healthy coronary risk men. In: Abstract book, Vth Int. Conf. Synthet. fibrinolytic agents, Malmö 1980, p. 104.

Arnesen, H., Nordby, E., Andersen, P. & Godal, H.C., A comparison between the euglobulin clot lysis time and the fibrin plate method for the estimation of fibrinolytic activity after venous stasis. Abstract book, Vth Int. Conf. Synthet. fibrinolytic agents, Malmö 1980, p. 124.

Kluft, C., Blood fibrinolysis. Thesis. Dutch Efficiency Bureau. Pijnacher 1978.

Mettinger, K.L., Nyman, D., Kjellin, K.G., Sidén, Å. & Søderstrøm, C.E., 1979, Factor VIII related antigen, antithrombin III, spontaneous platelet aggregation and plasminogen activator in ischemic cerebral disease. J. Neurol. Sci. 41:31-38.

Mettinger, K.L. et al.: (in press)

Nilsson, I.M., Åberg, M., Holmberg, L. & Vilhart, H., The release mechanism of plasminogen activator and F. VIII as studied by injection of DDAVP and venous occlusion. Abstract book, Vth Int. Conf. Synthet. fibrinolytic agents, Malmö 1980, p. 59.

Nilsson, I.M., Fibrinolysis in diabetes and obesity. Advances in coagulation, fibrinolysis, platelet aggregation and atherosclerosis. Proc. Europ. Symp., ed. Strano, A., C.E.P.I., Roma 1978, p. 95-105.

Stormorken, H. & Erikssen, J., 1979, Plasma antithrombin III and factor VIII antigen in relation to angiographic findings, angina and blood groups in middle aged men. Thrombos. Haemostas. 38:874-880.

Wahlberg, T.B., Blombäck, M. & Övermark, I., 1980, Blood coagulation studies in 45 patients with ischemic cerebrovascular disease and 44 patients with venous thromboembolic disease. Acta. Med. Scand. 27:385-390.

Walker, I.D., Davidson, J.F., Hutton, I. & Lawrie, T.D.V., 1977, Disordered "fibrinolytic potential" in coronary heart disease. Thromb. Res. 10:509-520.

LONG-TERM INDUCTION OF FIBRINOLYTIC ACTIVITY IN CHRONIC ARTERIAL VESSEL DISEASE

J.C.W. van de Loo

Department of Medicine
University of Münster
D-44 Münster, W-Germany

The purpose of this presentation is to answer the question of whether a long-term drug induction of hyperfibrinolysis in blood has convincingly been shown to influence the clinical course of arterial vessel disease and the outcome of patients affected by one of its manifestations. This answer, frankly spoken, is a simple "no".

We are talking here about months and years lasting oral application of drugs which are known to enhance a normal or to normalize a decreased plasma or tissue fibrinolytic activity. A big number of studies has been published in the last 15 years providing evidence that in human beings as well as in animals a stable state of slightly increased plasma fibrinolytic activity may be produced if one applies substances like the anabolic steroid hormones Stanazolol or Ethylestrenol without or in combination with one of the biguanides Phenformin or Buformin. From a pathogenetic point of view it is of major importance that in several studies a significant rise of activator activity after venous occlusion in treated patients could be demonstrated. This could indicate that these drugs act through an influence on the release of activators from the venous endothelial cells.

In contrast to these many observations on biochemical changes in blood and tissue after long-term induction of hyperfibrinolysis there are no prospective clinical trials - using a control group - available, in which a clear-cut clinical effect on signs, symptoms and outcome of patients with coronary, cerebral or peripheral arterial vessel disease could be demonstrated. This means - at the present state of knowledge - that the lack of reliable studies does not allow any conclusions on the clinical benefit of long-term induction of increased fibrinolytic activity in the blood of patients with one of the common manifestations of arteriosclerotic vessel disease.

In the trial of Bielawiec and coworkers 27 patients with coronary heart disease and 28 with occlusive peripheral vessel disease were treated with Stanozolol +Phenformin for 6 months. The authors report "a subjective improvement and a reduction of ECG-abnormalities" in the coronary patients and an "improvement in the walking distance" of the claudication patients. But no figures or data for validating these statements are given. The lack of a control group does not permit the conclusion that the observed effects may indeed be attributed to the drugs under discussion.

Some rare conditions of venous and arterial disease have been described in which long term induction of fibrinolytic activity seems to be clinically effective. Due to the small number of patients these reports are necessarily anecdotical in nature. Jarret et al, 1978 suggested Stanozolol treatment in liposclerosis which is a condition of induration, pigmentation, swelling and pain in the lower leg of patients with chronic venous post-thrombotic insufficiency. All their 15 patients stated improvement of pain and tenderness and a reduction of the affected skin area was noticed.

Isacson and Nilsson (1975) treated 33 patients presenting with idiopathic recurrent deep venous thombosis with a combination of Phenformin + Ethylestrenol for at least one year. All these patients had a low activator content in specimens of superficial skin veins before treatment and 11 out of the 33 patients responded with an abnormally low activator release after venous occlusion. The effect of the treatment on fibrinolytic activity was striking an all patients. Only one of these 33 patients had a new episode of thrombosis. Within the three months of treatment, the others remained free of recurrencies.

Another rare disease model for the application of drugs which enhance plasma fibrinolytic activity has been thought to be the Morbus Behcet. Some of the manifestations of this disease in skin, mucous membranes and in organs are known to be of thrombotic origin. Although a marked decrease of fibrinolytic activity in plasma and a reduced release of fibrinolytic activity after venous occlusion has been reported, anecdotical experiences of a treatment with anabolic steroids were not convincing.

All these rare conditions of disease are obviously not related to the chronic occlusive disease of arterial vessels. The fact that no reliable studies on the clinical effect of a long-term induction of fibrinolytic activity are available and that not one paper on this subject has been presented at the last three conferences of the International Society on Thrombosis and Haemostasis seems to indicate that the respective experts in the field do not expect intriguing clinical effects. In addition, from a pathogenetic point of view it seems to be more appropriate to manage secondary prevention of arterial vessel disease by influencing the primary processes of thrombotic complications, such as platelet activity or fibrin formation instead of activating the secondary repair mechanism.

Table 1. Long Term Induction of Fibrinolytic Activity in Patients with Liposclerosis (Jarret et al.).

No. of patients	14
Drugs given	2 x 5 mg Stanozolol for 3 months
Fibrinolytic effect	1. Shortening of lysis time (DBCLT) 2. Increase of the fibrin plate lysis 3. Decrease of fibrinogen
Clinical effect	Improvement of pain and skin softening in all patients Reduction of the area of induration

Table 2. Long Term Induction of Fibrinolytic Activity in Patients with Recurrent Deep Vein Thrombosis (Isacson and Nilsson, 1975).

No. of patients	33
Drugs given	2 x 50 mg Phenformin plus 2 x 4 mg Ethylestrenol for 1 year
Fibrinolytic effect	1. Increase of the low content of plasminogen activator in vein walls 2. Increased release of fibrinolytic activity after venous forearm occlusion
Clinical effect	One recurrence during the year of observation

REFERENCES

Asbeck, F., Meyer-Boernecke, D., van de Loo, J. 1977. Inhibition of the fibrinolytic system in Behcet disease? Haemostasis 6: 303.

Bielawiec, M., Mysliwiec, M., Perzanowski, A. 1978. Combined therapy with Phenformin plus Stanozolol in patients with occlusive arterial disease and recurrent venous thrombosis. In: Progress in chemical fibrinolysis and thrombolysis, Eds.: J.F. Davidson, R.M. Roman, M.M. Samama and P.C. Desnoyers, Raven Press, New York, p. 507.

Chajek, T., Aronowski, E., Izak, G. 1973. Decreased fibrinolysis in Behcet disease. Thromb. Diath. Hemorrh. 29: 610.

Isacson, S., Nilsson, I.M. 1975. Antithrombotic effect of a combined Phenformin-Ethylestrenol therapy medication. In: Synthetic fibrinolytic thrombolytic agents, K.N. von Kaulla, J.F. Davidson Eds.C. Thomas, Springfield, 314.

Jarret, P.E.M., Burnand, K.G., Morland,M., Browse, N.L. 1978. The treatment of venous liposclerosis of the legs by fibrinolytic enhancement. In: Progress in chemical fibrinolysis and thrombolysis, Eds.: J.F. Davidson, R.M. Roman, M.M. Samama and P.C. Desnoyers, Raven Press, New York, p. 507.

PART 6

HYPERTENSIVE VASCULAR DISEASE

FREE (UNCONJUGATED) CATECHOLAMINE CONCENTRATIONS IN PLATELETS: BIOLOGICAL SIGNIFICANCE AND CLINICAL IMPLICATIONS

G.B. Picotti, G.P. Bondiolotti, A.M. Cesura, C. Ravazzani, M.D. Galva and P. Mantegazza

Institute of Pharmacology, School of Medicine, University of Milan
Via Vanvitelli, 32, 20129 Milan, Italy

Introduction

Mammalian platelets do not contain monoamine synthesizing enzymes, but take up and accumulate in their "dense bodies", the serotonin (5-HT) organelles, monoamines present in plasma, e.g. 5-HT, catecholamines (CA), normetanephrine and p-octopamine (Da Prada et al., 1980; for review see Da Prada et al., 1981). The limits of sensitivity of the fluorimetric methods used in earlier studies (Weil-Malherbe and Bone, 1975; Markwardt, 1976) for measuring the low concentrations of plasma and platelet CA have recently been overcome by highly sensitive and specific radioenzymatic assays, which allow precise and simultaneous measurements of adrenaline (A), noradrenaline (NA) and dopamine (DA) in minute platelet (from 1 to 2.5 ml of platelet rich plasma) and plasma (<0.1 ml) samples(Da Prada and Picotti, 1979). These methods applied to platelet extracts submitted to acid hydrolysis have also made it possible to establish the presence of substantial amounts of conjugated CA in human but not in animal platelets (Da Prada et al., 1980).

In this paper data will be presented concerning free (unconjugated) CA concentrations in platelets from man and several laboratory animals, including albino patients and Fawn-Hooded rats with inherited storage pool deficencies (Hermansky and Pudlak, 1959; Tschopp and Weiss, 1974). The effects on rat platelet CA of treatments which enhance or lower plasma CA levels in rats will also be presented. Preliminary data suggesting for the utilization of platelet NA (and A)

Supported by CNR grant no. 80.01139.83 ("Progetto Finalizzato Medicina Preventiva").

concentrations in diagnosis of CA-secreting tumors will also be reported.

Methods

Blood was collected into EDTA or EGTA (1%, 1/10 v/v) and platelets isolated as previously described (Picotti et al., 1977; Da Prada and Picotti, 1979). The blood samples taken for plasma CA estimation from a patient with phaeochromocytoma were anticoagulated with heparin (10 NIH unit/ml), those from rats with either heparin or EGTA.

Plasma and platelet CA were measured by a sensitive radioenzymatic method (Da Prada and Zürcher, 1976; Da Prada and Zürcher, 1979), as previously described (Bühler et al., 1978; Da Prada and Picotti, 1979). Platelet proteins were measured colorimetrically (Lowry et al., 1951). Chlorisondamine .HCl was obtained from Ciba-Geigy. All other reagents were Analytical Grade.

Clinical data for two of the three albino patients with Hermansky-Pudlak syndrome have been reported elsewhere (Lorez et al., 1979), The third subject was a patient of Dr. F. Lattion (CHUV, Lausanne). The hypertensive subject with multiple phaeochromocytoma was a patient of Dr. G. Leonetti (Milan).

Albino rats of Wistar (SPF) and Sprague-Dawley (Nossan) origin, Fawn Hooded rats, Burgundian rabbits and guinea pigs of the Füllinsdorf strain were used. Chronic jugular or carotid catheterization and restraint stress, cold exposure (4° C) and chlorisondamine treatment of the rats were as previously described (Bühler et al., 1978; Picotti et al., 1981; Picotti et al., 1979).

Results

CA concentrations in normal and storage pool-deficient human and animal platelets

The contents of A, NA and DA in normal platelets from man and several laboratory animals are shown in Table 1. All three CA were detected consistently in the platelet samples examined, the highest concentrations being found in rabbit platelets. The level of NA in platelets, as in plasma (Bühler et al., 1978), always exceeded that of A and DA. The platelet CA concentrations were about one-thousandth those of 5-HT found in the same platelets (Da Prada and Picotti, 1979).

Storage pool-deficient platelets from albino patients, with biochemical and ultrastructural evidence of fewer and defective 5-HT storage organelles (Hermansky-Pudlak syndrome), exhibited markedly low contents of CA (Table 1, see also Lorez et al., 1979) confirming that CA are also stored in 5-HT organelles. The CA content in platelets of rodents with storage pool deficiencies, i.e. Fawn-Hooded rats (Table 1, see also Da Prada and Picotti, 1979) was also low.

Table 1. Concentrations of adrenaline (A), noradrenaline (NA) and dopamine (DA) in normal and storage pool-deficient (SPD) human and animal platelets.

	A	NA	DA	
Normal				
Man	0.05 ± 0.01	1.43 ± 0.34	0.08 ± 0.01	(10)
Rat (SPF)	0.28 ± 0.08	1.07 ± 0.26	0.27 ± 0.06	(6)
Guinea-pig	0.22 ± 0.04	1.56 ± 0.14	0.23 ± 0.06	(6)
Rabbit	1.46 ± 0.29	4.13 ± 0.77	1.22 ± 0.83	(8)
SPD				
Man (HPS)[x]	undetectable	0.02 ± 0.00	undetectable	(3)
Rat (FH)[xx]	0.04 ± 0.02	0.11 ± 0.03	0.01 ± 0.00	(6)

Values are means ± SEM and are expressed in pmols/mg protein. Number of subjects are shown in parenthesis. [x]HPS: Hermansky-Pudlak syndrome. [xx]FH: Fawn-Hooded.

Effects of cold exposure, restraint stress and ganglionic blockade on plasma and platelet CA concentrations in the rat

The effect of treatments that enhance or lower plasma CA levels in rats on platelet CA concentrations are shown in Tables 2 and 3. The concentrations of A and NA rose significantly in platelets of Wistar SPF rats exposed to 1 h restraint stress, a procedure which greatly increases the levels of plasma A and NA and, to a lesser extent, of DA (Table 2, see also Bühler et al., 1978). Cold exposure (5 h at 4° C), which induces a selective increase in plasma NA (Table 2, see also Picotti et al., 1981) also caused a selective, although not significant, increase of NA in platelets of SPF rats (Table 2).

Ganglionic blockade by chlorisondamine, which rapidly (within minutes, see Picotti et al., 1979) and persistently lowers plasma NA and A levels in Sprague-Dawley rats, was effective in inducing a decrease in platelet NA, which was however delayed by several hours after the plasma NA decrease in the same animals (Table 3).

Platelet and plasma CA concentrations in a patient with phaeochromocytoma

We have data (Picotti, in preparation) showing that patients with CA-secreting tumors have high levels of either A nad NA (phaeochromocytoma) or NA alone (phaeochromocytoma, neuroblastoma) in both plasma and platelets. In some instances,DA concentrations were also found to be elevated in plasma and platelets of patients with phaeochromocytoma and neuroblastoma tumors.

The CA concentrations in plasma and platelets from a patient with paroxysmally functioning multiple phaeochromocytoma taken during phases of both hypertension and normotension are shown in Table 4. The plasma concentrations of A nad NA were abnormally elevated during hypertensive crises, whereas during a normotensive phase they were less elevated (Table 4) and only slightly higher than those found in some non-tumor hypertensive patients (data not shown). By contrast, platelet A and NA (and DA) were persistently and unequivocally elevated, even during the normotensive phase (Table 4).

In the same patient, plasma NA concentrations were normal (data not shown) a few hours after surgical removal of the tumor (bilateral adrenalectomy), whereas the platelet NA concentration became normal only several days later (Fig.1). Due to the ablation of its peripheral source (i.e., adrenal medulla), A became undetectable in both plasma (data not shown) and paltelets (Fig.1), about four days after surgery.

Discussion

Blood platelets lack CA-synthesizing enzymes (Solomon et al., 1970) but take up CA from plasma (for review see Pletscher, 1978) and accumulate them mainly in the 5-HT granules, together with 5-HT and other amines (Da Prada et al., 1980; Da Prada et al., 1981). Extragranular CA may be metabolized by monoamine-oxidase (MAO; Pletscher et al., 1966), catechol-O-methyl-transferase (COMT; Stramenti-

Table 2. Effects of cold exposure and restraint stress on platelet and plasma adrenaline (A), noradrenaline (NA) and dopamine (DA) concentrations in Wistar SPF rats.

	PLATELETS (pmols/mg prot.)				PLASMA (pg/ml)			
	A	NA	DA		A	NA	DA	
Controls	0.22±0.08	1.07±0.26	0.27±0.06	(6)	83±24	429±96	42±7	(4)
Cold exposure	0.16±0.04	1.68±0.32	0.31±0.10	(4)	76±30	1234±178^{xx}	65±9	(4)
Restraint stress	2.53±0.66^{xx}	3.68±1.07^{x}	0.60±0.20	(3)	2968±447^{xx}	3228±290^{xx}	293±33^{xx}	(4)

Values are means ± SEM. Number of experiments shown in parenthesis. $^{x}P \leqslant 0.05$; $^{xx}P \leqslant 0.01$ vs controls (Dunnett t-test). Blood samples for platelets taken from abdominal aorta, for plasma from jugular catheter.

Table 3. Effect of ganglionic blockade by chlorisondamine on platelet and plasma noradrenaline (NA) concentrations in Sprague-Dawley rats.

	PLATELETS (pmols/mg prot.)		PLASMA (pg/ml)	
Time (h)	Rat 1	Rat 2	Rat 1	Rat 2
0	1.82	1.24	82	191
6	1.65	1.18	37	30
12	1.29	0.77	32	76

Chlorisondamine .HCl injections (20 mg/kg in 0.5 ml saline, at time 0 and 6) and sequential blood sampling (~ 0.8 ml with 1% EGTA 1/10 v/v, each time) for parallel platelet and plasma NA measurements through chronic carotid catheters.

Table 4. Adrenaline (A), noradrenaline (NA) and dopamine (DA) concentrations in plasma and platelets from a patient with multiple phaeochromocytoma.

	Sample	A	NA	DA
Plasma (pg/ml)	1	811	3537	68
	2	1045	5811	107
	3	120	870	63
Platelets (pmols/mg prot.)	3	1.55	7.81	0.20

Blood was collected by cubital venipuncture with the patient supine.
Samples 1 and 2 were taken during hypertensive crises, sample 3 during normotension.

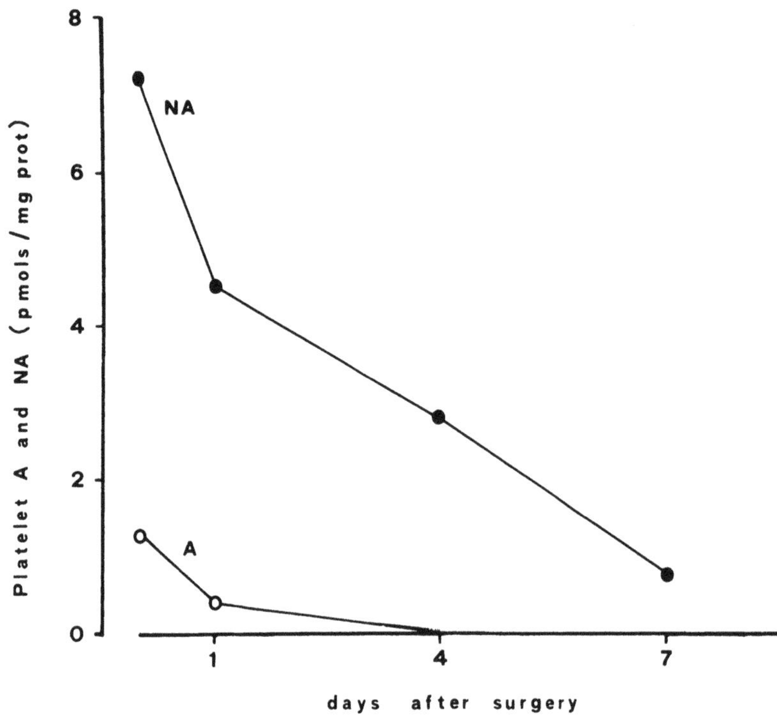

Fig. 1. Platelet adrenaline (A) and noradrenaline (NA) concentrations in a subject with multiple phaeochromocytoma, before and after bilateral adrenalectomy.

noli et al., 1978) and phenol sulphotransferase (PST; Hart et al., 1979). The concentrations of free CA in platelets, therefore, depend on several factors, e.g. the plasma concentrations of A, NA and DA and their relative affinities for platelet uptake processes, binding site(s) in storage organelles, and CA inactivating enzymes. However in platelets the active transport mechanism (the "5-HT pump") operates with low affinity for A and NA, so that these amines probably enter the platelets mainly by passive diffusion (Born and Smith, 1970; Gordon and Olverman, 1978; Da Prada and Picotti, 1979). Moreover, under physiological conditions only relatively small quantities of platelet CA undergo oxidative deamination (Pletscher et al., 1966); O-methylation or, as far as animal platelets are concerned, sulphoconjugation (Picotti and Da Prada, in preparation). Only in human platelets in which, due to the high content in PST, relatively large amounts of CA are sulphoconjugated, the CA conjugation process may be relevant to the free-CA distribution between platelets and plasma (Da Prada et al., 1980).

The importance of an efficient granular storage mechanism, which is an essential prerequisite for the formation and maintainance of a concentration gradient between platelet and plasma CA, is well established (for review see Da Prada, 1981). Platelets with inherited storage pool deficiencies, from albino patients (Hermansky-Pudlak syndrome) or Fawn-Hooded rats, which have few and atypical 5-HT organelles, with reduced capacity to store 5-HT, 5'-phosphonucleotides and mepacrine (Holmsen and Weiss, 1972; Weiss et al., 1974; Lorez et al., 1979; Tschopp and Weiss, 1974), are also extremely poor in free CA (the present study and Lorez et al., 1979), in spite of normal or not markedly low plasma CA concentrations (Da Prada and Picotti, 1979; Picotti and Da Prada,in preparation).

The present results indicate that under conditions of normally operant intraplatelet storage mechanisms plasma CA concentrations determine the levels of free CA in platelets (see also Da Prada and Picotti, 1979). NA, which in normal conditions is present in human and animal plasma in higher amounts than A and DA (Bühler et al., 1978), is also the CA which has the highest concentration in the platelets. The constantly higher levels of plasma NA than of A and DA available for uptake and/or diffusion and subsequent intracellular storage into the circulating platelet, explains why the contents of the three CA in the platelets in vivo reflect their relative concentrations in the plasma, in spite of the higher affinity in vitro of both platelets and 5-HT organelles for DA than for NA or A (Da Prada and Pletscher, 1969).

The plasma CA concentrations are maintained by the continuous release of these amines from the peripheral sympathetic nerves and adrenal medulla. It has been shown that increments in plasma NA essentially parallel increased neurosympathetic activity, whereas increases in plasma A directly reflect increased adreno-medullary secretion (for review see Callingham and Barrand, 1979). The present results show that in rats exposed to prolonged stress, long-lasting elevations of either A and NA (restraint stress; Popper et al., 1977: see also Bühler et al., 1978) or of NA alone (cold exposure; see Picotti et al., 1981) in plasma, result in increased A and/or NA in platelets. The increase in platelet CA is slower than the CA increase in plasma (Bondiolotti and Picotti, unpublished), most likely because of the low affinity of CA for the platelet transport system.

Moreover, in rats with sympatho-adrenal release of CA impaired by administration of the ganglion blocker chlorisondamine, plasma CA declined rapidly (see also Picotti et al., 1979), whereas platelet CA concentrations were lowered only several hours later. This demonstrates that, once accumulated in platelets, CA are released slowly from their stores and a new equilibrium between platelet and plasma CA levels reached. Thus, unlike the plasma CA concentrations which, due to the short half-life of CA in plasma (<60 sec; Picotti et al., 1979), immediately reflect the state of ongoing sympatho-adrenal activity, platelet CA concentrations appear to be a long-term index of the function of the peripheral sympathetic system.

An obvious clinical implication of these findings is the potential value of the assessment of platelet CA concentrations for the diagnosis of CA-secreting tumors. Assessment of plasma CA concentrations by sensitive and specific radioenzymatic assays is a most useful and reliable biochemical tool for the diagnosis of phaeochromocytoma and neuroblastoma tumors (Bravo et al., 1979). However, for tumor patients with paroxysmal hypertension, diagnostic uncertainty may arise when the blood sample for the plasma CA assay is not taken coincidentally with hypertensive crises. In fact, transient marked increases in plasma levels of CA may be followed by return to equivocally elevated CA values, as illustrated in the present study of a patient with phaeochromocytoma who secreted CA in paroxysmal bursts. In this patient the platelet CA, unlike the plasma CA, concentrations were persistently elevated even during a normotensive phase. Thus, it can be suggested that platelet CA concentrations are a reliable and useful index for detection of previous paroxysmal (and/or persistent) CA discharges into the blood streams of patients with phaeochromocytoma and neuroblastoma tumors.This is strengthened by the fact that in some of these patients the high plasma CA concentrations became normal a few hours after surgical removal of the tumor, whereas platelet CA are normal only after several days (the present study and Picotti, in preparation).

REFERENCES

Born, G.V.R., and Smith J.B., 1970, Uptake, metabolism and release of ^{3}H-adrenaline by human platelets, Br. J. Pharmac. 39: 765-778.

Bravo, E.L., Tarazi, R.C., Gifford, R.W., and Stewart, B.H., 1979, Circulating and urinary catecholamines in phaeochromocytoma. Diagnostic and pathophysiological implication, N. Engl. J. Med. 301: 682-686.

Bühler, U.H., Da Prada, M., Haefely, W., and Picotti, G.B., 1978, Plasma adrenaline, noradrenaline and dopamine in man and different animal species. J. Physiol. 276: 311-320.

Callingham, B.A., and Barrand, M.A., 1979, The catecholamines. Adrenaline, noradrenaline; dopamine, in: Hormones in blood (C.H. Gray and V.H.T. James, eds.), vol. 2, pp. 143-207, Academic Press, London.

Da Prada, M., and Pletscher, A., 1969, Differential uptake of biogenic amines by isolated 5-hydroxytryptamine organelles of blood platelets, Life Sci. 8: 65-72.

Da Prada, M., and Zürcher, G., 1976, Simultaneous radioenzymatic determination of plasma and tissue adrenaline, noradrenaline and dopamine within the fentomole range, Life Sci. 19: 1161-1174.

Da Prada, M., and Zürcher, G., 1979, Simultaneous radioenzymatic assay of adrenaline, noradrenaline and dopamine: recent improvements, Experientia 34: 928.
Da Prada, M., and Picotti, G.B., 1979, Content and subcellular localization of catecholamines and 5-hydroxytryptamine in human and animal blood platelets: monoamine distribution between platelets and plasma, Br. J. Pharmac. 65: 653-662.
Da Prada, M., Picotti, G.B., Kettler, L., and Launay, J.M., 1980, Serotonin, histamine, catecholamines, normetanephrine and octopamine in blood platelets, in: Platelets: cellular response mechanisms and their biological significance (A. Rotman, F.A. Meyer, C. Gitler and A. Silberberg, eds.), pp. 277-288, J. Wiley & Sons, London.
Da Prada, M., Richards, J.G., and Kettler, R., 1981, Amine storage organelles in platelets, in: Platelets in biology and pathology (J.C. Gordon, ed.), in press, Elsevier, Amsterdam.
Gordon, J.L., and Olverman, H.J., 1978, 5-Hydroxytryptamine and dopamine transport by rat and human blood platelets, Br. J. Pharmac. 62: 219-226.
Hart, R.F., Renskers, K.J., Nelson, E.B., and Roth, J.A., 1979, Localization and characterization of phenol sulfotransferase in human platelets, Life Sci. 24: 125-130.
Hermansky, F., and Pudlak, P., 1959, Albinism associated with hemorrhagic diathesis and unusual pigmented reticular cells in the bone marrow: report of two cases with histochemical studies, Blood 14: 162-169.
Holmsen, H., and Weiss, H.J., 1972, Further evidence for a deficient storage pool of adenine nucleotides in platelets from some patients with thrombocytopathia: storage pool disease, Blood 39: 197-209.
Lorez, H.P., Richards, J.G., Da Prada, M., Picotti, G.B., Pareti, F.I., Capitanio, A., and Mannucci, P.M., 1979, Storage pool disease: comparative fluorescence microscopical, cytochemical and biochemical studies on amine-storing organelles of human blood platelets, Br. J. Haematol. 43: 297-305.
Lowry, O.H., Rosebrough, N.J., Farr, A.L., and Randall, R.J., 1951, Protein measurement with folin phenol reagent, J. Biol. Chem. 193: 265-275.
Markwardt, F., 1976, Studies on the release of biogenic amines from blood platelets, in: Biochemistry of blood platelets (E. Kowalski and S. Niewiarowski, eds.), pp. 105-116, Academic press, London/New York.
Picotti, G.B., Carruba, M.O., Zambotti, F., and Mantegazza, P., 1977, Effects of mazindol and d-fenfluramine on 5-hydroxytryptamine uptake, storage and metabolism in blood platelets, Europ. J. Pharmacol. 42: 217-224.
Picotti, G.B., Carruba, M.O., Galva, M.D., Ravazzani, C., Bondiolotti, G.P., and Da Prada, M., 1979, Drug-induced changes of plasma catecholamine concentrations, in: Radioimmunoassay of drugs and hormones in cardiovascular medicine (A. Alber-

tini, M. Da Prada and B.A. Peskar, eds.), pp. 133-148, Elsevier, Amsterdam.

Picotti, G.B., Carruba, M.O., Ravazzani, C., Cesura, A.M., Galva, M.D., and Da Prada, M., 1981, Plasma catecholamines in rats exposed to cold: effects of ganglion and adrenoceptor blockade, European J. Pharmacol. 69: 321-329.

Pletscher, A., Bartholini, G., and Da Prada, M., 1966, Metabolism of monoamines by blood platelets and relation to 5-HT liberation, in: Mechanism of release of biogenic amines (V.S. Von Euler, S. Rosell and B. Uvnäs, eds.), pp. 165-175, Pergamon Press, Oxford.

Pletscher, A., 1978, Platelets as models for monoaminergic neurons, in: Essays in neurochemistry and neuropharmacology (M.B.H. Youdin, ed.), vol. 3, pp. 49-101, J. Wiley and Sons Ltd., London.

Popper, C.W., Chiueh, C.C., and Kopin, I.J., 1977, Plasma catecholamine concentrations in unanesthetized rats during sleep, wakefulness, immobilization and after decapitation, J. Pharmacol. Exp. Ther. 202: 144-148.

Solomon, H.M., Spirt, N.M., and Abrams, W.B., 1970, The accumulation and metabolism of dopamine by the human platelet, Clin. Pharmac. Therap. 11: 838-845.

Stramentinoli, G., Gualano, M., Algeri, S., De Gaetano, G., and Rossi, E.C., 1978, Catechol-O-methyl transferase (COMT) in human and rat platelets, Thrombos.Haemostas. 39: 238-239.

Tschopp, T.B., and Weiss, H.J., 1974, Decreased ATP, ADP and serotonin in young platelets of Fawn-Hooded rats with storage pool disease, Thrombos. Diathes. Haemorrh. 32: 670-677.

Weil-Malherbe, H., and Bone, A.D., 1957, The fluorimetric estimation of adrenaline and noradrenaline in plasma, Biochem. J. 67: 65-72.

Weiss, H.G., Tschopp, T.B., Rogers, J., and Brand, H., 1974, Studies of platelet 5-hydroxytryptamine (serotonin) in storage pool disease and albinism, J. Clin. Invest. 54:421-432.

PROSTAGLANDINS AND HYPERTENSION

P.C. Weber, B. Scherer, and W. Siess

Medizinische Klinik Innenstadt
Ziemssenstrasse 1
8 München 2, F.R.G.

Introduction

The level of arterial blood pressure is set by a complex interrelationship of several mechanisms which influence both blood flow in and resistance of the vascular system. An imbalance which favours those mechanisms that elevate vascular resistance or extracellular volume will result in hypertension. Such alterations may include increased activity of the adrenergic nervous system, of the renin angiotensin system, or excessive secretion of mineralocorticoids. Of equal importance may be an underactivity of blood pressure lowering factors, such as prostaglandins and the kallikrenin-kinin-system. A deficiency of the vasodepressor systems may lead to hypertension even without an increase in the activity of the blood pressure elevating systems. Beside a genetic predisposition, exogenous risk factors are assumed to play a major role in the natural history of essential hypertension and arterial vascular disease. The contribution of prostaglandins to the etiology of these cardiovascular disorders may be based on an inherent abnormality of the prostaglandin system as well as on the effects of major risk factors such as dietary intake of sodium and fat on prostaglandin formation.

Diet, precursor fatty acids and prostaglandin biosynthesis

A first step in the synthesis of prostaglandins and thromboxanes is the release of the polyunsaturated precursor fatty acids arachidonic acid (C20:4ω6), dihomo-γ-linolenic acid (C20:3ω6) and eicosapentaenoic acid (C20:5ω3) from storage in bound form, mainly membrane phospholipids. The incorporation of different essential fatty acids into storage sites depends on dietary intake, on the balance between chain elongation and desaturation and on their respective specificity for incorporation into different lipids. These metabolic balances may differ from one tissue to another. Under our nutritional conditions, arachidonic acid (C20:4ω6) is generally the most abundant within the ω6-family. The total amount in the tissues of the fatty acids from the ω6- and ω3-families, respectively, is dependent on the dietary supply, since the human organism is unable to produce fatty acids having ω6- and ω3 double bonds (for review see 20,28, 46).

Beside their role as precursors for the biologically active prostaglandins, prostacyclin and thromboxanes and the leukotrienes, the polyunsaturated fatty acids have important functions maintaining cell membrane structure and fluidity which in turn influence e.g. membrane bound receptors and hormone receptor-adenylate cyclase coupling.

Following the appropriate stimulus the release of the prostaglandin precursors fatty acids is brought about by a group of enzymes, acylhydrolases, such as phospholipase A_2 and triglyceride-lipase. After the precursor fatty acid is released from tissue lipids, a concentrated series of reactions transforms it into prostaglandins, prostacyclin or thromboxanes. After cyclisation and incorporation of molecular oxygen into the fatty acid the prostaglandin endoperoxides are formed as common intermediates in the prostaglandin cascade. These unstable compounds are then metabolised into the classical prostaglandins (PG) PGE, PGD and PGF_{α}, as well as thromboxane A (TXA) and prostacyclin (PGI) (28).

Prostaglandins, prostacyclin and thromboxane from arachidonic acid-derived PG endoperoxides retain two double bonds in their alkyl side chains, denoted by subscript 2, as e.g. PGE_2, PGI_2 and TXA_2, as shown in Figure 1. Prostaglandins and thromboxanes derived from dihomo-γ-linolenic and eicosapentaenoic acids have one and three double bonds, respectively, and are designed for example PGE_1 and PGE_3, TXA_1 and TXA_3. In contrast to PGG_2/PGH_2- or PGG_3/PGH_3 - the dihomo-γ-linolenic acid derived PG endoperoxides PGG_1 and PGH_1 are not substrates for prostacyclin synthesis. Usually, the number of double bonds in the side chains does not qualitatively alter the characteristic biological properties of prostaglandins and prostacyclin; e.g. PGE_1, PGE_2 and PGE_3, or PGI_2 and PGI_3 have similar effects on vascular smooth muscle cells. However,whereas TXA_2 is a potent vasoconstrictor and strong aggregator of platelets, TXA_1 and TXA_3 are reported to be unable to aggregate plates (Table 1).

Effects of prostaglandins within the cardiovascular-renal system

Each tissue may possess different enzymes using the PG endoperoxides as substrate and, therefore, produce different amounts and types of prostaglandins. In the blood vessels, PGI_2 is the predominant product of prostaglandin synthetase (20). Both, vascular endothelial and smooth muscle cells have the capacity to produce this vasodilatory and platelet aggregation inhibiting compound. Vascular smooth muscle cells produce, to a lesser degree, also PGE_2

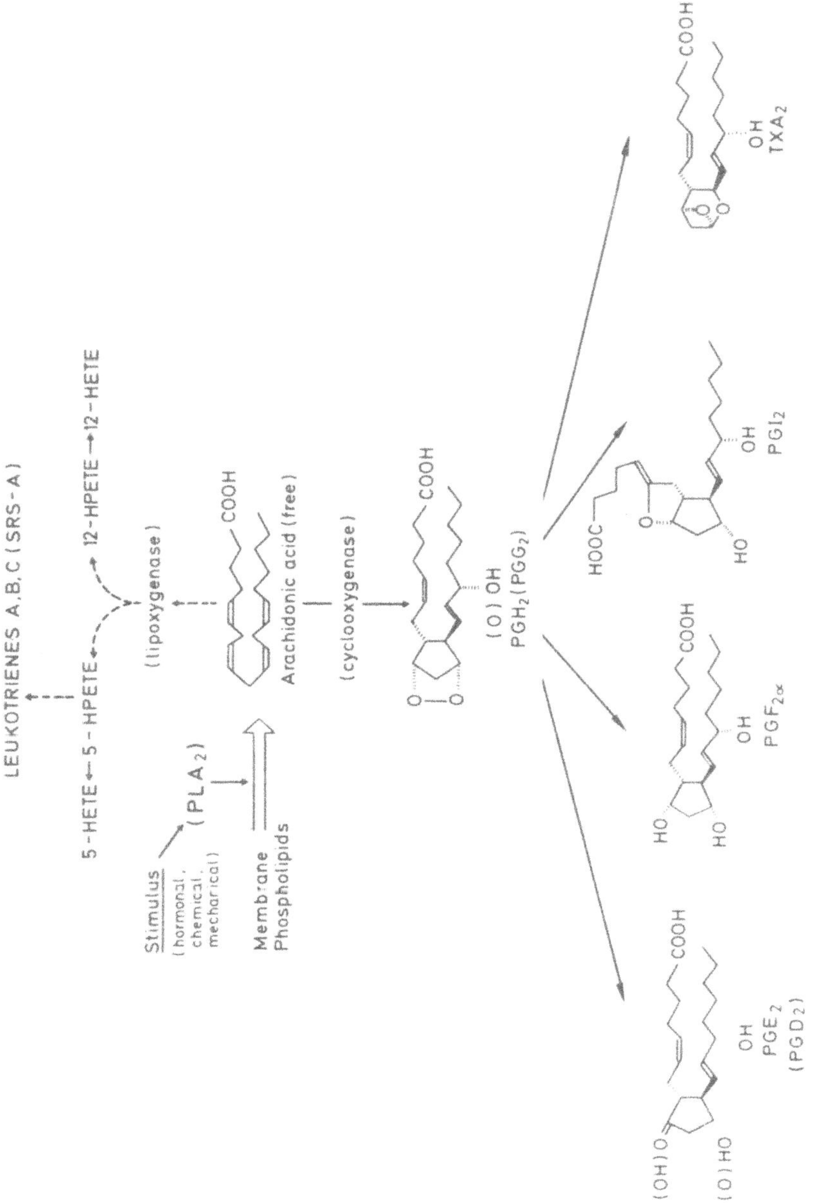

Fig. 1. The prostaglandin cascade

and $PGF_2\alpha$ (for review see 21). In the blood platelets, PGG_2 is metabolised mainly to the vasoconstrictive and platelet aggregating TXA_2 (12) and, to a lesser extent, to PGD_2, an inhibitor of platelet aggregation (25). The kidney has a high capacity to form prostaglandins. Predominant production of PGI_2 in the cortical and vascular compartment and high levels of PGE_2 and $PGF_{2\alpha}$ in the medulla support the assumption of several roles of the renal PG's for vascular and tubular functions of the kidney: renal blood flow and glomerular filtration rate, renin release and the tubular handling of water and electrolytes (for reviews see 9, 45).

The activity of phospholipase A_2 and the rate of prostaglandin formation is under the control of a veriety of factors. Potent vasoactive hormones, such as angiotensin, norepinephrine and bradykinin, but also thrombin or collagen, as well as mechanical stimuli such as perfusion pressure increase prostaglandin synthesis by activation of PLA_2 which is supposed to be the rate limiting step of PG synthesis (3, 18, 49).

The possible significance of prostaglandins as antihypertensive principle received support mainly from the demonstration of synthesis of prostaglandins in the blood vessels and in the kidney. In addition to their direct effects on smooth muscle cells they interact with a series of other systemic hormonal and neurogenic factors contributing to the control of vascular resistance and blood volume (for review see 40). Thus, locally produced PGE_2 and PGI_2 dilate arterial blood vessels and reduce the vasoconstrictor action of angiotensin II and norepinephrine. In addition, PGE_2 mediates the vasodilation following bradykinin (21) and it reduces norepinephrine release upon nerve stimulation (13). In contrast, $PGF_{2\alpha}$ seems to be vasoconstrictive (predominantly on the venous side of the circulation) as it enhances the vasoconstrictor response following nerve stimulation (13) and mediates the venoconstriction of bradikinin (21). Prostacyclin reduces vascular resistance most probably by a direct action, since - in contrast to PGE_2 - it does not inhibit norepinephrine release upon nerve stimulation. Platelet TXA_2 formed upon aggregation during endothelial cell repair is vasoconstrictive and could contribute to vascular resistance. Thus, the modulator action of prostaglandins on the effects of vasoactive hormones may be one basis for the antihypertensive effect, i.e. inhibition of pressor hormones and augmentation of the action of depressor hormones.

Renal cortical formation of prostaglandins contributes to the regulation of renal blood flow, glomerular filtration rate and renin release. By these actions prostaglandins are involved in the major renal mechanisms controlling extracellular volume and blood pressure. Abundant evidence suggests that, in the intact kidney, arachidonic acid, and PGI_2 stimulate renin release (44). The mechanisms seem to involve a direct effect on the juxtaglomerular apparatus, as well as an interaction of locally produced prostaglandins with the baroreceptor, the β-adrenergic and the macula densa receptor for renin release. Also, the tubulo-glomerular feedback system, contributing to the control of electrolyte excretion, seems to be dependent on an intact prostaglandin system. Inhibition of PG synthesis attenuates the feedback response observed after changes of loop of Henle flow rates by 50%. This diminution of feedback response can be restored by PGI_2 infusion (33). There is good evidence that the state of electrolyte balance influences renal prostaglandin formation and that renal prostaglandin formation effects renal electrolyte excretion. PGE_2, PGD_2, PGI_2 and intraarterial arachidonic acid increase the urinary excretion of sodium, most probably as a result of changes in renal hemodynamics (for reviews see 9, 45). On the other hand, and despite some evidence to the contrary, the bulk of the published data suggests that chronic salt depletion increases PGE_2 production and release into the urine, whereas chronic high sodium intake suppresses PGE_2 production (for reviews see 9, 45 and 8, 41). This decrease of the vasodilatory PGE_2 at high NaCl intake could contribute to the decrease of renin secretion and to the increase of vascular responsiveness to vasoconstrictors at high NaCl intake. The findings suggest that one of the known risk factors for high blood pressure - high NaCl intake - may operate through a mechanism involving a reduction in the formation of vasodilatory prostaglandins.

Manipulation of prostaglandin formation and blood pressure

If a deficiency of vasodilatory prostaglandins increases blood pressure or contributes to the development of hypertension, inhibition of prostaglandin production or dietary deprivation of precursor fatty acids should result in elevated blood pressure. On the other hand, manipulation of the precursor fatty acid pool or pharmacological maneuvers leading to an increased synthesis of vasodilatory prostaglandins should reduce blood pressure.

Previous animal studies had demonstrated that indomethacin pretreatment enhanced the pressor response to angiotensin and norepinephrine by inhibition of the vascular synthesis of counteracting, vasodilatory prostaglandins (for review see 40). Recently it has been reported that chronic inhibition of PG synthesis by more than 80% resulted in a sustained elevation of blood pressure in the rabbit (6). Studies in man showed an increase of blood pressure and an increased pressor response to angiotensin and norepinephrine after acute blockade of prostaglandin production by indomethacin (19, 48). The blood pressure changes in the latter experiments were associated with a reduced renin secretion, significantly lowered plasma norepinephrine levels and a reduced heart rate (19). Chronic deprivation of prostaglandin precursors in rats and rabbits by feeding an essential fatty acid-deficient diet elevated blood pressure, increased the pressor response to angiotensin and norepinephrine and reduced the ability of the kidney to excrete sodium after loading (24, 27, 37).

In accordance with the interpretation that vascular and renal formation of vasodilatory prostaglandins may play a significant role in modulating the vascular response to pressor hormones and thus exert an antihypertensive function are studies in normotensive and spontaneously hypertensive rats (34) and in essential hypertensive patients (7) in which a diet supplemented with linoleic acid, the ultimate precursor fatty acid of the prostaglandins of the 1- and 2-series reduced blood pressure. In the experiments in the rat, the linoleic acid-supplemented diet which lowered blood pressure not only induced an increased prostaglandin production, but shifted the pathway of prostaglandin synthesis away from the vasoconstrictor $PGF_{2\alpha}$ to the vasodilatory PGE_2 (34). This observation suggests that the ratio in the formation of different acting prostaglandins in the cardiovascular system may be as critical for blood pressure control as the absolute amounts of vasodilatory prostaglandins produced. Studies from this and other laboratories support indeed the idea that an alteration in the pathway of prostaglandin formation from PGE_2 to $PGF_{2\alpha}$, or from prostacyclin to thromboxane A_2 may lead to an increase of blood pressure and may be one mechanism by which genetic or exogenous risk factors contribute to the hypertensive vascular disease.

In essential hypertensive patients we found an increased ratio of $PGF_{2\alpha}$: PGE_2 under basal conditions as well as after stimulation with furosemide (43). High sodium-chloride intake - one of the risk factors for essential hypertension - reduced PGE_2 production in the rabbit and, thereby, shifted the ratio of $PGF_{2\alpha}$: PGE_2 in urine from 1 to about 4 (41). In addition, we found in newborns during the first week of life a positive correlation between blood pressure and $PGF_{2\alpha}$ excretion (31), and an association between an increased $PGF_{2\alpha}$: PGE_2 ratio in urine at birth and higher blood pressure during the first year of life (32).

In the spontaneously hypertensive rat, an increased renal $PGF_{2\alpha}$ formation was observed even before overt hypertension developed (2). Very recently, an increased renal production of the vasoconstrictor TXA_2 was reported in the spontaneously hypertensive rat (35). Other studies have shown that development of hypertension in rats receiving saline drinking without and in combination with indomethacin treatment was paralleled by a relative excess in the vascular production of PGF_{α} over PGE associated with an increased ratio of vascular cGMP: cAMP, possibly contributing to the sensitation of the vessel to pressor hormones (23). Preliminary results in feline cerebral cortex showed a stimulatory effect of norepinephrine on $PGF_{2\alpha}$ production which was paralleled by a reduction in the synthesis of 6-keto-$PGF_{1\alpha}$, the stable hydrolysis product of PGI_2 (4).

Evidence for impaired prostaglandin formation in essential hypertension

The hemodynamic situation in the most frequent form of uncomplicated essential hypertension is characterized by elevated blood pressure, unchanged cardiac output, and marked increase in systemic and renal vascular resistance. At the same time, catecholamine levels are reported to be in the normal range (17) and mineralocorticoids are not elevated, but the pressor response to angiotensin and norepinephrine is increased (26). In addition, the increase of vascular resistance in essential hypertension has been reported to be associated with a reduction of renin secretion (5, 29).

As mentioned above, vasodilatatory prostaglandins are critically involved in the mechanisms regulating renin release, in controlling vascular resistance, renal blood flow, and modulating the pressor response to vasoactive hormones. Therefore, a defect in the formation of vasodilatory prostaglandins could contribute to the following abnormalities in established essential hypertension: Increase of vascular resistance, associated with a reduction of renin secretion and increased responsiveness to norepinenephrine and angiotensin at normal endogenous levels of these pressor hormones.

We, as others, have indeed demonstrated a reduction of urinary PGE_2 excretion in patients with essential hypertension (1, 38, 47). In addition, we showed in patients with essential hypertension a a reduced response of plasma renin activity initially (10 - 15 min) after furosemide which was paralleled by a blunted response of urinary PGE_2 (but not of $PGF_{2\alpha}$) and of kallikrenin excretion (43). Previous studies had indicated that furosemide very rapidly and transiently stimulates renal PG formation and thereby increases renin release and renal blood flow (30, 42). The results in essential hypertensive patients point, therefore, to a reduced capacity of the kidney in essential hypertension to produce vasodilatory PGE_2 (and possibly PGI_2) upon challenge with furosemide. Prostaglandins seem physiologically to be produced upon demand (e.g. by increased levels of norepinephrine or angiotensin during stressful conditions). Therefore, the results with furosemide, showing a reduced capacity for PG formation fit into the concept that the increased pressor responsiveness of essential hypertensive patients to pressor agonists could partly be the result of a reduced capacity of the vasculature to produce vasodilatory prostaglandins.

The afore-mentioned evidence of an impairment of prostaglandin formation in essential hypertension may include (1) a reduced pool of prostaglandin precursor fatty acids, (2) a reduced activity of acylhydrolases making the precursor fatty acid available for prostaglandin production, (3) a reduced formation of vasodilatory prostaglandins such as PGE_2 or PGI_2, or (4) a relative or absolute predominance of $PGF_{2\alpha}$ or TXA_2.

Prostaglandins, hypertension and arteriosclerosis

There exists a complex interrelationship between diet, blood pressure and arterial disease. Hypertension increases the susceptibility of the blood vessels to arteriosclerosis. Considerable evidence suggests that endothelial dysfunction and alterations in the platelet-vessel wall interaction could play an initiating role in arteriosclerotic vascular disease (for review see 14).

Recent insight into the mechanisms by which thromboxane and prostacyclin contribute to the platelet-vessel wall interaction, the vascular integrity and to vascular tone suggests an involvement of these counteracting prostaglandin endoperoxide-derived compounds in the natural history of hypertension involving arteriosclerosis. In addition to promoting platelet aggregation, TXA_2 constricts blood vessels at the site of its release from the aggregating platelets.

It has been suggested that deficiency of prostacyclin formation is characteristic of arteriosclerosis. On the other side, cholesterol seems to increase platelet aggregability by stimulating platelet TXA_2 production (for references see 36). Consequently, an imbalance in the formation of the vasoconstrictor TXA_2 and the vasodilator PGI_2 could both, facilitate thrombus formation and increase vascular tone and hence blood pressure. Therefore, one strategy for the prevention and control of arteriosclerotic and hypertensive vascular disease by non-pharmacological intervention may be based on the potential benefit to be derived from modifying thromboxane-prostacyclin interactions by nutritional means involving a special spectrum of prostaglandin precursor fatty acids (10, 16, 22, 36).

Ones of these approaches originated from epidemiological studies in Eskimos. Greenland Eskimos, beside having a low salt intake and practically no hypertension have, in addition a bleeding tendency and a low incidence of myocardial infarction which was attributed to the platelet inhibitory effect of high levels of eicosapentaenoic acid in their maritime diet and consequently in their tissue lipids (10). In subsequent studies (36) we demonstrated in white men that a mackerel diet containing high levels of eicosapentaenoic acid (the precursor fatty acid for prostaglandins of the $\omega 3$-series) reduces platelet aggregability and inhibits the formation of proaggregatory and vasoconstrictive TXA_2. Previous in vitro studies had indicated that eicosapentaenoic acid leaves the vascular formation of a potent antiaggregatory and vasodilatory agent, presumably PGI_3, unaffected (10, 22). In addition to the reduction of platelet aggregation and thromboxane formation we demonstrated a blunted pressor response to pressor hormones during the mackerel diet (19). Interestingly, these effects were associated with high plasma renin levels which could be an expression of unopposed, even enhanced, vascular formation of vasodilatory prostaglandins such as PGI_2 and PGI_3.

These other studies point to a decisive role played by unsaturated fatty acid precursors to prostacyclin and thromboxane as determinants of antagonistic acting cyclooxygenase products. They represent a basis for therapeutic or preventive approaches in hypertensive vascular disease including prostaglandin precursors such as eicosapentaenoic acid which inhibits thromboxane formation and favours the production of vasodilatory and platelet inhibiting prostaglandins.

Acknowledgment: Mrs. S. Havenstein helped in preparing the manuscript.

Table 1. Prostaglandin precursor fatty acids, major active prostaglandins and primary actions

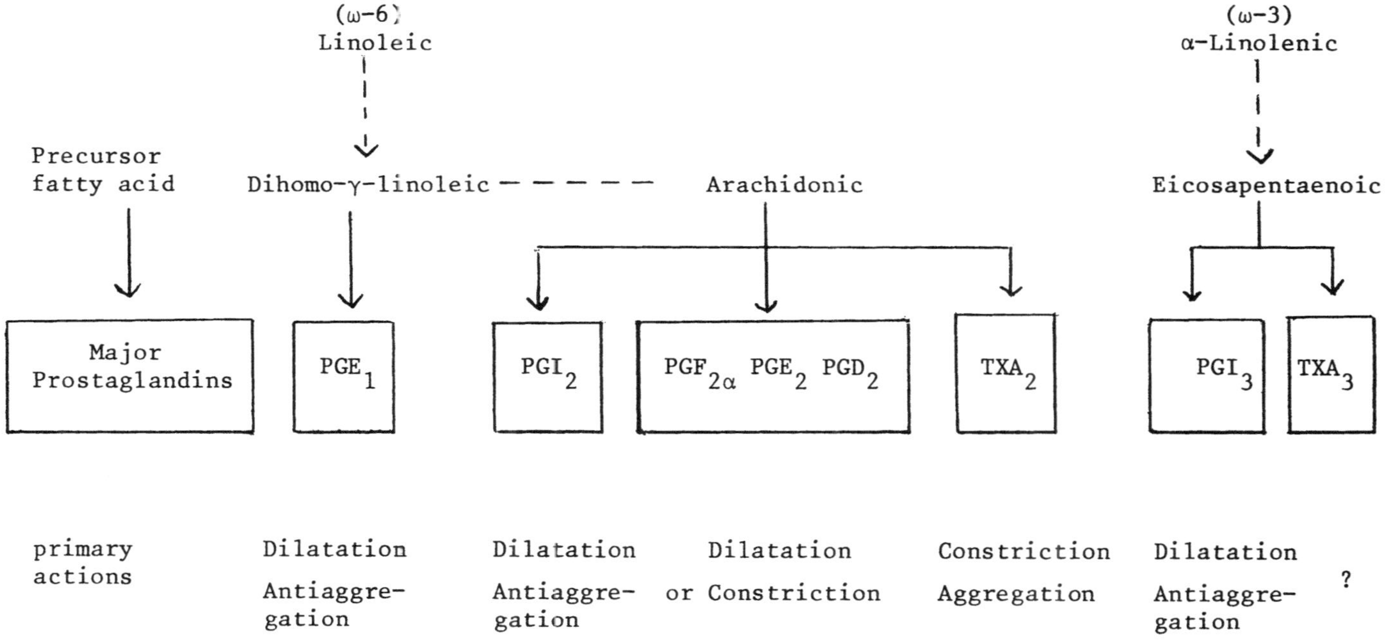

	(ω-6) Linoleic				(ω-3) α-Linolenic	
Precursor fatty acid	Dihomo-γ-linoleic	Arachidonic	Arachidonic	Arachidonic	Eicosapentaenoic	Eicosapentaenoic
Major Prostaglandins	PGE_1	PGI_2	$PGF_{2\alpha}$ PGE_2 PGD_2	TXA_2	PGI_3	TXA_3
primary actions	Dilatation Antiaggregation	Dilatation Antiaggregation	Dilatation or Constriction	Constriction Aggregation	Dilatation Antiaggregation	?

REFERENCES

1. K. Abe, M. Yasujima, N. Irokawa, M. Seino, S. Chiba, Y. Sakurai, M. Sato, Y. Imai, K. Saito, T. Ito, T. Haruyama, Y. Otsuka and K. Yoshinaga, 1978, The role of intrarenal vasoactive substances in the pathogenesis of essential hypertension. Clin. Sci. Mol. Med. 55:363s-366s.
2. I. Ahnfelt-Ronne and E. Arrigoni-Martelli, 1978, Increased $PGF_{2\alpha}$ synthesis in renal papilla of spontaneously hypertensive rats. Biochem. Pharmacol. 27:2363-2367.
3. T.K. Bills, J.B. Smith and M.J. Silver, 1976, Metabolism of ^{14}C arachidonic acid by human platelets. Biochem. Biophys. Acta 424:303-314.
4. D.L. Birkle, C.K. Ellis and E.F. Ellis, 1980, Norepinephrine inhibits 6-keto-$PGF_{1\alpha}$ synthesis and stimulates $PGF_{2\alpha}$ synthesis in feline cerebral cortex homogenates. Fed. Proc. 39:1103.
5. D.B. Case, W.J. Casarella, J.H. Laragh, D.L. Flower and P.J. Canon, 1978, Renal cortical blood flow and angiography in low- and normal-renin essential hypertension. Kidney Int. 13:236.
6. J. Colina-Chourio, J.C. McGiff and A. Nasjletti, 1979, Effect of indomethacin on blood pressure in the normotensive unanaesthetized rabbit: Possible relation to prostaglandin synthesis inhibition. Clin. Sci. 57:359-365.
7. H.U. Comberg, S. Heyden, C.G. Hames, A.J. Vergroesen and A.I. Fleischman, 1978, Hypotensive effect of dietary prostaglandin precursor in hypertensive man. Prostaglandins 15:193-197.
8. D. Davila, T. Davila, E. Oliw and E. Ånggard, 1977, The influence of dietary sodium on urinary prostaglandin excretion. Acta Physiol. Scand. 103:100-106.
9. M.J. Dunn and V.L. Hood, 1977, Prostaglandins and the kidney. Am. J. Physiol. 233:F-169-F-184.
10. J. Dyerberg, H.O. Bang, E. Stoffersen, S. Moncada and J.R. Vane, 1978, Eicosapentaenoic acid and prevention of thrombosis and atherosclerosis? The Lancet 2:117-119
11. M. Esler, S. Julius, A. Zweifler, O. Randall, E. Harburg, H. Gardiner and V. DeQuattro, 1977, Mild high-renin essential hypertension: Neurogenic human hypertension? N. Engl. J. Med. 296:405-411.
12. M. Hamberg, J. Svensson and B. Samuelsson, 1975, Thromboxanes: a new group of biologically active compounds derived from prostaglandin endoperoxides. Proc. Natl. Acad. Sci. USA 72:2994-2998.
13. P. Hedquist, 1976, Prostaglandin action on transmitter release at adrenergic neuroeffector junctions. In: Advances in prostaglandin and thromboxane research, Vol. 1, B. Samuelsson, R. Paoletti edit., Raven Press, New York, pp. 357-363.
14. W. Hollander, 1976, Role of hypertension in atherosclerosis and cardiovascular disease. Am. J. Cardiol. 38:786-800.

15. S. Julius and M. Esler, 1976, Increased central blood volume: a possible pathophysiological factor in mild low-renin essential hypertension. Clin. Sci. Mol. Med. 51:207s-210s.
16. P.B.A. Kernoff, A.L. Willis, K.J. Stone, J.A. Davies and G.P. McNicol, 1977, Antithrombotic potential of dihomo-gamma-linolenic acid in man. Br. Med. J. 2:1441-1444.
17. C.R. Lake, M.G. Ziegler, M.D. Coleman and I.J. Copin, 1977, Age-adjusted plasma norepinephrine levels are similar in normotensive and hypertensive subjects. N. Engl. J. Med. 296:208-209.
18. L. Levine and M.A. Moskowitz, 1979, α- and β-adrenergic stimulation of arachidonic acid metabolism in cells in culture. Proc. Natl. Acad. Sci. USA 76:6632-6636.
19. R. Lorenz, U. Spengler, W. Siess, P.C. Weber, 1980, Einfluss veränderter Prostaglandin-Bildung auf die sympathoadrenerge Aktivität und die Blutdruckregulation. Verhdl. Deutsch. Ges. für Inner Medizin, Wiesbaden 1980, in press.
20. S. Moncada and J.R. Vane, 1979, The role of prostacyclin in vascular tissue. Fed.Proceedings 38:66-71.
21. A. Nasjletti and K.U. Malik, 1979, Relationships between the Kallikrenin-kinin and prostaglandin systems. Life Sci. 25: 99-110.
22. Ph. Needleman, M.O. Whitaker, A. Wyche, K. Watters, H. Sprecher and A. Raz, 1980, Manipulation of platelet aggregation by prostaglandins and their fatty acid precursors: Pharmacological basis for a therapeutic approach. Prostaglandins 19: 165-181.
23. A.A. Nekrasova, R.N. Sokolova, Yu. Levitskaya, N.V. Speranskaya, V.P. Kulagina and N.P. Leghonkays, 1980, Prostaglandins of blood vessels and vessel reactivity in rats receiving sodium chloride and indomethacin. In: Advances in prostaglandin and thromboxane research, Vol. 7, B. Samuelsson, R. Paoletti edit., Raven Press. New York, pp. 1139-1143.
24. P.M.S. O'Brien and F.B. Pipkin, 1979, The effects of deprivation of prostaglandin precursors on vascular sensitivity to angiotensin II and on the kidney in the pregnant rabbit. Br. J. Pharmac. 65:29-34.
25. O. Olez, R. Olez, H.R. Knapp, B.J. Sweetman and J.A. Oates, 1977, Biosynthesis of prostaglandin D_2: formation by human platelets. Prostaglandins 13:225-234.
26. Th. Philipp, A. Distler and U. Cordes, 1978, Sympathetic nervous system and blood-pressure control in essential hypertension. The Lancet 2:959-963.
27. J. Rosenthal, P.G. Simone and A. Silbergleit, 1974, Effects of prostaglandin deficiency on natriuresis, diuresis, and blood pressure. Prostaglandins 5:435-440.
28. B. Samuelsson, M. Goldyne, M. Granström, M. Hamberg, S. Hammarström and C. Malmsten, 1978, Prostaglandins and thromboxanes. Ann. Rev. Biochem. 47:997-1029.

29. M.A.D.H. Schalekamp, M.P.A. Schalekamp-Kuyken and W.H. Birkenhäger, 1970, Abnormal renal haemodynamics and renin suppression in hypertensive patients. Clin. Sci. 38:101-110.
30. B. Scherer and P.C. Weber, 1978, Time dependent changes in prostaglandin excretion in response to furosemide in man. Clin. Sci. 56:77-81.
31. B. Scherer and P.C. Weber, 1980, Urinary prostaglandins in the newborn: Relationship to urinary osmolality, urinary potassium, and blood pressure. In: Advances in prostaglandin and thromboxane research, Vol. 7, B. Samuelsson, P.W. Ramwell and R. Paoletti, edit., Raven Press, New York, pp.1033-1038.
32. B. Scherer and P.C. Weber, 1980, Renal factors in juvenile hypertension. Klin. Wschr. 58:1099-1104.
33. J. Schnermann and P.C. Weber, 1980, A role of renal cortical prostaglandins in the control of glomerular filtration rate in rat kidneys. In: Advances in prostaglandin and thromboxane research, Vol. 7, B. Samuelsson, P.W. Ramwell and R. Paoletti edit., Raven Press, New York, pp. 1047-1052.
34. N.W. Schoene, V.B. Reeves and A. Ferretti, 1980, Effects of dietary linoleic acid on the biosynthesis of PGE_2 and $PGF_{2\alpha}$ in kidney medullae in spontaneously hypertensive rats. In: Advances in prostaglandin and thromboxane research, Vol.8, B. Samuelsson, P.W. Ramwell and R. Paoletti edit., Raven Press, New York, pp. 1791-1792.
35. Y. Shibouta, Y. Inada, Z. Terashita, K. Nishikawa, S. Kikuchi and K. Shimamoto, 1979, Angiotensin-II-stimulated release of thromboxane A_2 and prostacyclin (PGI_2) in isolated, perfused kidneys of spontaneously hypertensive rats. Biochem. Pharmacol. 28:3601-3609.
36. W. Seiss, P. Roth, B. Scherer, I. Kurzmann, B. Böhlig and P.C. Weber, 1980, Platelet-membrane fatty acids, platelet aggregation, and thromboxane formation during a mackerel diet. The Lancet 1:441-444.
37. L. Somova, P. Hoffmann and W. Förster, 1980, The reactivity of isolated blood vessels of salt-loaded rats fed with low or high linoleic acid diets. Europ. J. Pharmacol. 64:79-83.
38. S.Y. Tan, P. Sweet and P.J. Mulrow, 1978, Impaired renal production of prostaglandin E_2: A newly identificated lesion in human essential hypertension. Prostaglandins 15:139.
39. M. Ulrych, 1976, The role of vascular capacitance in the genesis of essential hypertension. Clin. Sci. Mol. Med. 51: 203s-205s.
40. J.R. Vane, J.C. McGiff, 1975, Possible contributions of endogenous prostaglandins to the control of blood pressure. Circ. Res. 36 and 37, suppl. I, 1-68 and 1-75.
41. P.C. Weber, C. Larsson and B. Scherer, 1977, Prostaglandin E_2-9-ketoreductase as a mediator of salt intake-related prostaglandin-renin interaction. Nature 266:65-66.
42. P.C. Weber, B. Scherer and C. Larsson, 1977, Increase of free arachidonic acid by furosemide in man as the cause of

prostaglandin and renin release. Europ. J. Pharmacol. 41: 392-332.

43. P.C. Weber, B. Scherer, E. Held, W. Siess and H. Stoffel, 1979, Urinary prostaglandins and kallikrenin in essential hypertension. Cli. Sci. 57:295s-261s.

44. P.C. Weber, B. Scherer, W. Siess, E. Held and J. Schnermann, 1980, Possible significance of renal prostaglandins for renin release and blood pressure control. In: Advances in prostaglandin and thromboxane research, Vol. 7, B. Samuelsson, P.W. Ramwell and R. Paoletti edit., Raven Press, New York, pp. 1067-1077.

45. P.C. Weber, B. Scherer, W. Siess, E. Held and J. Schnermann, 1979, Formation and action of prostaglandins in the kidney. Klin. Wochenschr. 57:1021-1029.

46. P.C. Weber, W. Siess and B. Scherer, 1979, Prostaglandins in cardiovascular and renal function: Biochemical, physiological and clinical findings. Klin. Wochenschr. 57:425-444.

47. P.C. Weber, W. Siess and B. Scherer, 1980, Possible significance of renal prostaglandins in essential hypertension. Clin. and Expt. Hypertension 2:(3 and 4), 741-760.

48. A. Wennmalm, 1978, Influence of indomethacin on the systemic and pulmonary vascular resistance in man. Clin. Sci. Mol. Med. 54:141-145.

49. R.M. Zusman, and H.R. Keiser, 1977, Prostaglandin E_2 biosynthesis by rabbit renomedullary interstitial cells in tissue culture. J. Biol. Chem. 252:2069-2071.

EFFECTS OF ANTIHYPERTENSIVE TREATMENT ON PERIPHERAL FLOW OF THE LOWER LIMBS

A. Pinto, F. Riolo, A.M. Notarbartolo, G. Avellone,
D. Galati, F. Clemenza, D. Gullotti, and A. Strano

Institute of Clinical Medicine and Medical Therapy I°
University of Palermo - Piazza della Cliniche, 2
Palermo, Italy

INTRODUCTION

The clinical pattern determined in subjects that undergo a high and prolonged pressure regime is defined as "hypertensive disease".

Arterial hypertension, whatever its etiology may be, is an abnormal situation for the organism because: a) it determines complications in vital organs and apparatuses (heart, brain, kidney, eye); b) it facilitates and worsens the progressive deterioration of the vascular system which undergoes wear because of high pressure regime.

The aim of antihypertensive therapy must be therefore to bring back and maintain the arterial blood pressure to values considered normal so as to reduce or eliminate organic complications. Even now it is impossible to ascertain the "ideal" antihypertensive therapy, in fact on the one hand it is possible to bring back the arterial blood pressure within normal values, on the other hand the tensive values reduction is not able to eliminate alone some of the most frequent complications (acute myocardial infarction, arterial vascular disease, etc.); this is perhaps because arterial hypertension is not the only cardiovascular risk factor[5,8,19,52,53,54].

MATERIAL AND METHODS

As we do not yet know the effects of antihypertensive therapy on the district circulation of the lower limbs, we carried out, by strain-gauge plethysmography[14,16,45], a study on the peripheral arterial flow at the calf in subjects with essential hypertension examining:

I°) subjects with essential hypertension (H) at 1st stage W.H.O. in comparison with control subjects (C);
II°) hypertensive arteriopathic subjects (AH) in comparison with normotensive arteriopathics (A);
III°) the effect of antihypertensive drugs in the peripheral arterial flow in the lower limbs.

The drugs studied were:

- Captopril: recently introduced in the therapy of arterial hypertension, it acts by inhibiting the conversion of angiotensin I into angiotensin II, inducing an important reduction of systemic vascular resistances and a significant decrease of tensive systo-diastolic values[1,2,3,7,15,18,28,29,30,31,32,35,60].

- Indapamide: it acts by reducing the calcium ion influx inside the plain muscle fibrocells of vessels and reducing the vascular reactivity to the aminovasopressor action (angiotensin II, adrenalin, noradrenalin)[6,24,61].

- Labetalol: this alpha-beta blocking agent exerts its antihypertensive action mainly by a reduction of systemic vascular resistances without any significant changes of the cardiac output and myocardial contractility indices[17,26,27,36,39,40,46,49,59].

- Clonidine Hydrochloride: this drug is thought to act by stimulating central post-synaptic alpha-receptors in the cardiovascular control center of the medulla oblongata. Clonidine, furthermore, suppresses renin release, but the antihypertensive role of this mechanism is not yet clear[11,13,21,22,25,41,43,48,57].

The parameters studied were as follows:

RF = rest flow = ml/min100 gr of tissue;
PF = peak flow = ml/min/100 gr of tissue;
PF/RF= ratio;
BVR = basal vascular resistances $(\frac{MAP}{RF})$
MVR = minimal vascular resistances $(\frac{MAP}{PF})$
tPF = time to reach peak flow in seconds;
$tT\frac{1}{2}$ = time until 50% reduction of the peak flow in seconds;
tT = total time of recovery of reactive hyperemia in seconds;
SBP = systolic blood pressure in mmHg;
DBP = diastolic blood pressure in mmHg;
SBPC = systolic blood pressure at the calf in mmHg;
MAP = mean arterial pressure = $\frac{SBP+2DBP}{3}$ in mmHg;

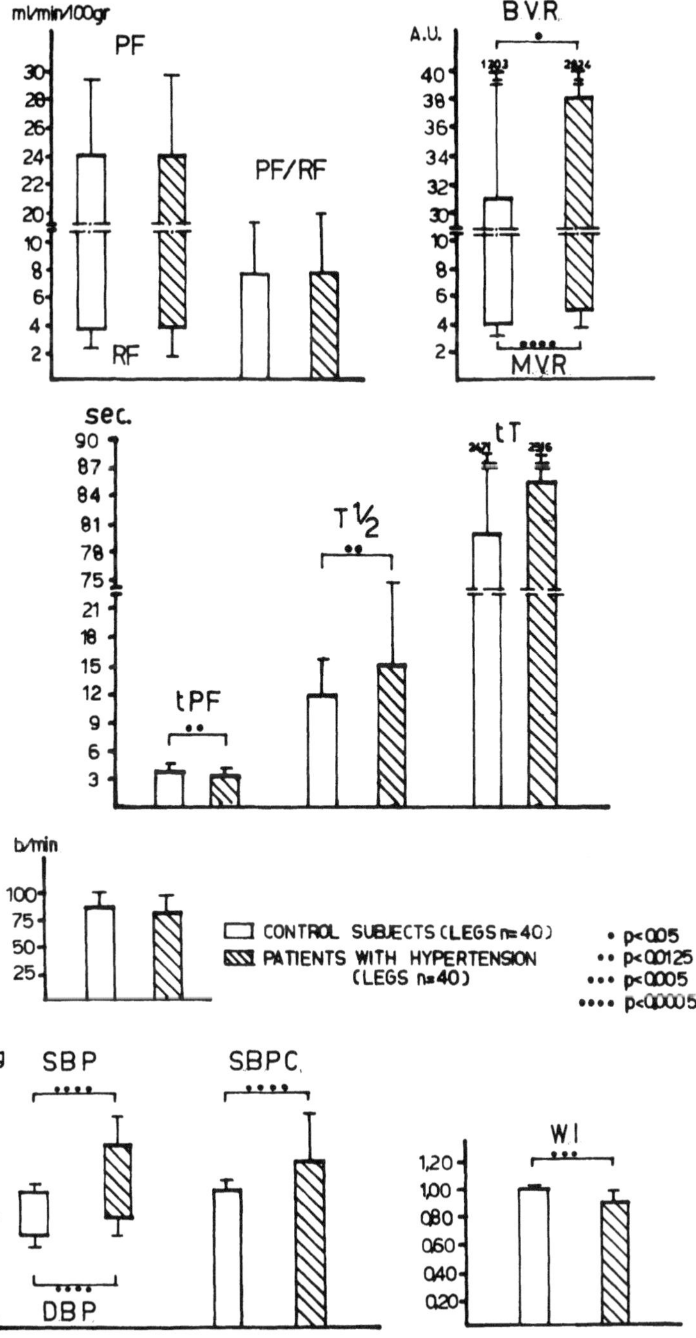

Fig. 1. Behaviour of arterial blood flow and vascular reactivity in control subjects (C) and in patients with essential hypertension (H).

HR = heart rate in beats/minute;
WI = Windsor's index i.e. ratio of SBPC/SBP.

The results were evaluated statistically using Student's "t" test for paired data.

RESULTS

I° study. "Behavior of the flow of the lower limbs, at rest and after reactive hyperemia, in patients with arterial hypertension, in comparison with control subjects".

No changes of RF, PF and PF/RF ratios were observed between the two groups of subjects studied; instead the BVR and MVR were obviously higher in the hypertensive subjects. The arterial wall reactivity times showed a greater increase also in the hypertensive subjects in comparison with the control ones. The SBP, DBP and SBPC were higher in the hypertensive subjects, while WI was slightly higher in the controls in comparison with the hypertensive subjects. No statistic changes of HR were observed in the groups of subjects studied (Figure 1).

II° study. "Arterial hypertension and blood flow of the lower limbs in patients with and without claudicatio intermittens".

RF showed a statistically significant decrease in group A in comparison with groups C and H, and in group A in comparison with group AH, while no differences were noticed between groups H and C. Besides, we found no changes in the post-ischaemic hyperemia between groups H and C, while groups AH and A showed a decrease of post-ischaemic hyperemia values in comparison with groups H and C.

PF/RF ratio was higher in group C in comparison with group AH, in group H in comparison with group AH and in group A in comparison with group AH. BVR were higher in group AH compared to groups A, H and C. Group A also, compared to groups H and C, showed higher BVR values; in the same way, in group H we observed higher BVR values compared to group C. MVR were higher in group AH in comparison with groups H and C, in group A compared to groups H and C and finally in group H compared to group C. tPF, tT½ and tT, indirect indices of arterial wall reactivity, were statistically higher in groups H, A and AH compared to group C.

SBP and DBP were obviously higher in groups H and AH in comparison with groups C and A. SBPC was higher in the hypertensive subjects (H) compared to the controls (C), arteriopathics (A) and to the hypertensive subjects with arterial vascular disease of the lower limbs (AH). The control subjects showed higher systolic tensive values at the calf compared to the subjects with arterial vascular

AH = PATIENTS WITH ARTERIOSCLEROSIS OBLITERANS OF THE LOWER LIMBS AND HYPERTENSION (legs 36)
A = PATIENTS WITH ARTERIOSCLEROSIS OBLITERANS OF THE LOWER LIMBS (legs 22)
H = PATIENTS WITH HYPERTENSION ONLY (legs 40)
C = CONTROL SUBJECTS (legs 40)

• p<0,01
•• p<0,0125
••• p<0,025
•••• p<0,05
••••• p<0,0025
•••••• p<0,005
••••••• p<0,0005

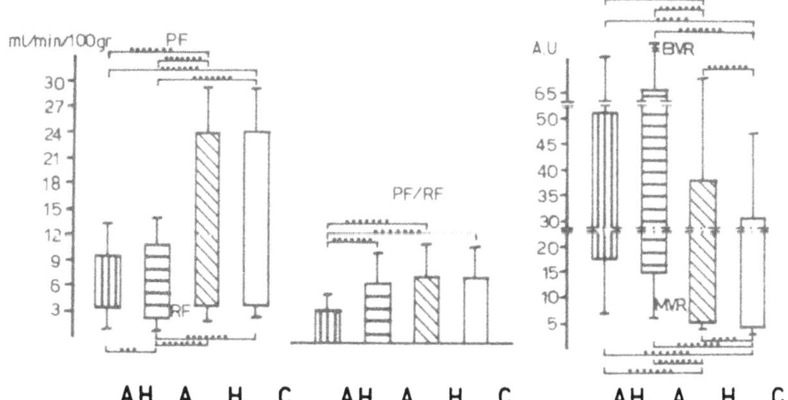

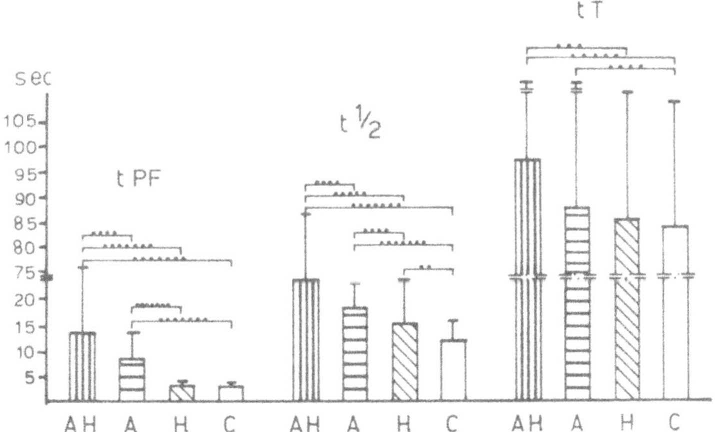

Fig. 2. Non-invasive haemodynamic recordings in control subjects (C) and in patients with arteriosclerosis obliterans of the lower limbs (A) in relation to patients with hypertension only (H) and in patients with arteriosclerosis obliterans of the lower limbs and hypertension (AH).

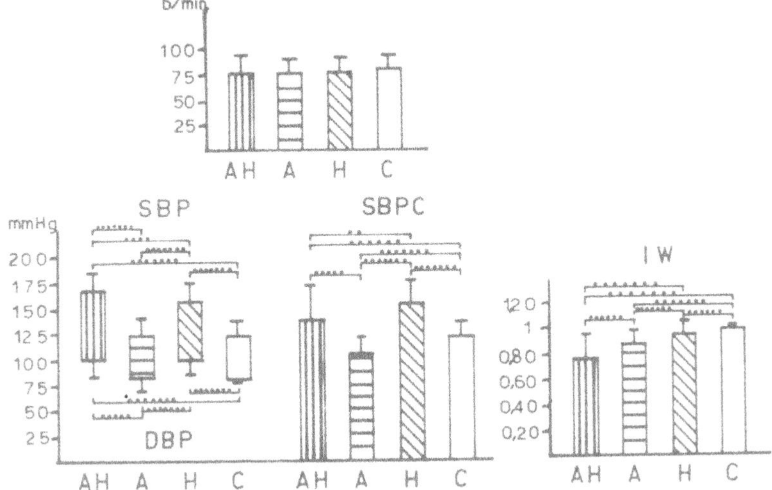

Fig. 2. Continued

disease of the lower limbs. WI was statistically higher in the controls in comparison with the other groups. No statistical change of HR was observed in all groups examined (Figure 2).

III° study. "The effect of antihypertensive drugs in the peripheral arterial flow in the lower limbs".

- Captopril: after the posological research period, in which captopril was gradually increased from 75 mg/die to a maximum of 450 mg/die in relation to the therapeutic answer, the patients were treated for 28 days with the most suitable drug dosage (450 mg/die for 6 patients and 150 mg/die for 3 patients).

Table 1 shows a significant reduction of MAP, BVR, and MVR with a statistical increase of RF and PF.

- Indapamide: the peripheral arterial flow changes at the calf were evaluated after 10 days of 2.5 mg/die of indapamide.

Table 2 shows how after 10 days of treatment, all parameters considered presented a statistical increase.

- Labetalol: the effects of prolonged administration of labetalol (for 6 months at 600 mg/die) are shown in Figure 3. It can be seen, labetalol determined a statistical reduction of BVR and MVR; an increase of RF without changes of PF. Furthermore, an evident reduction of SBP, DBP and HR was observed.

Table 1

Parameters	Run-in	Posological Research	Chronic Treatment
M.A.P. (mmHg)	131.83±17.35	111.33±16.59**	104.57±14.12****
R.F. (ml/min/100 gr. tissue)	2.489± 1.05	3.159± 1.17*	3.7± 1.7**
P.F. (ml/min/100 gr. tissue)	21.03± 7.28	24.22± 6.02	28.1± 6.78*****
B.V.R. (U.A.)	52.96±19.29	34.94±16.91***	27.1±13.59*****
M.V.R. (U.A.)	6.26± 3.12	4.61± 3.8*	3.64± 2.55***

Significance in relation to the run-in period
*p 0.05; **p 0.025; ***p 0.01; ****p 0.005; *****p 0.0005

Table 2

	Run-in	After 10 Days Treatment	(Legs = 20)
R.F. =	3.19± 1.58	4.05± 1.88	p < 0.05
P.F. =	16.18± 8.97	23.80± 9.65	p < 0.005
B.V.R. =	45.93±22.17	29.61±13.01	p < 0.005
M.V.R. =	8.85± 4.90	5.04± 3.35	p < 0.005
M.A.P. =	143.93±14.07	119.95±12.02	p < 0.0005
W.I. =	0.90± 0.04	1.07± 0.13	p < 0.0005

- Clonidine Hydrochloride: after 3 weeks of treatment with 0.45 mg/die of clonidine hydrochloride we observed (Figure 4):

- a statistical decrease of BVR and MVR;
- no changes of RF and PF;
- a statistical decrease of SBP, DBP, SBPC and HR;
- no statistical changes of WI.

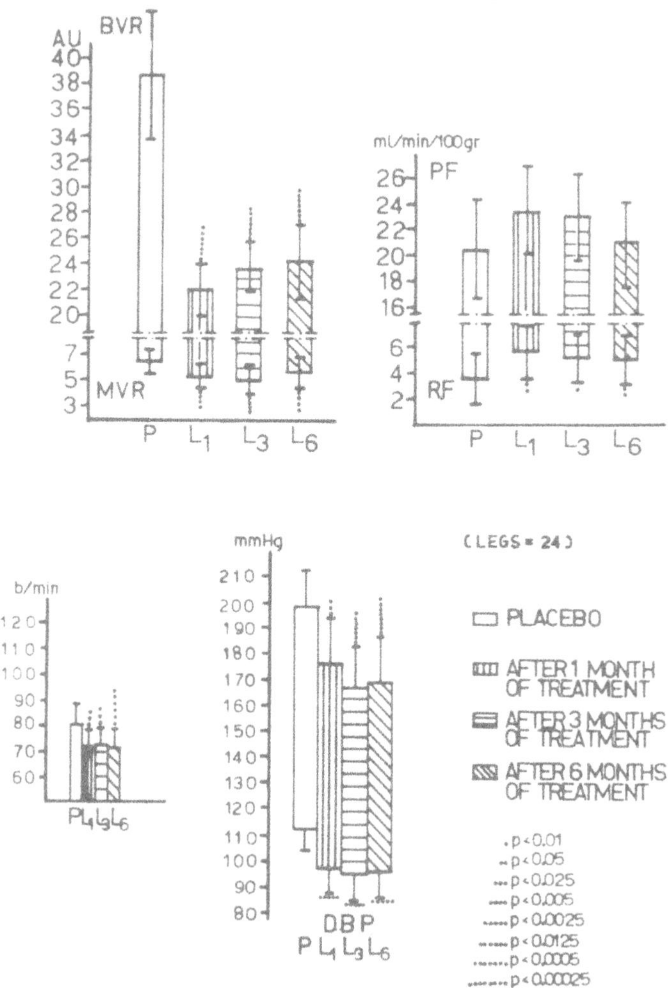

Fig. 3. Behaviour of arterial blood flow of the lower limbs and of some haemodynamic parameters after chronic treatment with labetalol in patients with arterial hypertension (H).

CONCLUSIONS

The study we have carried out on the haemodynamic district of the lower limbs, showed that in uncomplicated essential arterial hypertension there are no changes of arterial blood flow, while there is a change of arterial wall reactivity (1st study) to be assigned

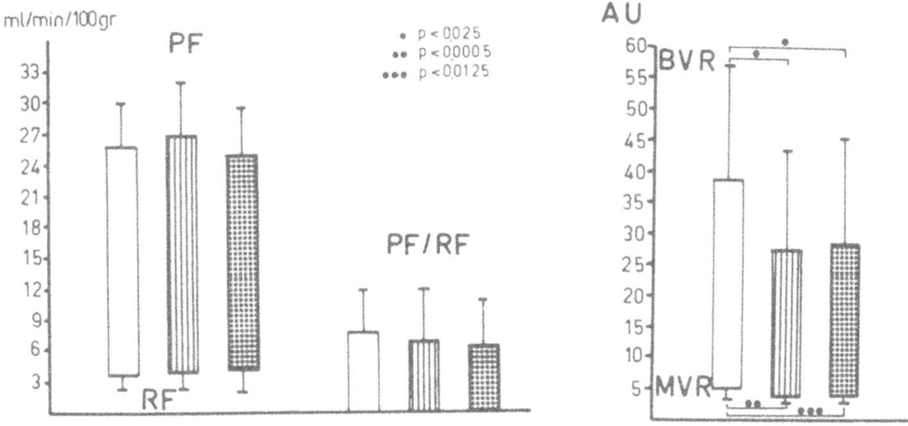

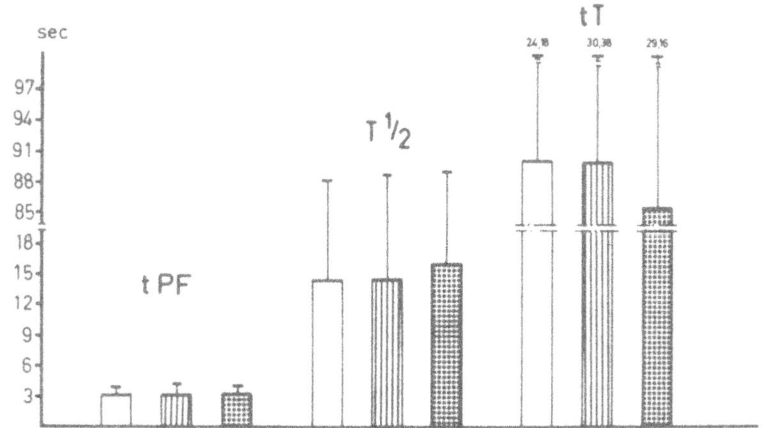

Fig. 4. Behaviour of arterial blood flow of the lower limbs and of some haemodynamic parameters after a short time treatment with clonidine hydrochloride in patients with arterial hypertension (H).

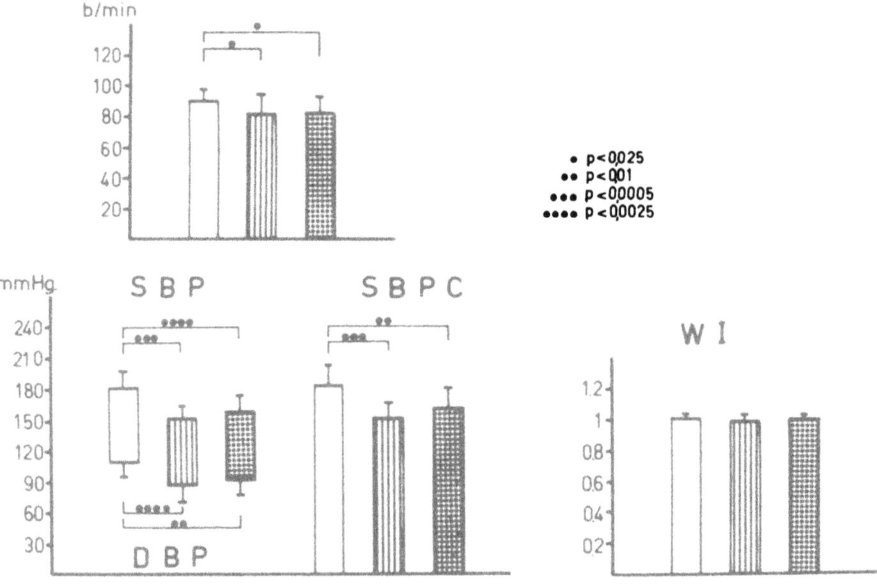

Fig. 4. Continued

probably to the decrease of elasticity modulus for the high tensive regime existing in the arterial tree. This concept has been confirmed by the second study in which a remarkable decrease of the haematic flow corresponded to the wall changes, that were more severe in the subjects with arterial vascular disease of the lower limbs and concomitant arterial hypertension compared to the hypertensive subjects alone. This also confirms that arterial hypertension going on for a long time determines a severe worsening of the haemodynamic district. Because of this it is necessary to evaluate if the antihypertensive treatment can influence the peripheral flow conditions negatively; in fact, some antihypertensive drugs are known to worsen rather than to improve the general clinical situation, above all when arterial hypertension is complicated, as has happened, for instance, using the thiazide diuretic drugs in renal insufficiency, or for the vasodilating drugs, such as hydralazine in hypertensive-ischaemic heart disease, or for non-cardioselective beta blocking drugs in subjects that, together with heart diseases, suffer also from a concomitant arterial vascular disease of the lower limbs. For this reason it is necessary to arrange clinical and methodological bases to use rationally the great number of antihypertensive drugs at our disposal. Our third study showed how the antihypertensive treatments that were employed (captopril, indapamide, labetalol, clonidine) have influenced positively the haemodynamics of the lower limbs in spite of the reduction in the tensive systo-diastolic values. For this reason, our opinion is that the choice of the drug to be employed in the antihypertensive therapy must be in relation to the possible presence of organic complications, and above all requires a fairly good knowledge of the possible effects of the drugs on the haemodynamic system

REFERENCES

1. A. B. Atkinson, J. Brown, A. F. Lever, J. I. S. Robertson, Combined treatment of severe intractable hypertension with captopril and diuretic. Lancet 8186:105 (1980).
2. A. B. Atkinson, J. J. Morton, J. Brown, D. L. Davies, R. Fraser, P. Kelly, B. Leckie, A. F. Lever, J. I. S. Robertson, Captopril in clinical hypertension. Changes in componentes of renin-angiotensin system and in body composition in relation to fall in blood pressure with a note on measurement of angiotensin II during converting enzyme. Br.Heart J. 44:290 (1980).
3. S. A. Atlas, D. B. Case, J. E. Sealey, J. H. Laragh, D. N. McKinstry, Interruption of the renin-angiotensin system in hypertensive patients by captopril induces sustained production in aldosterone secretion, potassium retention and natriuresis. Hypertension 1:274 (1979).
4. C. L. Berry, Hypertension and arterial development. Long-term consideration. Br.Heart J. 40:709 (1978)
5. C. A. Bloxham, D. G. Beevers, J. M. Walker, Malignant hypertension and cigarette smoking. Br.Med.J. 1:581 (1979.
6. C. Brater, S. Anderson, C. Muckleroy, Effects in normal subjects of long term administration of azosenide. Clin.Pharmacol. Ther. 26:437 (1979).
7. H. R. Brunner, H. Gavras, B. Waeber, S. C. Textor, G. A. Turini, J. P. Wanters, Clinical use of an orally acting converting enzyme inhibitor: captopril. Hypertension 2:558 (1980).
8. C. J. Bulpitt, L. J. Beilin, P. Clifton, C. T. Dollery, G. S. Harper, E. C. Coles, J. S. S. Gear, B. F. Johnson, A. D. Munro-Faure, Risk factors for death in treated hypertensive patients. Report from the D.H.S.S. hypertension care computing project. Lancet 8134:134 (1979).
9. C. Cavallaro, Modificazioni della parete arteriosa nell'aterosclerosi. In: "Cardiologia d'Oggi", Vol.. 1 p. 193, Mediche Scientifiche, ed., Torino, 1975).
10. A. W. Jr. Cowley, The concept of autoregulation of total blood flow and its role in hypertension. Am.J.Med. 68:906 (1980).
11. D. S. Davies, J. L. Reid, Central cardiovascular actions of clonidine. In: "Central Action of Drugs in Blood Pressure Regulation", The Whitefriers Press, ed., London, (1975).
12. C. De Mey, D. Wellens, P. M. Vanhoutte, Fisiopathology and pharmacotherapy of occlusive arterial disorders. Angiology 30:433 (1979).

13. A. Ebringer, A. E. Doyle, T. R. Dawborn, Clonidine in the treatment of hypertension. Br.Med.J. 1:402 (1971).
14. B. Fagrell, Digital pulse plethysmography and digital blood pressure measurement in the evaluation of arterial circulation in the lower limbs. Scand.J.Clin.Lab.Invest. 31:128 (1973).
15. K. Roger, R. K. Ferguson, H. Peter, J. Vlasses, D. Pharm, R. Janice, R. N. Kojlin, B. S. Anne Shirinian, F. James, J. Burke, C. John, R. Alexander, Captopril in severe treatment-resistant hypertension. Am.Heart J. 99:579 (1980).
16. S. Forconi, A. Jagenau, M. Guerrini, S. Pecchi, R. Cappelli, Strain-gauge plethysmography in the study of circulation of the limbs. Angiology 30:487 (1979).
17. W. I. Frishman, S. Halprin, Clinical pharmacology of the new beta-adrenergic blocking drugs. VII. New Horizons in beta-adrenoceptor blockade therapy: Labetalol. Am.Heart J. 98:660 (1979).
18. H. Gravas, Antihypertensive effects of the oral angiotensin converting-enzyme inhibitor. New Engl.J.Med. 298:991 (1978).
19. R. M. Greenhangh, D. S. Rosengarten, I. Mervert, B. Lewis, J. S. Colman, P. Martin, Serum lipids and lipoproteins in peripheral vascular desease. Lancet 2:947 (1971).
20. B. Gribbin, T. G. Pickerilg, P. Sleight, Arterial distensibility in normal and ipertensive man. Clin.Sci. 56:413 (1979).
21. L. Hansson, S. N. Hunyor, S. Julius, S. W. Hobler, Blood pressure crisis following withdrawal of clonidine. Am.Heart J. 85:605 (1973).
22. S. W. Hoobler and E. Sagastume, Clonidine hydrochloride in the treatment of hypertension. Am.J.Cardiol. 28:67 (1971).
23. W. G. Hughson, J. Mann and A. Garrod, Intermittent claudication: prevalence and risk factors. Br.Med.J. 1:1379 (1978).
24. K. Hutchinson and H. Williams, Calf blood flow and ankle systolic blood pressure in intermittent claudication monitored over five years. Angiology 29:719 (1978).
25. R. G. Hutchinson, Medical management of hypertension. Angiology 30:558 (1979).
26. G. Koch, Haemodynamic effects of combined alpha and beta-adrenoceptor blockade after intravenous labetalol in hypertensive patients at rest and during exercise. Br.J.Clin. Pharmacol. 3(Suppl.):725 (1976).
27. G. Koch, Effetti emodinamici del blocco alfa e beta-recettoriale acuto con somministrazione di labetalolo e.v. e variazioni in corso di trattamento orale protratto in pazienti affetti da ipertensione essenziale. in: "Atti Convegno Venezia", p.65 (1978).
28. H. Koffer, P. H. Vlasses, R. K. Ferguson, M. Weiss and A. G. Abler, Captopril in diuretic treated hypertensive patients. J.A.M.A. 244:2532 (1980).

29. B. O. Kristensen and J. Skork, Captopril or frusemide in drug-resistant hypertension (Letter) Lancet 8196:699 (1980).
30. D. W. Johns, K. M. Baker, C. R. Ayers, E. D. Vanghau Jr., R. M. Carey, M. J. Peach, M. R. Yancey, E. M. Ortt and S. C. Williams, Acute and chronic effect of captopril in hypertensive patients. Hypertension 2:567 (1980).
31. C. L. Johnson, B. P. McGrath, J. A. Miller and P. G. Mathews, Long term effects of captopril (SQ 14 225) on blood pressure and hormone levels in essential hypertension. Lancet 8141:493 (1979).
32. P. Lijnen, R. Fagard, J. Staessen, L. J. Verschueren and A. Amery, Dose response in captopril therapy of hypertension. Clin.Pharmacol.Ther. 28:310 (1980).
33. G. M. London, M. E. Safar, Y. A. Weiss and A. Simon, Total effective Compliance of the vascular bed in essential hypertension. Am.Heart J. 95:325 (1978).
34. G. A. McGregor, N. D. Markandu, J. E. Roulston and J. C. Jones, Essential hypertension: effect of an oral inhibitor of angiotensin converting enzyme. Br.Med.J. 2:1106 (1979).
35. A. Maruyama, T. Ogihara, T. Naka, H. Mikami, T. Hata, M. Nakamaru, K. Iwanaga and Y. Kumahara, Long term effects of captopril in hypertension. Clin.Pharmacol.Ther. 28:316 (1980).
36. G. Mattioli, S. Ricci and P. Bertoncelli, Haemodynamics of hypertension. Changes caused by beta blocking agents. Minerva Cardioangiol. 27:463 (1979).
37. P. Mayer, J. L. Elghozi and J. P. Grünfield, The physiological basis of the treatment of arterial hypertension. Nouv.Presse Med. 8:2325 (1979).
38. F. Messerly, J. De Carvalho, B. Christie and B. Fröhlich, Systemic and regional haemodynamics in low, normal and high cardiac output borderline hypertension. Circulation 58:441 (1978).
39. J. Metha and J. N. Cohn, Haemodynamic effects of labetalol, an alpha and beta-adrenoceptor blocking agent, in hypertensive subjects. Circulation 55:370 (1977).
40. C. Alicandri, E. Agabiti-Rosci, R. Fariello, L. Corea and B. Muiesan, Effetti emodinamici della somministrazione acuta e cronica del labetalolo nell'ipertensione arteriosa. in: "Atti Convegno Venezia", p.31 (1978).
41. K. D. Boch, P. Merguet and V. H. Heimsoth, Effect of clonidine on regional blood flow and its use in the treatment of hypertension, in: "Hypertension: Mechanisms and Management", G. Onesti, K.E. Kim and J.A. Mayer eds., Grune and Stratton Inc. p.395 New York, (1973).
42. L. H. Opie, Drugs and the heart. III Calcium antagonist. Lancet 8172:806 (1980).
43. W. A. Pettinger, Clonidine a new antihypertensive drug. New.Engl.J.Med., 293:1179 (1975).

44. G. Thomas, T. G. Pickering, H. John and P. Laragh, Autoregulation as a factor in peripheral resistance and flow: clinical implications for analysis of high blood pressure (editorial). Am.J.Med. 68:801 (1980).
45. A. Pinto, La semeiotica strumentale delle arteriopatie obliteranti degli arti inferiori. Collana di quaderni monografici a cura di E. Massari. in: "Patologia arteriosa distrettuale", E.S.I. Redaz. Stampa Medica.
46. B. N. C. Pichard, Beta-adrenoceptor blocking agents in the management of hypertension
47. L. E. Ramsay, Intermittent claudication in hypertensive men. Journal of the Royal College of Physicians of London 13:100 (1979).
48. J. L. Reid, H. J. Dargie and C. T. Dollery, Clonidine withdrawal in hypertension. Lancet 2:1171 (1977).
49. D. A. Richards and E. P. Wooding, The effects of oral AH 5158, a combined alpha and beta-adrenoceptor antagonist in healthy volunteers. Br.J.Clin.Pharmacol. 1:505 (1974).
50. A. Simon, B. Levy, Y. Weiss, M. Kheder and J. Levenson, Arterial compliance in permanent essential hypertension. Angiology 29:402 (1978).
51. A. Simon, M. A. Safar, J. Levenson, A. Kheder and B. Levy, Systolic hypertension: haemodynamic mechanism and choice of anti-hypertensive treatment. Am.J.Cardiol. 44:505 (1979).
52. J. Stamler, Prevenzione primaria e secondaria delle malattie aterosclerotiche. in: "Arteriosclerosi", Vol.II, R. Paoletti and C.R. Sirtori (Coord.), Ambrosiana, Milano, (1977).
53. R. Stamler, J. Stamler, W. F. Riedlinger, G. Algera and R. H. Roberts, Family (parental) history and prevalence of hypertension. Results of a nationwide screening program. J.A.M.A. 241:43 (1979).
54. A. Strano, S. Novo, G. Davì, A. Pinto and R. P. Riolo, Aspetti epidemiologici delle arteriopatie degli arti. in: "Giornate Angiologiche Fiorentine", Firenze 14 Giugno (1979).
55. A. Strano, Fattori emodinamici nell'aterosclerosi. in: "Aterosclerosi: problemi di patologia e terapia". Incontri con i medici 1977-1979, a cura della Direzione Medica Janssen.
56. A. Takeshita and A. L. Mark, Decreased vasodilator capacity of forearm resistance vessels in borderline hypertension. Hipertension 2:610 (1980).
57. P. A. Van Zwieten, The central action of antihypertensive drugs, mediated via central alpha-receptors. J.Pharm.Pharmacol. 25:89 (1973).
58. J. K. Vyden, J. Thorner, K. Nagasewa, T. Takano, M. F. Groseth-Dittrich, R. Perlow and M. J. Swen, Metabolic and cardiovascular abnormalities in patients with peripheral arterial disease. Am.Heart J. 90:703 (1975).
59. P. Weidmann, R. De Chatle, W. H. Ziegler, J. Flammer and F. Reubi, Alpha and beta-adrenergic blockade with orally admin-

plasma renin and catecholamine excretion. Am.J.Cardiol. 41:570 (1978).
60. M. J. Wendeburg, Prolonged treatment of high renin hypertension with a converting enzyme inhibitor. Br.Med.J. 2:866 (1978).
61. L. Werkö, Vascular adaptation to long term blood pressure reduction (Letter). Acta Med.Scand. 207:207 (1980).
62. A. Zanghetti, Overview of cardiovascular reflexes in hypertension. Am.J.Cardiol. 44:912 (1979).

HAEMODYNAMIC AND ANTIHYPERTENSIVE EFFECT OF PROSTACYCLIN

A. Szczeklik, R.J. Gryglewski, J. Szczeklik, and
R. Nizankowski

Departments of Internal Medicine and Pharmacology
Copernicus Academy of Medicine
Skawinska 8
31-066 Krakow, Poland

Prostacyclin (2) is a natural product of blood vessels, synthetized predominantly in endothelium and released in minute amounts into circulation (3). Besides its potent antiplatelet activity (1,4, 6), prostacyclin is also a powerful vasodilator. The vasodilating properties were noticed already during first administration of prostacyclin to man (7), and were subsequently studied in detail in 10 subjects without evidence of coronary heart disease or cardiac failure (11, 12). Prostacyclin was infused in three dose levels (2, 5 and 10 ng/kg/min) leading to following effects:

1) Distinct fall in peripheral and total pulmonary vascular resistances;
2) Drop in intra-arterial blood pressure;
3) Acceleration of the heart rate;
4) Increase in muscle blood flow;
5) Stroke volume, mean right atrial pressure and left ventricular end-diastolic pressure showed no significant changes.

We have now extended our haemodynamic observations to 27 patients with cardiovascular diseases. Of these, 12 patients had peripheral vascular disease without evidence of cardiac involvement, 7 had effort angina, 7 secondary pulmonary hypertension due to mitral stenosis, and one pulmonary hypertension due to ventricular septal defect. The results obtained in these 27 patients are presented in Figures 1-3, and in Table 1.

Conclusions which can be drawn from these studies are as follows:

1) Prostacyclin in a dose of 2-10 ng/kg/min strongly dilates arterioles and precapillary sphincters, but does not affect peripheral venous circulation.
2) The fall in peripheral nad pulmonary vascular resistances

induced by prostacyclin is accompanied by a decrease in arterial blood pressure and acceleration of heart rate.

3) In a dose 5 ng/kg/min prostacyclin has no direct inotropic effects.

In comparison to prostaglandin E_1 (PGE_1) prostacyclin has a stronger action in man. Doses of PGE_1 (10) at least twice as high were necessary to reduce pulmonary vascular resistance to the range observed during prostacyclin administration. Prostacyclin was also better tolerated than PGE_1. We have not observed abdominal cramps or back pain, which were frequently recorded in subjects receiving PGE_1, and which had necessitated interruption of the infusion (5).

Our results suggest that prostacyclin could be of interest not only in treatment of peripheral (8) and coronary (9) vessel disease, but also in clinical conditions associated with significant rise in vascular resistance, including pulmonary hypertension, hypertensive emergencies and cardiogenic shock.

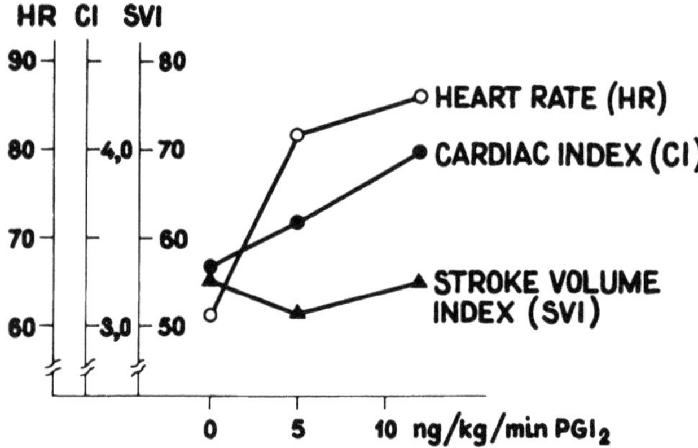

Fig. 1 Heart rate, cardiac index and stroke volume index (means) in 27 patients with cardiovascular diseases during consecutive infusion of two doses of prostacyclin. Measurements were taken at the end of the infusion periods, each lasting 45 minutes.

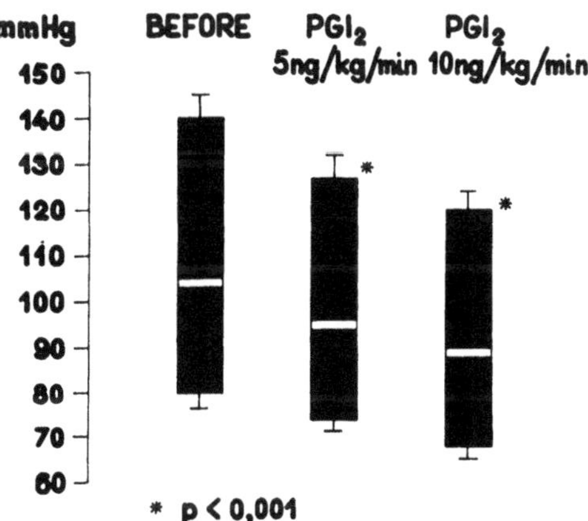

Fig. 2 Behaviour of the blood pressure in aorta during infusion of prostacyclin to 27 patients with cardiovascular disease. Two doses of PGI_2 were given, one after another, each lasting 45 minutes.

Table 1. Haemodynamic indices in 27 patients with cardiovascular disease. The results were recorded initially and at the end of 45 minute infusion periods of two doses of prostacyclin.

Parameters studied		Initial values	During 5 ng/kg/min PGI_2	During 10 ng/kg/min PGI_2
A_o m mmHg	max	140.0 ± 5.1	127.2 ± 4.8^{xxx}	119.8 ± 4.7^{xxx}
	min	79.8 ± 2.3	74.7 ± 3.0^{xx}	68.0 ± 2.8^{xx}
	mean	104.1 ± 2.9	95.3 ± 3.3^{xxx}	88.8 ± 3.1^{xxx}
RA_m mmHg		4.3 ± 0.6	3.8 ± 0.5	3.6 ± 0.6
HR		72.3 ± 2.9	83.0 ± 3.7^{xxx}	85.2 ± 3.5^{xxx}
PAP mmHg	max	32.4 ± 3.6	29.1 ± 3.6^{xx}	28.2 ± 3.7^{xxx}
	min	15.0 ± 1.8	13.5 ± 1.8xx	13.6 ± 2.1x
	mean	21.0 ± 2.5	18.4 ± 2.3^{xxx}	19.0 ± 2.7^{xx}
PWP_m mmHg		10.9 ± 1.3	9.7 ± 1.2^{xx}	8.9 ± 1.3^{xx}
CI $l/min/m^2$		3.39 ± 0.14	3.60 ± 0.12^{x}	3.97 ± 0.15^{xxx}
SVI $ml/beat/m^2$		52.9 ± 4.5	51.6 ± 4.1	55.2 ± 4.3
LVSWI $gm/beat/m^2$		60.0 ± 3.9	62.9 ± 5.6	57.4 ± 4.9^{xxx}

PWR dynes $s.cm^{-5}$	117.8 ± 17.4	102.6 ± 14.9^{xx}	83.5 ± 14.4^{xxx}
TPR dynes $s.cm^{-5}$	310.0 ± 49.8	248.8 ± 39.8^{xxx}	234.7 ± 40.2^{xxx}
PVR dynes $s.cm^{-5}$	1410.6 ± 75.5	1199.5 ± 67.8^{xxx}	1030.5 ± 56.3^{xxx}

A_o m = mean aortic blood pressure; RA_m = mean right atrial pressure; HR = heart rate; PAP = pulmonary artery pressure; PWP = pulmonary wedge pressure; CI = cardiac index; SVI = stroke volume index; LVSWI = left ventricular stroke volume index; PWR = pulmonary wedge resistance; TPR = tctal pulmonary resistance; PVR = peripheral vascular resistance.

x = $p<0.05$; xx = $p<0.01$; xxx = $p<0.001$.

All statistical computations were made in comparison to initial values.

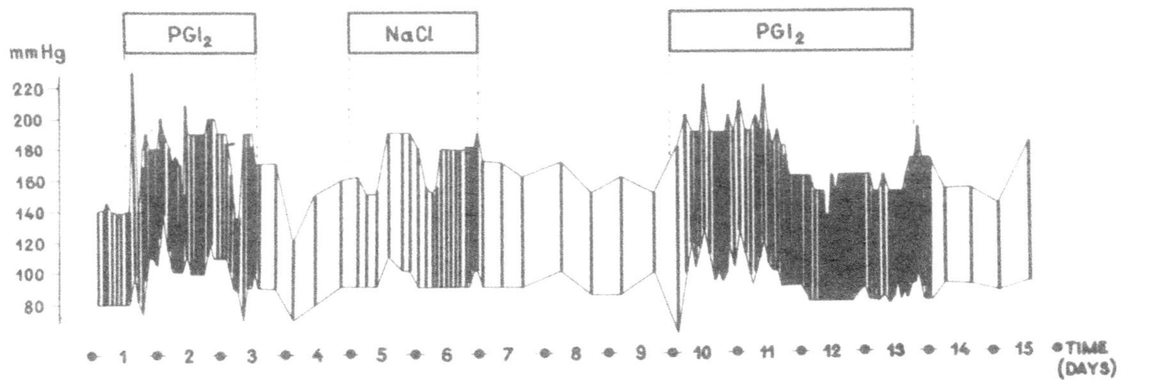

Fig. 3 Paradoxical response of blood pressure to prostacyclin infusions (5-10 ng/kg/min) in a 60-year-old patient with angina at rest and a history of hypertension. This type of reaction, characterized by elevation of blood pressure during PGI_2 administration, was observed in 4 of 85 subjects studied by us. All these four subjects have been known to be hypertensive. In the remaining 81 patients, prostacyclin invariably lowered blood pressure.

REFERENCES

1. R.J. Gryglewski, Prostaglandins, platelets and atherosclerosis. CRC Series in Biochemistry 7: 291 (1980).
2. R.J. Gryglewski, S. Bunting, S. Moncada, R.J. Flower, J.R. Vane, Arterial walls are protected against deposition of platelet thrombi by a substance (Prostaglandin X) which they make from prostaglandins endoperoxides. Prostaglandins 12: 685 (1976).
3. R.J. Gryglewski, R. Korbut, A. Ocetkiewicz, Generation of prostacyclin by lungs in vivo and its release into arterial circulation. Nature 273: 765 (1978).
4. R.J. Gryglewski, A. Szczeklik, R. Nizankowski, Anti-platelet action of intravenous prostacyclin in man. Thrombos. Res. 13: 153 (1978).
5. A. Ollson, L.A. Carlson, Clinical, haemodynamic and metabolic effects of intraarterial infusion of prostaglandin E_1 in patients with peripheral vascular disease. Adv. Prostagl. Thrombox. Res. 1: 429 (1976).
6. A. Szczeklik, R.J. Gryglewski, E. Nizankowska, R. Nizankowski, J. Musial, Pulmonary and anti-platelet effects of intravenous and inhaled prostacyclin in man. Prostaglandins, 16: 651 (1978).
7. A. Szczeklik, R.J. Gryglewski, R. Nizankowski, J. Musial, R. Pieton, J. Murk, Circulatory and antiplatelet effects of intravenous prostacyclin in healthy men. Pharmacol. Res. Commun. 10: 545 (1978).
8. A. Szczeklik, R. Nizankowski, S. Skawinski, J. Szczeklik, P. Gluszko, R.J. Gryglewski, Succesful therapy of advanced arteriosclerosis obliterans with prostacyclin.Lancet 1: 1111 (1979).
9. A. Szczeklik, J. Szczeklik, R. Nizankowski, P. Gluszko, Prostacyclin for unstable angina. N. Engl. J. Med. 303: 881 (1980).
10. J. Szczeklik, J.S. Dubiel, M. Mysik, Z. Pyzik, R. Krol, R. Horzela, Effects of prostaglandin E_1 on pulmonary circulation in patients with pulmonary hypertension. Br. Heart J. 40: 1397 (1978).
11. J. Szczeklik, A. Szczeklik, R. Nizankowski, Haemodynamic effects of prostacyclin in man. Adv. Prostagl. Thrombox. Res. 7: 769 (1980).
12. J. Szczeklik, A. Szczeklik, R. Nizankowski, Haemodynamic changes induced by prostayclin in man. Br. Heart J. 44: 254 (1980).

PART 7

PULMONARY VASCULAR DISEASES

MECHANISMS UNDERLYING PULMONARY HYPERTENSION BY HYPOXEMIA

M. Condorelli, F. Rengo, B. Trimarco, D. Bonaduce, F. Iodice, F. Piscione, C. Vigorito, and G. Marone

Istituto di Patologia Speciale Medica e Metodologia Clinica
II Policlinico Napoli
Napoli, Italy

Mechanisms underlying pulmonary hypertension are not completely clarified. However, it has been shown that pulmonary blood flow, alveolar pressure or left atrial pressure and blood viscosity do not change at all during hypoxia. Furthermore, it has been reported that alveolar hypoxia produces an increase in pulmonary pressure by a vasoconstrictive response although the mechanisms responsible for this phenomenon remain unclear (1-4).

The possibility to elicit the hypoxic pressor response in isolated lung without sympathetic connections, in sympathectomized man and animals (5, 6), and in animals after adrenergic depletion (7) or after adrenergic blocking agents (8-10), counteracts the role of the sympathetic nervous system in pulmonary hypoxic vasoconstrictor response. Although the weight of evidence seems to be against a pre minent role for the autonomic nervous system in the pressor response to acute hypoxia, more subtle participation of this system cannot be ruled out.

Both alpha- and beta-adrenergic receptors are present in pulmonary vessels, but alpha receptors are numerically and functionally preeminent (11). Recently renewed interest has concerned the effects of pharmacologic blockade on hypoxic and hypercapnic pulmonary vasoconstrictor responses. Both responses are susceptible to alpha and beta blockade, in particular in isolated lungs the vasoconstriction is markedly enhanced by beta blockade and reduced by alpha blockade (12). Nevertheless, this effect in intact animals is less clear.

Over the years serious attention has been given to the question of whether alveolar hypoxia only or also the exaggeration of normal pre-capillary hypoxemia elicits pulmonary arterial and arteriolar constriction. Small pulmonary veins too contribute to hypoxic pressor response even if such a role seems to be subsidiary.

Fishman schematically proposed that both alveolar and blood hypoxia could affect smooth muscle of the small pulmonary arteries and venules (Fig. 1). The precapillary vessel is subdivided into two segments: a proximal conducting part (A) in which the mixed venous PO_2 is the major determinant, and a terminal one (B) in which alveolar PO_2 ordinarily is the major determinant. Breathing air the low mixed venous PO_2 is responsible for the marked vasoconstrictor tone of the proximal pulmonary vascular segments, while the high alveolar PO_2 is responsible for the slight vasoconstrictor tone of the distal segment. During hypoxia, the proximal segment undergoes little change whereas there is an increase in the vasoconstrictor tone in the distal segment. Actually the alveolar PO_2 decreases to reach a level that is not appreciably different from blood PO2 in the distal segment; to the high tone of the proximal segment is added the increase in tone of the distal segment which therefore is the main component of the pressor response to hypoxia (13)

Moreover hypoxia could directly increase the tension of pulmonary arterial smooth muscle by affecting the mechanisms that control membrane excitation, excitation-contraction coupling or the chemomechanical transducer. According to Duke's hypothesis hypoxia impairs the cellular energy supply of the membrane sodium pump of the pulmonary vascular smooth muscle and thus depolarizes the cell and induces electrical activation (14). But Detar and Bohr have demonstrated that, in contrast to systemic vascular smooth muscle, in which hypoxia depresses oxidative production of ATP, hypoxia accelerates ATP production in pulmonary vascular smooth muscle by accelerating the glycolytic pathway.

Bergofsky and Holtzman, without excluding an effect on the contractile process or an excitation-contraction coupling, hypothesized that hypoxia depolarizes the membrane of vascular smooth muscle cells and brings them closer to the threshold for excitation (15). Finally, Liljestrand, suggested that hypoxia exerts its pulmonary pressor effect by releasing lactic acid in pulmonary smooth muscle (16).

It has been postulated that chemical mediators might play a significant role in the control of pulmonary hypertension. In particular prostaglandins (P s) and histamine (H) have been implicated in the control of pulmonary circulation. It has been proposed that $PGF_{2\alpha}$ elicit a vasoconstrictor response through cyclic GMP increase; in contrast, PGs of E series show a vasodilatator response by mean of cyclic AMP increase. However, unless new supporting evidence is adduced, it seems unlikely that any of PGs will emerge as a unique chemical mediator (17, 18).

Table I summarizes the characteristics of possible humoral mediators of pulmonary vasoconstrictor response to hypoxia or hypercapnia. Histamine seems to be the front-runner of humoral agents which might play a regulatory role on lung vasculature. Thus in isolated perfused rat lungs large doses of antihistamines and H depletors diminish the pulmonary pressor response to hypoxia, whereas a

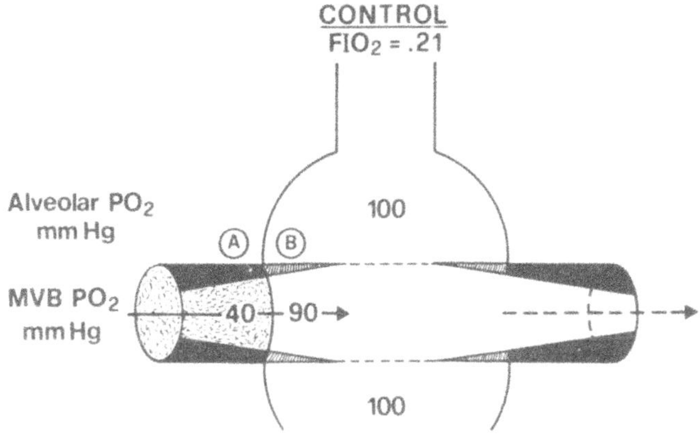

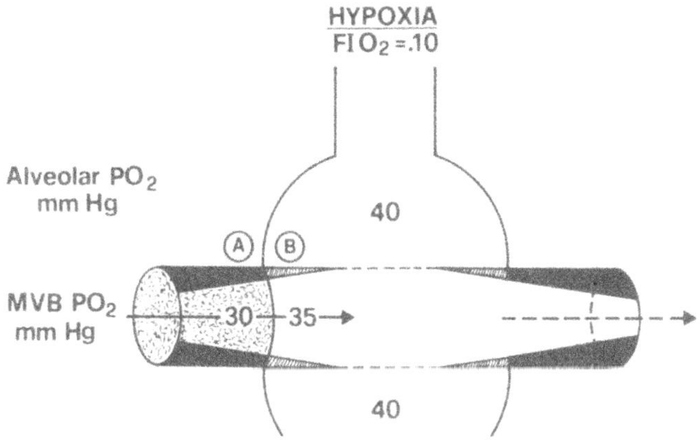

Fig. 1. Fishman hypothesis

histaminase inhibitor potentiates it. (19-21).

Moreover during hypoxia the concentration of the H in the effluent from the lungs increases. In addition the periarterial mast-cells in the lungs degranulate in the rat and guinea pig during hypoxia (22). However the hypothesis of H mediated hypoxic pulmonary hypertension was questioned in a number of recent reports. Some have had difficulty in reproducing the blunting and blocking effects of antihistamines and H depletors on the pulmonary pressor response.

Table I. Characteristics of possible humoral mediators of pulmonary vasoconstrictor response to hypoxia or hypercapnia (Bergofsky).

Agent	↓ Hypoxic response by inhibitor	Strong Pulmonary Vasopressor	Strategically stored	Activated released in lung	Consistent * α β adrenergic profile
Histamine	+	++	++	++	+
Serotonin	?	++	+	+	0
Norepinephrine	0	++	++	++	+
Angiotensin	?	++	0	++	+
$PGF_{2\alpha}$	?	+	0	++	0
Vasopressin	?	± **	0	0	?
Bradykinin	± **	0	0	?	?

* i.e., vasoconstrictor response enhanced and blunted by beta and alpha blockade, respectively, as occurs with hypoxia and hypercapnic acidosis.

** Pulmonary vasoactive response variable; often vasodilator.

Some doubt exists about the specificity for H of the antihistamines and H releasers. Dowson and Delano utilizing the H depletor compound 48/80 found that H depletion was not necessary for inhibition of hypoxic vasoconstriction by this compound (23). In order to investigate the mechanisms of hypoxic pulmonary hypertension and the role of the H we have administered chlorpheniramine (0,3 mg/Kg) to 8 normal subjects and 20 patients with chronic obstructive lung disease. Pulmonary artery pressure (PAP), pulmonary capillary pressure (PCP), cardiac output (CO) and pulmonary vascular resistances (PVR) were evaluated together with PO_2 and PCO_2. Chlorpheniramine reduced only in chronic obstructive lung disease patients (COLD) PAP and PVR while PO_2 increased and PCO_2 decreased; CO and HR remained unchanged. In normal subjects chlorpheniramine failed to modify these parameters (24).

These results seem to lead further support to the hypothesis that H plays an important role as mediator of pulmonary vasoconstrictive response. Moreover, in dogs pulmonary artery pressure (PP) and systemic arterial pressure (AP) were recorded and H content was measured in aorta, pulmonary artery, distal inferior vena cava and hepatic vein. In 5 animals, which served as controls, the data were collected after 20 minutes of breathing room air; in the other 7 dogs, the measurements were repeated after 5 minutes of breathing a mixture contianing 8% oxygen. Histamine content was significantly increased in the pulmonary artery blood while it was unchanged in the aorta: the difference between the H content in the pulmonary artery and in the aorta increased. Moreover the inferior vena cava content of the agent rose significantly and it did not change in the hepatic vein (Fig. 2). Simultaneously, PP increased and AP was only slightly changed (Fig. 3). Therefore H is probably released by skeletal muscle during hypoxia, since it is increased in the distal vena cava and uptaken by the lung as shown by the increase in PA-Ao difference (Fig. 4). More recent studies seem to indicate that H acts as a modulator rather than as a mediator of the pulmonary hemodynamic response to hypoxia (25).

A study performed in our laboratory by the use of disodium-cromoglycate (DSCG) is in agreement with this hypothesis. Key and Grover showed that acute hypoxic pulmonary vasoconstriction could be prevented in dogs by the administration of DSCG so, it seemd likely that hypoxic pulmonary hypertension could be mediated by the release of some humoral agents and that H may be such a substance. Our study was assigned to accertain whether or not this drug possesses such an effect and also to clarify the mechanism of action of DSCG. Accordingly, in dogs hypoxia was induced and hemodynamic measurements performed. Histamine blood concentration was also assessed. Hypoxia significantly increased mean pulmonary artery pressure while blood H content in the pulmonary artery and in inferior vena cava rose. Pretreatment with 8 mg/Kg of DSCG was able to abolish both hypoxia induced responses. To asses whether or not the pulmonary hypertension and the increase in blood H levels were linked by a cause-effect relationship, the effects of hypoxia after intravenous administration of 1, 2.5, 5 and

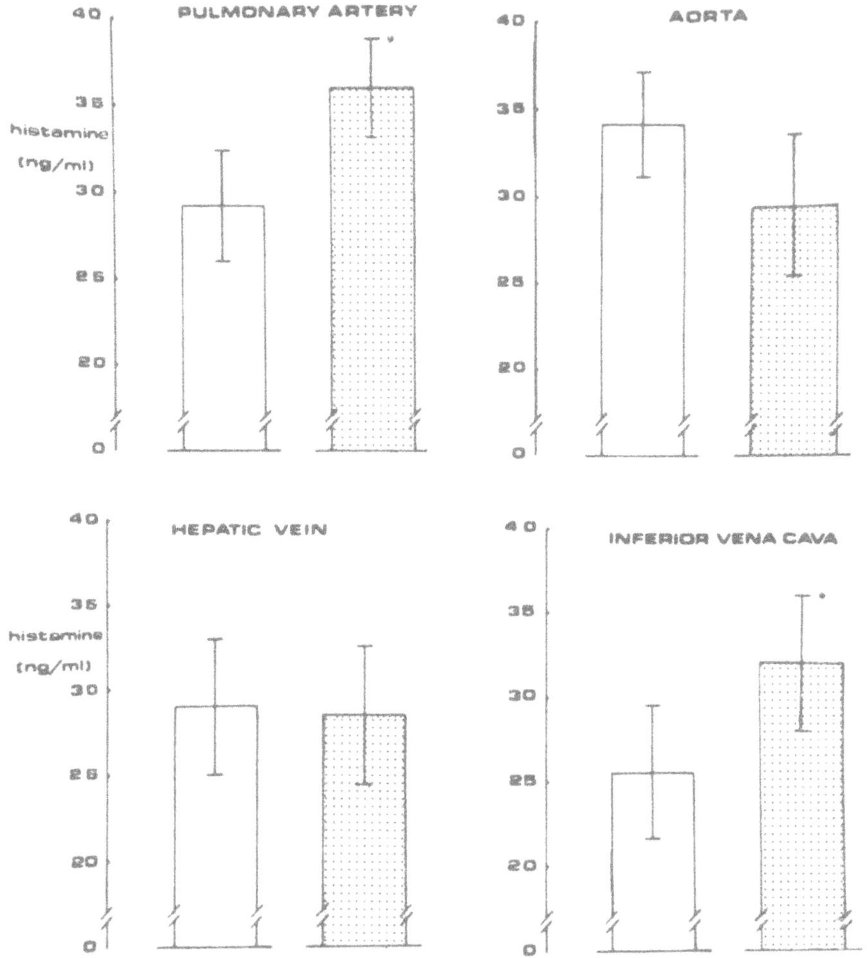

Fig. 2. Changes in histamine content induced by 5 min hypoxia in the pulmonary artery, distal inferior vena cava, and hepatic vein. The solid columns represent the control values, the dotted columns the values measured after hypoxia. Note the significant increase of histamine content in the pulmonary artery and inferior vena cava.
* = different from control, $P < 0.05$
All numbers represent mean ± 1 SE

8 mg/Kg of DSCG were investigated. The administration of DSCG was able to abolish completely the hypoxia induced increase in blood H levels at a dose as low as 1 mg/Kg. In contrast, to achieve the complete inhibition of hypoxic pulmonary hypertension, 8 mg/Kg of DSCG were needed. Moreover, in dogs pretreated with atropine, DSCG (8 mg/Kg) was unable to block hypoxia induced pulmonary hypertension

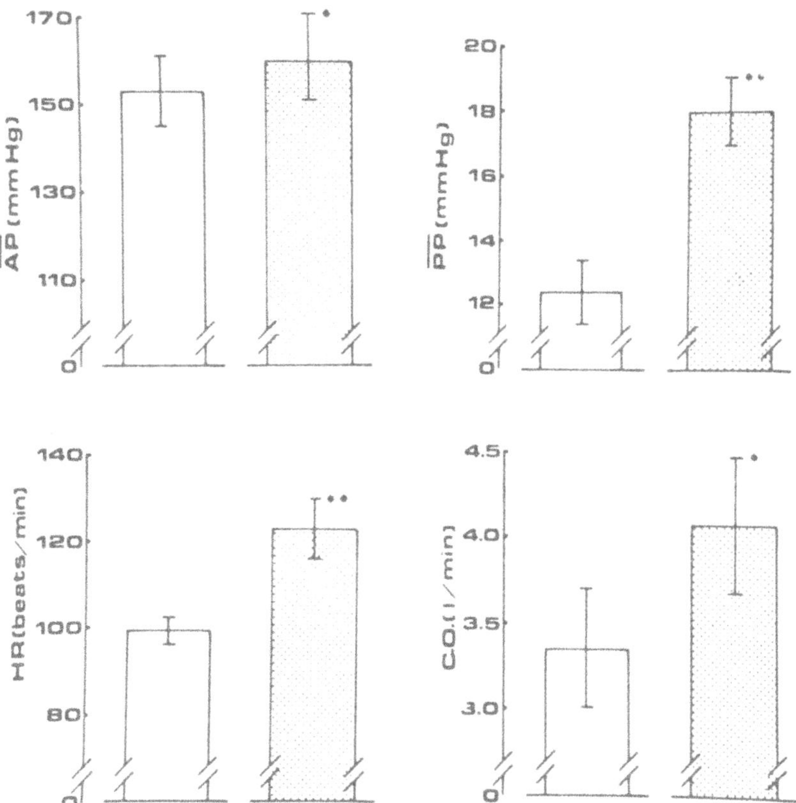

Fig. 3. Changes in hemodynamic parameters induced by 5 min hypoxia. The solid columns represent the control values obtained after 5 min of breathing a gas mixture containing 8% oxygen and 92% nitrogen.
AP = Systemic arterial pressure (kPa)
PP = Pulmonary pressure (kPa)
HR = Heart rate (beats x min $^{-1}$)
CO = Cardiac output (litres x min $^{-1}$)
* = Different from control, P < 0.005
** = Different from control, P < 0.01
All numbers represent mean ± 1 SE n = 7.

although atropine did not exert any effect on H concentration; actually the hypoxia induced increase in H content was inhibited similarly when DSCG was given alone as well as after atropine (Fig. 5). The results of this study suggest that the DSCG is able in dogs to prevent pulmonary hypertension induced by hypoxia and that this effect is related to a sharp increase in vagal tone due to pulmonary chemo-

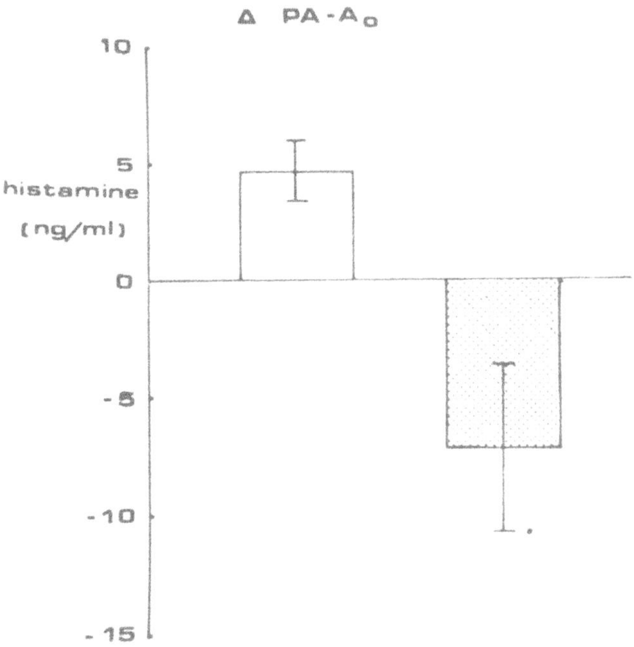

Fig. 4. Difference in histamine content of pulmonary artery and aorta before (solid column) and after (dotted column) 5 min hypoxia. Note that, while in the control period there is a histamine release, hypoxia induces uptake of the agent by the lungs.
All numbers represent mean ± 1 SE n 7
*Different from control, $P < 0.05$

reflexes (26).

Furthermore, we have studied the effect of chlorpheniramine on some spirometric parameters in patients affected by chronic obstructive lung disease. In these patients the administration of this drug decreased the airways resistances and the residual volume/total lung volume ratio and improved the maximum breathing capacity (Fig. 6) and the forced expiratory volume (Fig. 7) while it had no effect in normal subjects (27). This study could suggest a direct effect of chlorpheniramine on smooth muscle. So it is possible that chlorpheniramine

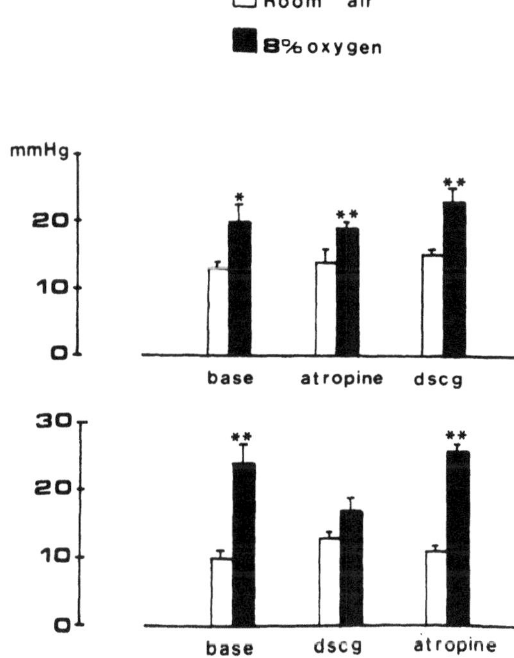

Fig. 5. Changes in mean pulmonary artery pressure induced by 5 min of hypoxia under control conditions and after i.v. administration of atropine (0,5 mg) and atropine plus DSCG (8 mg/Kg) (upper pannel) and before and after i.v. administration of DSCG 8 mg/Kg and DSCG plus atropine (0,5 mg) (lower pannel). Statistical analysis was performed by comparing data collected before and after each hypoxic period.
* = Different from control, $P < 0.05$
** = Different from control, $P < 0.01$
Each bar represents mean ± 1 SE

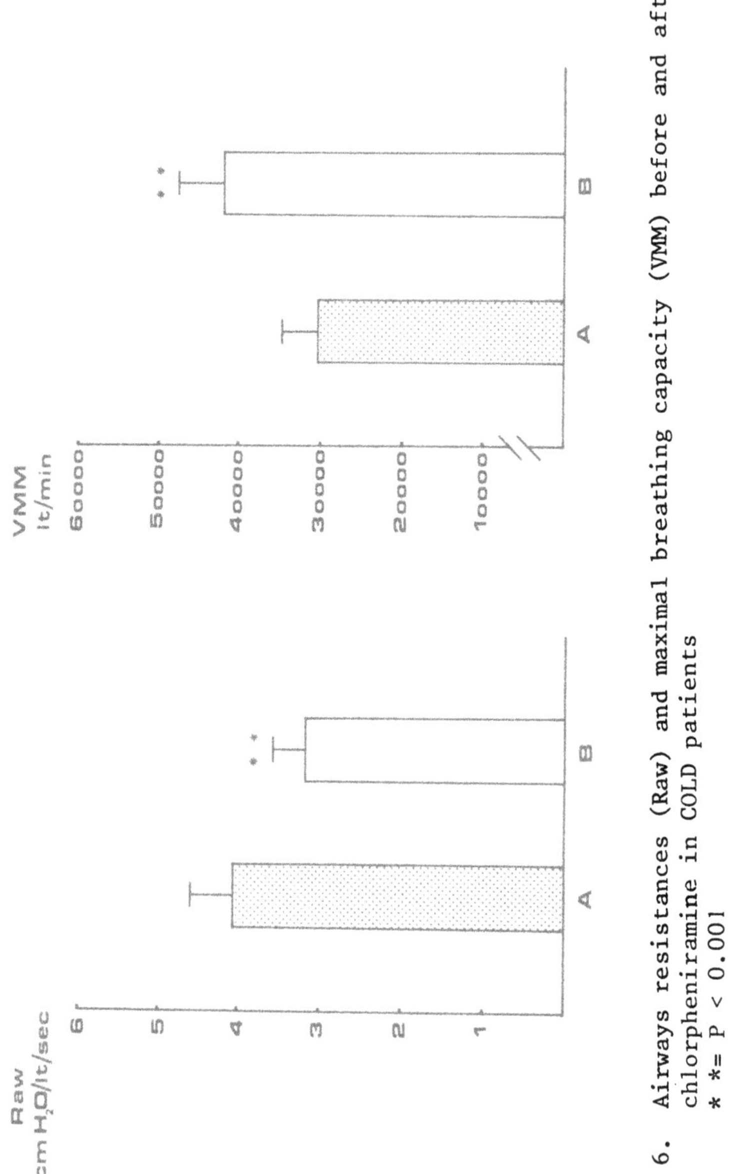

Fig. 6. Airways resistances (Raw) and maximal breathing capacity (VMM) before and after chlorpheniramine in COLD patients
* *= $P < 0.001$

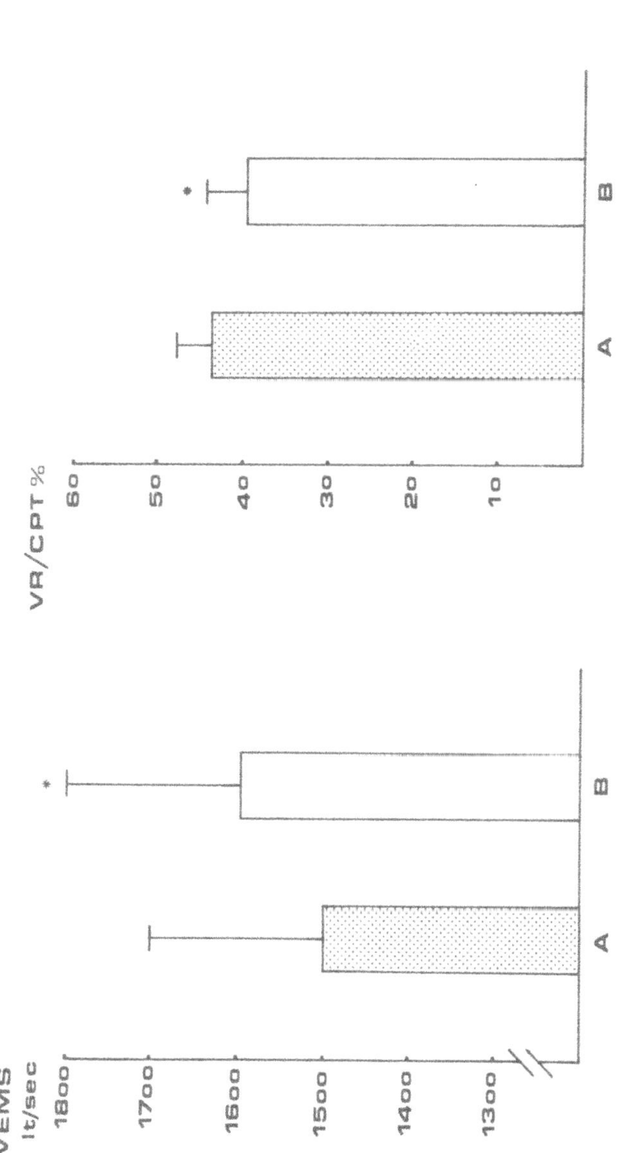

Fig. 7. Maximal second expiration velocity (VEMS) and residual volume/total lung volume ratio before and after chlorpheniramine in COLD patients
* *= P < 0.001

Table II. Effect of histamine infusion (0,4 ng/Kg/min) on the cardiovascular system

EFFECT OF HISTAMINE INFUSION (0.4 ng/Kg/min) ON THE CARDIOVASCULAR SYSTEM			
	CONTROL	HISTAMINE INFUSION	POST INFUSION
HEART RATE (BEATS/MIN)	68±7	97±7	70±7
SYSTOLIC AORTIC PRESSURE (mm Hg)	130±13	101±13	126±6
DIASTOLIC AORTIC PRESSURE (mm Hg)	70±7	48±5	69±7
CARDIAC INDEX (L/min/m^2)	3.5±.3	4.2±.3	3.2±.3
STOKE INDEX (ml/m^2)	51±1	46±3	48±6
SYSTEMIC VASCULAR RESISTANCE (dyne-sec-cm^{-5})	1170±113	724±57	1237±42
LV/dP/dT MAX (mm Hg/sec)	1589±146	1860±165	1639±22
LVEDP (mmHg)	8.3±.1	3.0±.6	8.3±.7
MEAN PULMONARY ARTERIAL PRESSURE (mmHg)	13±3	10±1.5	15.6±3.2
PULMONARY VASCULAR RESISTANCE (dynes-sec-cm^{-5})	43±12	25±5	77±22
PLASMA HISTAMINE (ng/ml)	0.3±.01	6±1	0.2
PLASMA EPINEPHRINE (pg/ml)	28.8±9	79.6±17	34.3±6
PLASMA NOREPINEPHRINE (pg/ml)	332.6±11	534.8±20	314±64

improves pulmonary function in COLD patients by means of a precise action on bronchial smooth muscle. On the other hand it is possible that chlorpheniramine reduces pulmonary vascular resistances in COLD patients causing a general depression of vascular reactivity. Recently, Altura and Altura have shown that antihistamines exhibit numerous pharmacologic properties that can affect blood vessels (28). Finally, we have studied the cardiovascular effect of intravenous H infusion (0,4 mg/Kg/min) in subjects with normal left ventricular function undergoing diagnostic cardiac catheterization. After 2-5 min of H infusion we observed a significant increase in heart rate, cardiac index, LV dp/dT and decrease of systolic, diastolic and mean aortic pressure, LV end diastolic pressure, stroke index and systemic vascular resistances. H infusion failed to produce any significant changes in mean pulmonary arterial pressure and pulmonary vascular resistances. Truly, there was an increase in plasma catecholamines during H infusion, however such an increase is unable to produce in man hemodynamic variation in amount observed in our study (Tab II).

In conclusion, so far the mediator of pulmonary hypoxic hypertension remains still unkown and the response of pulmonary vessels to hypoxia is more complex and moreover one or more humoral mediators concur together with changes in autonomic nervous system tone in the genesis of pulmonary hypertension by hypoxia.

REFERENCES

1. D.M. Aviado, The lung circulation, vol 1. Oxford Pergamon Press, 1965.
2. U.S. von Euler, G. Liljestrand, Observation on the pulmonary arterial blood pressure in the cat. Acta Physiol. Scand. 12:301 (1964).
3. G.G. Nahas, M.B. Visscher, G.W. Mather, F.J. Haddy, H.R. Warner, Influence of hypoxia on the pulmonary circulation in nonarcotized dogs. J. Appl. Physiol. 6:467 (1954).
4. D.M. Aviado, The pharmacology of the pulmonary circulation. Pharmacol. Rev. 12:159 (1960).
5. T.C. Lloyd Jr., The role of nerve pathways in the hypoxic vasoconstriction of lung. J. Appl. Physiol. 21:1351 (1961).
6. A.P. Fishman, H.W. Fritts, A. Cournand, Effects of acute hypoxia and exercise on the pulmonary circulation. Circulation 22: 220 (1960).
7. R.M. Goldring, G.M. Turino, G. Cohen, A.G. Jamieson, B.G. Bass, A.P. Fishman, the catecholamines in the pulmonary arterial pressor response to acute hypoxia. J. Clin. Invest. 41:1211 (1962).
8. E. Housley, S.W. Clarke, R.B. Hedworth-Whitty, J.M. Bishop, Effect of acute and chronic acidemia and associated hypoxia on the pulmonary circulation of patients with chronic

bronchitis. Cardiovasc. Res. 4:482 (1970).
9. E.H. Bergofsky, Mechanisms underlying vasomotor regulation of regional pulmonary blood flow in normal and disease states. Am. J. Med. 57:378 (1974).
10. E.D. Silove, R.F. Grover, Effects of alpha adrenergic blockade and tissue catecholamine depletion on pulmonary vascular response to hypoxia. J. Clin. Invest. 47:274 (1968).
11. R.J. Porcelli, E.H. Bergofsky, Adrenergic receptors in pulmonary vasoconstrictor response to gaseous and humoral agents. J. Appl. Physiol. 34:483 (1973).
12. R.J. Porcelli, A. Viau, M. Demeny, E. Naftchin, E.H. Bergofsky, Relation between hypoxic pulmonary vasoconstriction, its humoral mediators and alpha-beta adrenergic receptors. The 19th Aspen lung conference. The pulmonary circulation. Chest 71 (Suppl.) 310 (1977).
13. A.P. Fishman, Hypoxia on the pulmonary circulation. How and where it acts. Circ. Res. 38:221 (1976).
14. H.N. Duke, E.M. Kollock, J.V. Marchant, Changes in pH of the perfusate during hypoxia in isolated perfused cat lungs. J. Physiol. (London) 157:90 (1960).
15. R. Detar, D.F. Bohr, Contractile responses of isolated vascular smooth muscle during prolonged exposure to anoxia. Am. J. Physiol. 2:1269 (1972).
16. G. Liljestrand, Chemical control of the pulmonary blood flow. Acta Physiol. Scand. 44:216 (1958).
17. J.L. Walker, The regulatory function of prostaglandins in the release of histamine and SRS A from passively sensitized human lung tissue. Advances in Biosciences 253:9 (1973).
18. A.A. Mathè, Studies on actions of prostaglandins in the lung. Acta Physiol. Scand. Suppl. 441 (1976).
19. A. Hague, K.L. Melmon, Role of histamine in hypoxic pulmonary hypertension in the rat. II depletion of histamine, serotonin and catecholamins. Circ. Res. 22:385 (1968).
20. A. Hague, N.C. Staub, Prevention of hypoxic vasoconstriction in cat lung by histamine-releasing agent 48/80. J. Appl. Physiol. 26:693 (1969).
21. A. Susmano, R.A. Carleton, Prevention of hypoxic pulmonary hypertension by chlorpheniramine. J. Appl. Physiol. 31: 531 (1971).
22. F. Haas, E.H. Bergofsky, role of the mast-cell in the pulmonary pressor response to hypoxia. J. Clin. Invest. 51:3154 (1972).
23. C.A. Dowson, F.A. Delano, L.H. Hamilton and W.J. Stekiel, Histamine releasers and hypoxic vasoconstriction in isolated cat lungs. J. Appl. Physiol. 17:670 (1974).
24. F. Iodice, F. Piscione, G. Giuffrida, G. De Michele, Les effects des antihistaminiques sur l'hypertension pulmonaire par hypoxie chronique chez l'homme.
25. F. Rengo, B. Trimarco, M. Chiariello, B. Ricciardelli, M. Volpe, R. Violini, G. Rasetti, Histamine and hypoxic pulmonary hypertension. A quantitative study. Cardiovasc. Res. 12:

752 (1978).

26. F. Rengo, B. Trimarco, B. Ricciardelli, M. Volpe, R. Violini, L. Saccà, M. Chiariello, Effects of disodium cromoglycate on hypoxic pulmonary hypertension in dog. J. Pharmacol. Exper. Ther. 211:686 (1979).

27. D. Bonaduce, P. Scarafile, L. De Caprio, M. Petretta, G. De Fabrizio, A. Carlomagno. Effetti della clorfeniramina sulle resistenze bronchiali in soggetti affetti da broncopneumopatia ostruttiva. In: Atti Internacional Conference on Pneumology and of European Specialist Physicians. Eolian Islands, Messina 1977.

28. B.M. Altura, B.T. Altura, Effects of local anesthetics antihistamines and glucocorticoids on peripheral blood flow and vascular smooth muscle. Anesthesiology 41:197 (1974).

PLATELETS, HYPOXEMIA AND PULMONARY HYPERTENSION

Giuseppe G. Nenci

Institute of Semeiotica Medica
University of Perugia Medical School
Policlinico Monteluce
06100 Perugia, Italy

The capacity of hypoxia to induce pulmonary hypertension (PH) in animals and in man has been known for many years (von Euler and Liljestrand, 1974; Motley et al., 1974). Some evidence exists that platelets may undergo changes in function and in number because of an altitude hypoxemia (Sharma et al., 1979; Sharma, 1980). This, together with altitude decompression, may even lead to a pulmonary sequestration of platelets (Gray et al., 1975). Nevertheless, it seems doubtful that platelets significantly contribute to the enhancement of pulmonary vascular resistance induced by hypoxia.

In hypoxemic patients, on the other hand, many parallel facts which are verified in the lungs and platelets (Table 1) suggest that an important part of PH in patients with chronic obstructive pulmonary disease (COPD) is mediated through the activation of platelets and the release from them of powerful pulmonary vasoconstrictor substances, such as serotonin (Rickaby et al., 1980) or thromboxane A_2 (TXA_2) (Svensson et al., 1977; Dusting et al., 1979).

Steel et al. (1977) and more recently Tremoli et al. (1980) and we ourselves (fig. 1) have demonstrated that in patients with severe COPD and PH, hypoxemia is associated with a shortened platelet survival or regeneration time as well as with enhanced plasma levels of β-thromboglobulin (fig. 2), a protein that is released from platelets when they are activated or destroyed.

Results obtained in experimental acute respiratory failure suggest that damaged endothelium and not damaged platelets produce the entrapment and activation of platelets induced by hypoxemia (Hechtman et al., 1978). In fact, hypoxemia has shown to produce breaks in the endothelium (Kjeldsen, 1975) which might result in an increased platelet-surface interaction. This would cause a release of platelet vasoconstrictor agents in the blood circulating in the pulmonary

Table 1. HYPOXEMIC PULMONARY HYPERTENSION

FACTS

In Lung	In Platelets
(Hypoxia induces PH)	(Hypoxia may lead to platelet consumption or segregation)
Hypoxemia induces or worsens PH in patients with COPD	Hypoxemia is associated with shortened PST in patients with COPD
Hypoxemic PH is, at least in part, reversible	Platelets release substances that evoke a pulmonary vasoconstriction

HYPOTHESIS

Antiplatelet Drugs Could

Avert or Reverse

Hypoxemic Pulmonary Hypertension

vascular bed. It has indeed been demonstrated that it is a pulmonary vasoconstriction rather than an intravascular obstruction that causes the platelet-mediate PH (Rådegran et al., 1971; Bo and Hognestad, 1972), and this is also true when a microembolisation of the lung is produced by the infusions of platelet aggregating substances or even of glass beads (Mlczoch et al., 1978).

It is interesting to note that an increase in arterial PO_2 produces an increase in platelet survival time in patients with hypoxemia (Johnson et al., 1978), exactly as their pulmonary vascular resistance is lowered by continuous oxygen therapy, as was established many years ago by Levine et al. (1967) and Abraham et al. (1968). The liability and reversibility of PH is also suggested by the demonstration that initially, PH is only nocturnal in patients with COPD and oxygen desaturation limited to the sleep, and that this nocturnal PH may be abolished with low-flow oxygen administration during the night (Boysen et al., 1979). In addition, the observation of Kirby (1980) of the strong correlation between PH and indices of pulmonary gas exchange, but not between PH and lung volumes leaves little doubt about the relationship existing between PH and hypoxemia in patients with COPD. From what has been said, it may be inferred that it should be possible to revert hypoxemic pulmonary hypertension,

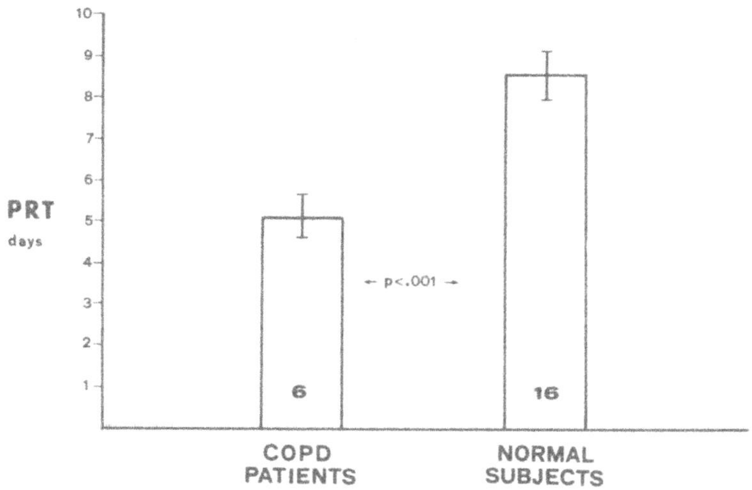

Fig. 1. Platelet regeneration time (PRT) in normal subjects and in patients with hypoxemic pulmonary hypertension.

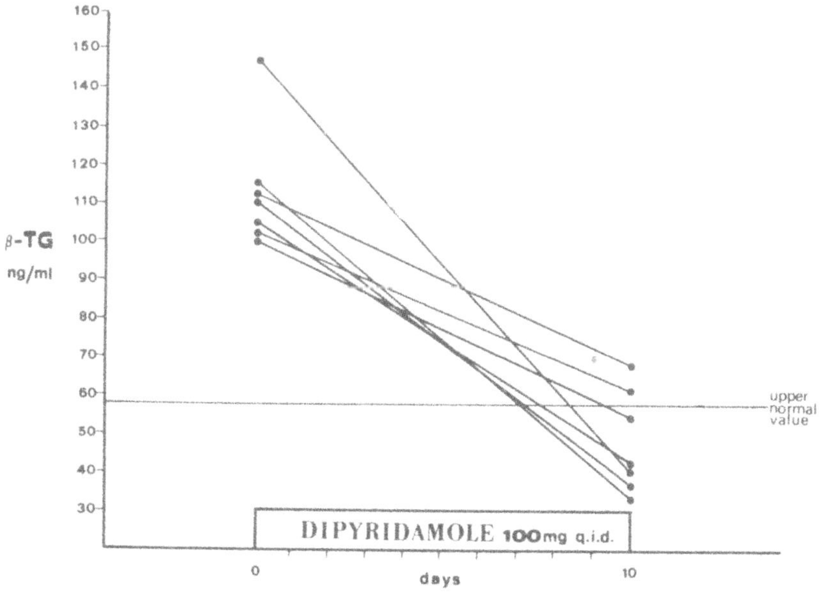

Fig. 2. Plasma levels of β-thromboglobulin (β-TG) in seven patients with COPD: effect of dipyridamole.

or at least a part of it, not only by oxygen therapy but also by drugs that inhibit platelet functions. One could, in fact, not only suppose that platelets may be involved in the thromboembolic complications that develop in patients with hypoxemia, as Steel et al. (1977) have suggested, but also that they could be responsible in providing the smooth muscle contracting substances that consolidate and aggravate hypoxemic PH. The hypothesis that we shall deal with and which we intend to verify is thus that the use of appropriate antiplatelet drugs allows us to obtain a slowing down, or even a regression, in the evolution of hypoxemic PH.

Primary PH has been treated with some success with many vasodilators, including hydralazine (Rubin and Peter, 1978) and diazoxide (Wang et al., 1978). When indomethacin, an inhibitor of cyclooxigenase, and therefore a powerful antiplatelet agent was tried, it was reported to be both ineffective by Nagasaka et al. (1978) and effective, by Person and Proctor (1979). Clearly, patients with primary PH are not the best models to test the hypothesis here considered, because their arterial haemoglobin saturation is usually normal both at rest and during exercise. Moreover, primary PH is probably not a distinct disorder but a non-homogeneous group of disorders with varying etiology (Wagenvoort and Wagenvoort, 1970). As the lung is the main organ of prostaglandin synthesis and degradation, the possibility that some cases may be related to a disorder of these functions must be considered. Perhaps the contrasting responses evoked by prostaglandin antagonists reflect this underlying non-homogeneity, as Person and Proctor (1979) pointed out.

On the contrary, patients with COPD and PH are usually hypoxemic and often the decrease in arterial oxygen tension is pronounced so that they may constitute an ideal tool for challenging our working hypothesis.

In choosing the drugs that could be useful in improving hypoxemic PH through an inhibition of platelet functions, it must be considered that many of them interfere more or less directly with the synthesis or the action of prostaglandins, and mention must be made of the fact that major active end products in the prostaglandin synthesis from arachidonic acid in the two districts, of lung and platelets, show distinctly opposite properties.

Prostacyclin (PGI_2) is a normal product of pulmonary vessels which is released from the lungs into the circulating blood (Gryglewski et al., 1978; Watkins et al., 1980). PGI_2 acts as a powerful pulmonary vasodilator and inhibitor of platelet aggregation, while platelet-derived thromboxane A_2 (TXA_2) stimulates platelet aggregation and may be associated with pulmonary vasoconstriction and bronchoconstriction (Dusting et al., 1979; Svensson et al., 1977). The administration of PGI_2 could then lower pulmonary vascular resistance and relieve PH both by dilating pulmonary vascular smooth muscle and by contemporaneously inhibiting the aggregation of platelets and release of vasoactive substances. In effect, PGI_2 infusions have recently proven to be effective in a case of severe chronic idiopathic PH described by Watkins et al. (1980).

The drugs that inhibit platelet and vessel-wall cyclooxygenase (such as aspirin, indomethacin and, to a lesser extent, sulfinpirazone) contrast platelet release reactions but may contemporaneously impair the formation of prostaglandins in the lung. Since the physiological and pharmacological properties of PGI_2 and PGE_1 are opposite to those of PGG_2, PGH_2, TXA_2, TXB_2 and $PGF_{2\alpha}$ in the lung and in platelets (Hyman et al., 1978), the effect of these drugs on hypoxemic PH may produce unpredictable results. Although it has been shown that vessel-wall cyclooxygenase is less sensitive than platelet cyclooxygenase to these drugs, it is not yet well defined which doses can affect platelet thromboxane synthesis without impairing the vessel-wall production of prostaglandins in the majority of patients (Moncada and Korbut, 1978). Additional difficulties also arise from the considerable between-persons difference in the response to aspirin (O'Brien, 1980).

In effect, prostaglandin synthesis inhibitors have not proven able to decrease hypoxic pulmonary vasoconstriction (Weir et al., 1976), indomethacin causes an inhibition of the hydralazine-induced attenuation of hypoxic PH (Rubin, 1980), and both aspirin and indomethacin have ever been shown by Hales et al. (1978) to induce a fourfold increase of alveolar hypoxic pulmonary vasoconstriction in weak-reactor dogs. Furthermore, these drugs have been proven able to produce the constriction of a patent ductus arteriosus in the newborn (F riedman et al., 1976), and when given in the treatment of preterm labour, they inhibit fetal prostaglandin synthesis, thus causing the constriction of the ductus arteriosus in utero, PH, and the growth of pulmonary smooth muscle (Rudolph, 1978). Although sulfinpyrzone has been shown able to lengthen platelet survival in one-half of the patients with hypoxemia and PH, this drug did not alter either arterial oxygen tension, or pulmonary artery pressure, as stated by Steel et al. (1977).

Only in the very different case when PH or bronchoconstriction is experimentally evoked by direct activation of the platelets, do aspirin and sulfinpyrazone, when preliminarily administered, exert a preventive effect which may result to the same extent as platelet depletion (Rådegran et al., 1971; Mlczoch et al., 1978). This clearly occurs through the inhibition of platelet response to the action of stimulators.

In contrast to cyclooxygenase inhibitors, that lower the vessel-wall production of PGI_2, phosphodiesterase inhibitors, such as dipyridamole, seem to act through the potentiation (Moncada and Korbut, 1978) and prolongation (Jorgensen et al., 1978) of the effect of prostacyclin and/or stimulation of its biosynthesis (Blass et al., 1980; Neri Serneri et al., 1980). The data of Neri Serneri, however, suggest that this last effect is unique for dipyridamole and not for other phosphodiesterase inhibitors.

Dipyridamole has been demonstrated by Tremoli et al. (1980) to prolong the short platelet regeneration time in the COPD patients and additionally, we have shown that the increased plasma level of β-htromboglobulin in hypoxemic patients is also corrected by dipyri-

Table 2. The PHPH Trial a double-blind corssover study

Aim	Verify if dipyridamole (100 mg q.i.d.) can contain or reverse the PH of patients with COPD
Treatments	3mo. on drug + 3mo. on placebo (random sequence) Acetylcysteine 100 mg q.i.d. added to both treatments 10 days of treatment with other drugs toletated in first 2 mo. of each treatment
Patients	20 male subjects aged 30 to 70 yrs with COPD and: Ppa > 30/15 mmHg PaO_2 < 60 mmHg informed consent
Evaluation of at { entry, crossover, end }	lung volumes and airway dynamics (whole body plethysmography) blood gas tensions and pH right atrium, right ventricel and pulmonary artery pressure responsiveness to acute normobaric hyperoxia platelet activation (β-thromboglobulin) and consumption (PRT)

Table 3. The PHPH Trial in 1980 Patients entered and completed: 6

Main base-line data		
Ppa s/d	mean 49/23·(39-56/16-30)	mmHg
PaO	mean 50.8 (46-59)	mmHg
FEV %Pred.	mean 37.0 (28-49)	%
PRT	mean 5.08 (3.9-6.0)	days
MDA basal v.	mean 3.09 (2.4-3.4)	nM/10 Plts

damole (fig. 2).

With the aim of verifying whether dipyridamole, through its prostacyclin adjuvant activity, is able to revert some of the PH of patients with COPD, we have initiated a double-blind crossover study, and have called it the Persantin Hypoxemic Pulmonary Hypertension Trial (Table 2).

Of the six patients who have entered and completed the trial this year, main data at entry are here presented (Table 3). As may be seen, all patients were hypoxemic, had a pulmonary hypertension and a very significant shortening of platelet regeneration time. Of course, no interim results can be given, because of the double-blindness of this trial, which will end October 1981.

REFERENCES

Abraham, A.S., Cole, R.B., Bishop, J.M., 1968, Reversal of pulmonary hypertension by prolonged oxygen administration to patients with chronic bronchitis. Circ. Res. 23:147.

Blass, K.E., Block, H.U., Förster, W., Pönicke, K., 1980, Dipyridamole, a potent stimulator of Prostacyclin (PGI_2) biosynthesis. Br. J. Pharmacol. 68:71.

Bø, G., Hognestad, J., 1972, Effects on the pulmonary circulation of suddenly induced intravascular aggregation of blood platelets. Acta Physiol. Scand. 85:523.

Boysen, P.G., Block, A.J., Wynne, J.W., Hunt, L.A., Flick, M.R., 1979, Nocturnal pulmonary hypertension in patients with chronic obstructive pulmonary disease. Chest 76:536.

Dusting, J.D., Moncada, S., Vane, J., 1979, Prostaglandins, their intermediates and precursors: cardiovascular actions and regulatory roles in normal and abnormal circulatory systems. Prog. Cardiovasc. Dis. 21:405.

von Euler, V.S., Liljestrand, G., 1947, Observation on the pulmonary arterial blood pressure in the cat. Acta Physiol. Scand. 12:301.

Friedman, W.F., Hirschklau, M.G., Printz, M.P., Pitlik, P.T., Kirkpatrick, S.E., 1976, Pharmacological closure of patent ductus arteriosus in the premature infant. N. Engl. J. Med. 295:526.

Gray, J.W., Bryan, A.C., Freedman, M.H., Houston, C.S., Lews, W.F., McFadden, D.M., Newell, G.,1975, Effect of altitude exposure on platelets. J. Appl. Physiol. 39:648.

Gryglewski, R.J., Korbut, R., Ocetkeiwicz, A., 1978, Generation of prostacyclin by lungs in vivo and its release into the arterial circulation. Nature 273:765.

Hales, C.A., Rouse, E.T., Slate, J.L., 1978, Influence of aspirin and indomethacin on variability of alveolar hypoxic vasoconstriction. J. Appl. Physiol. 45:33.

Hechtman, H.B., Lonergan, E.A., Staunton, H.P.B., Dennis, R.C., Shepro, D., 1978, Pulmonary entrapment of platelets during acute respiratory failure. Surgery 83:277.

Hyman, A.L., Spannhake, E.W., Kadowitz, P.F., 1978, Prostaglandins and the lung. Am. Rev. Resp. Dis. 117:111.

Johnson, T.S., Ellis, J.H., Steele, P.P., 1978, Improvement of platelet survival time with oxygen in patients with chronic obstructive airways disease. Am. Rev. Resp. Dis. 117:255.

Jorgensen, K.A., Dyerberg, J., Stoffersen, E., 1979, Prostacyclin (PGI_2) and the effect of phosphodiesterase inhibitors on platelet aggregation. Pharm. Res. Commun. 11:605.

Kirby, B.J., 1980, Relationship between pulmonary gas exchange and pulmonary hypertension in chronic obstructive lung disease. Bull. Europ. Physiopath. Resp. 16:74.

Kjeldsen, K., 1975, The effect of hypoxia on the fine structure of the aortic intima of rabbits. Lab. Invest. 33:533.

Levine, B.E., Bigelow, D.B., Hamstra, R.O., er al., 1967, The role of long term continuous oxygen administration in patients with chronic airway obstruction with hypoxemia. Ann. Intern. Med. 66:639.

Mlczoch, J., Tucker, A., Weir, E.K., Reeves, J.T., Grover, R.F., 1978, Platelet-mediated pulmonary hypertension and hypoxia during pulmonary microembolism. Reduction by platelet inhibition. Chest 74:684.

Moncada, S., Korbut, R., 1978, Dipyridamole and other phosphodiesterase inhibitors act as antithrombotic agents by potentiating endogenous prostacyclin. Lancet 1:1286.

Motley, H.L., Cournand, A., Werko, L. et al., 1947, The influence of short periods of induced acute anoxia upon pulmonary artery pressure in man. Am. J. Physiol. 150:315.

Nagasaka, Y., Hiroshi, A., Lee, Y.S., et al., 1978, Long-term favourable effect of oxygen administration on a patient with primary pulmonary hypertension. Chest 74:299.

Neri Serneri, G.G., Masotti, G., Poggesi, L., Galanti, G., Castellani, S., Dipyridamole stimulates prostacyclin biosynthesis in man and in vitro. In: 6th International Congress on Thrombosis, Mediterranean League Against Thromboembolic Diseases, Monte-Carlo, October 23-25, 1980.

O'Brien, J.R., 1980, Platelets and the vessel wall: how much aspirin? Lancet 1:372.

Person, B., Proctor, R., 1979, Primary pulmonary hypertension: response to indomethacin, terbutaline and isoproterenol. Chest 76:601.

Rådegran, K., Bergentz, S.E., Lewis, D.H., Ljungquist, U., Olsson, P., 1971, Pulmonary effects of induced platelet aggregation. Intravascular obstruction or vasoconstriction? Scand. J. Clin. Lab. Invest. 28:423.

Rickaby, D.A., Dawson, C.A., Maron, M.B., 1980, Pulmonary inactivation of serotonin and site of serotonin pulmonary vasoconstriction. J. Appl. Physiol. 48:606.

Rubin, L.J., 1980, The influence of prostaglandin synthesis inhibition on the effects of hydralazine in dogs with hypoxic pulmonary hypertension. Am. Rev. Resp. Dis. 121:444.
Rubin, L.J., Peter, R.H., 1978, Oral hydralazine therapy for primary pulmonary hypertension. N. Engl. J. Med. 302:69.
Rudolph, A.M., 1978, Effects of prostaglandins and synthetase inhibitors on the fetal circulation. In: Preterm labour, A. Anderson, R. Beard, M. Brudenell, P. Dunn, Eds. Royal College of Obstetricians and Gynaecologists, p. 231-242.
Sharma, S.C., 1980, Platelet count on acute induction to high altitude. Thrombos. Haemostas. 43:29.
Sharma, S.C., Balasubramanian, V., Chadha, K.S., 1979, Platelet adhesiveness in permanent residents of high altitude. Thrombos. Haemostas. 42:1508.
Steele, P., Ellis, J.H., Wiley, H.S., Genton, E., 1977, Platelet survival time in patients with hypoxemia and pulmonary hypertension. Circulation 55:660.
Svensson, J., Strandberg, T., Tuveno, T., Hamberg, M., 1977, Thromboxane A_2: effects on airway and vascular smooth muscle. Prostaglandins. 14:426.
Tremoli, E., Bertoli, L., Maderna, P., Conti, F., Merlini, R., Mantero, O., 1980, Platelet anti-aggregating therapy in chronic obstructive lung disease. Clin. Resp. Physiol. 16:84.
Wagenvoort, C.A., Wagenvoort N., 1970, Primary pulmonary hypertension: a pathologic study of the lung vessels in 156 clinically diagnosed cases. Circulation 42:1163.
Wang, S.W.S., Pohl, J.E.F., Rowlands, D.J., Wade, E.G., 1978, Diazoxide treatment of primary pulmonary hypertension. Brit. Heart J. 40:572.
Watkins, W.D., Peterson, M.B., Crone, R.K., Shannon, D.C., Levine, L., 1980, Prostacyclin and Prostaglandin E_1 for severe idiopathic pulmonary artery hypertension. Lancet 1:1083.
Weir, E.K., McMurty, I.F., Tucker, A., Reeves, J.T., Grover, R.F., 1976, Prostaglandin synthetase inhibitors do not decrease hypoxic pulmonary vasoconstriction. J. Appl. Physiol. 41:714.

THE DIAGNOSIS AND MANAGEMENT OF PULMONARY EMBOLISM

Graham A.H. Miller

Brompton Hospital
Fulham Road
London SW3 6HP
England

The first essential when discussing the diagnosis and management of pulmonary embolism is to distinguish between different types of embolism since the presentation, physical signs and prognosis are profoundly influenced by, in particular, the duration and severity of embolism. In the past much confusion has been caused by the use of imprecise terms such as "symptomatic embolism" and by failure to distinguish between signs that are due to embolism per-se and those due to co-existing cardio-respiratory disease. In this presentation I will confine my remarks to the effects of embolism occurring in patients without other cardiorespiratory disease. We recognise four clinical syndromes resulting from pulmonary thromboembolism. These can be distinguished on the clinical history and are (1) Acute minor embolism (2) Acute massive embolism (3) Sub-acute massive embolism and (4) Chronic thrombo-embolic pulmonary hypertension.

In acute minor embolism the symptoms are of pleuritic pain and haemoptysis due to pulmonary "infarction". There is no haemodynamic disturbance and no specific treatment is required. Spontaneous recovery without sequelae is the rule. In acute massive pulmonary embolism there is a profound haemodynamic disturbance which dominates the presentation. The patient presents with "collapse" or syncope and acute-onset dyspnoea but pleuritic pain is only a feature in a minority. Urgent treatment is required and can be life-saving. In sub-acute massive embolism the history is of gradually increasing breathlessness over days or weeks, episodes of pleurisy and haemoptysis and symptoms due to deep-vein thrombosis (painful, swollen leg) are common. Such patients have a significantly higher pulmonary artery pressure than those with acute massive embolism but treatment is the same. Finally patients with chronic thrombo-embolic pulmonary hypertension present with a history of gradually increasing breathlessness and of effort syncope. A history of deep vein thrombosis or of pleurisy/haemoptysis is often lacking. Such patients have the highest pulmonary artery pressures of all. The prognosis is grave and there is no effective treatment. For the remainder of this presentation I shall discuss the diagnosis and management of massive pulmonary embolism since this is the one condition which is life-threatening and for which treatment is effective. The symptoms and signs of acute massive embolism are due to the haemodynamic disturbance and can be categorized under three headings; (1) Acute right ventricular failure (2) Acute disturbance of pulmonary ventilation and perfusion and (3) Acute reduction of cardiac output.

(1) Acute right ventricular failure and dilatation may be responsible for central chest pain (angina) present in one third of patients and important since it may lead to an erroneous diagnosis of myocardial infarction. Right ventricular failure is detected by (a) elevation of central venous pressure, (b) a gallop rhythm (summation gallop) at the left sternal edge and, (c) delayed, but usually inaudible, pulmonary valve closure sound. The acutely stressed, previously normal, right ventricle is unable to generate a pressure of more than 50 mmHg. Thus there are no signs of pulmonary hypertension. At cardiac catheterisation we detect a raised right atrial and right ventricular end-diastolic pressure and a pulmonary artery pressure of 40-50 mmHg.

(2) Acute disturbance of pulmonary ventilation and perfusion. This is responsible for the symptoms of acute dispnoea and the observed tachypnoea and hyperventilation. Arterial desaturation (average saturation 85%) present in almost all patients may only be detectable clinically in about 2/3 of patients and is probably due to some continuing perfusion of collapsed non-ventilated alveoli. This together with hyperventilation is responsible for the typical blood-gas picture of a low $pO2$ and a low $pCO2$.

(3) Acute reduction of cardiac output is the result of reduced pulmonary venous return to the left heart which is otherwise unaffected. The low output is responsible for syncope or cardiac arrest and for the signs of shock. Thus the diagnosis of massive pulmonary embolism is made when the signs of right ventricular failure are detected in a shocked patient with dispnoea of acute onset.

If I have laboured the clinical diagnosis of pulmonary embolism it is because it is still our experience that the diagnosis is frequently missed or made in patients who do not have massive embolism. The condition which is most frequently miss-diagnosed as pulmonary embolism is septicaemic shock but such patients do not have the signs of right ventricular failure.

Turning now to management our first concern is with the rescussitation of a collapsed patient. Here the conventional measures of correction of acidosis, oxygen administration and external cardiac massage are appropriate. In addition there is one important consideration in massive embolism - the need to maintain right ventricular function. Right ventricular function is critically dependant on filling pressure - venous return; and this is maximal in the supine position. Thus the patient must be nursed flat and no drugs should be given which can cause vasodilatation. Morphine and diuretics are contraindicated. Nor should anything else be done which might reduce venous return - there is thus no place for operations on the inferior vena cava in the management of acute embolism.

The next step in the management of such patients is to establish the diagnosis beyond doubt. Combined pulmonary ventilation and perfusion scanning can do this but we prefer to visualise the emboli directly by cardiac catheterisation and pulmonary arteriography. We now have experience of over 100 patients with massive embolism studied in this way without mortality or morbidity.

Specific treatment with either thrombolysis (streptokinase) or emergency pulmonary embolectomy can now be started. It has been shown that streptokinase accelerates the resolution of pulmonary emboli. Whether or not this actually saves lives is difficult to prove - though I have no doubt that it does. Certainly when we look at the "treatment failure rate" - that is to say the numbers of patients in each treatment group (embolectomy, streptokinase or heparin) who deteriorate on treatment or suffer a complication of treatment. We find that streptokinase or embolectomy appear equally effective but heparin treatment alone certainly results not only in much slower resolution but also in a higher "treatment failure rate". Our policy today is to use streptokinase in all cases of massive embolism unless there is a contraindication to thrombolytic therapy. When thrombolysis is contra indicated we employ emergency pulmonary embolectomy on cardio-pulmonary bypass. In either case the mortality and morbidity in patients who have survived long enough for specific treatment to have been started should be much less than 25%.

Finally there is the question of the long-term outlook. Many people imagine that recurrent embolism and the development of pulmonary hypertension are significant complications of acute pulmonary embolism. Our experience is that these complications rarely, if ever, occur in energetically treated patients; as a result we see no place for the frequently performed procedures for placing a "filter" in the inferior vena-cava.

PLATELET ACTIVITY IN RELATION TO SMOKE AND EXERCISE IN PATIENTS WITH CHRONIC OBSTRUCTIVE LUNG DISEASE: EFFECTS OF PLATELET ANTIAGGREGATING DRUGS

S. Novo, G. Davì, G. Caimi[**], F. Castello, L. Valdes[***], S. Marino, A. Romano[**], M. Fazio, B. La Menza, A. Mazzola, G. Carpentiere, A. Sarno[*], and A. Strano

Institute of Clinical Medicine and Medical Therapy I°, [*]Respiratory Function Service, [**]Institute of Clinical Medicine III, [***]Institute of pharmacology - University of Palermo - Piazza delle Cliniche, 2 - Palermo, Italy

Lung tissue is involved in the synthesis and/or metabolism of many vasoactive substances such as histamine, serotonin, dopamine, norepinephrine, bradikinin, angiotensin II and prostaglandins (1).

Prostaglandins, in the lung, have the ability to increase or decrease the tone of respiratory tract smooth muscle (2).

Some reports indicate that the endoperoxide intermediates (PGG_2 -PGH_2), endoperoxide analogs PGE_2, $PGF_{2\alpha}$ and PGD_2, increase pulmonary vascular resistances in a variety of species (3).

The endoperoxide analogs $PGF_{2\alpha}$ and PGD_2 increase lung resistance and decrease dynamic compliance like arachidonic acid (3).

Moreover, from clinical studies in asthmatics it is confirmed that PGE_1, given intravenously, and PGE_1 and PGE_2, given as inhalation aerosols, produce bronchodilation (2), but PGE_1 occasionally and PGE_2 frequently determine bronchoconstriction (4).

The pulmonary vascular effects of TxA_2 are uncertain, but this substance has potent smooth muscle stimulating and platelet aggregating activity and its breakdown product, TxB_2, has modest pressor activity in the pulmonary vascular bed (5).

In contrast to the effects of PGH_2, PGG_2, PGD_2, $PGF_{2\alpha}$ and TxB_2, PGI_2 has pulmonary vasodilator activity (5), determines relaxation of respiratory tract smooth muscle in guinea pig and in human (2).

The lungs in vivo generate continuously PGI_2 and can certainly regulate their own production of prostacyclin and a theory stating that PGI_2 is a circulating hormone and that the endocrine function of the lung represents an important mechanism for the control of platelet aggregation in the arterial circulation has been developed recently (1, 6).

Hyperventilation is followed by an increase in PGI_2 secretion by the lungs (7). On the other hand tobaco smoking may diminish the PGI_2 generation capacity of the lungs and pathological situations, such as lung diseases, can also influence the production or release of PGI_2 by pulmonary endothelium (7).

A condition favouring thrombosis has been reported in patients with chronic obstructive lung disease (C.O.L.D.), characterized by coagulation activation (8, 9) and by enhanced platelet activity (10) with shortened platelet regeneration time (11, 12, 13) and increased beta-thromboglobulin levels (14).

Furthemore, in patients with COLD, platelets, through serotonin (15) or TxA_2 (16,17,18) release, could increase pulmonary hypertension and thus pulmonary hypertension could be consequent to the platelet mediated vasoconstriction rather than to intravascular obstruction (19,20).

Platelets could be involved not only in the thromboembolic complications of patients with COLD but also be responsible of contracture of smooth muscle cells of pulmonary vasculature (11).

These observations demonstrate that it is very useful to know the platelet function state in patients with COLD.

The purpose of this study was to investigate the changes of platelet function induced by smoke and dynamic exercise in patients with COLD and to evaluate the influence of dipyridamole infusion on platelet activity and on some indices of pulmonary function before and after cyclooxygenase inhibition by ASA.

In fact, dipyridamole, a phosphodiesterase inhibitor, acts through the increase of the effect of prostacyclin (21,22) and/or the stimulation of its biosynthesis (23,24), whereas aspirin, a cyclooxygenase inhibitor, at low dose, inhibits TxA_2 production by platelets without influencing the endothelium prostacyclin production, while, at high dose, inhibits the synthesis of both (25, 26, 27).

Preliminary results of this study are reported.

MATERIALS AND METHODS

Ten patients (6 males and 4 females) with COLD aged 50 to 64 years, with an average age of 57.1 years, without respiratory failure but still in a compensation stage were studied.

All patients had suspended for at least two weeks all drug therapy acting on platelets.

The patients were subdivided in two groups, A and B.

The following parameters were evaluated in patients of group A:

1. Plasmatic betathromboglobulin (RIA) (28).
2. Circulating plasmatic TxB_2 (29).
3. Plasmatic 6-keto $PGF_{1\alpha}$ (30).
4. Actual pH.

5. Carbon dioxide tension (PCO_2 = mmHg).
6. Actual plasmatic bicarbonate (mEq/l).
7. FEV_1.
8. MEF 25 - 50 - 75. Spirometric evaluation of expiratory flow normalized at 75%, 50%, 25% of the forced vital capacity was done with Repotest-Dargatz closed circuit.

The above parameters from 1 to 6 were recorded before and after exercise and 30 minutes in the recovery phase.

The following parameters were evaluated in patients of group B:

1. Plasmatic betathromboglobulin (RIA) (28).
2. Plasmatic 6-keto $PGF_{1\alpha}$ (30).
3. Actual pH.
4. Carbon dioxide tension.
5. Actual plasmatic bicarbonate, before, at the end and 15 minutes after two Marlboro cigarettes.

The blood samples for A 1, 2, 3 and B 1, 2 were obtained from antecubital vein; the samples for A 4, 5, 6 and B 3, 4, 5 from the brachial artery.

The study was carried out in three days. On the 1st day all parameters were evaluated in basal conditions and after exercise or smoking in group A and B respectively.

The 2nd day all parameters were evaluated in basal conditions, after dipyridamole infusion and after exercise or smoking.

The 3rd day all parameters were evaluated after ASA pretreatment 2400 mg in 36 hours and dipyridamole infusion (8ng/min/kg/2h) followed by smoking or exercise.

Exercise was performed by Jaeger Ergometer Bicycle, with patient supine, using work load of 20 W for three minutes and of 40 W for three minutes.

Student's t test for paired data was used for statistical evaluation.

RESULTS

1. Patients of group A (exercise)

In patients of group A dynamic exercise induced a slight but not significant increase of FEV_1 (Table I) in basal conditions like after dipyridamole infusion and ASA pretreatment plus dipyridamole. MEF 25 (Table II) and MEF 50 (Table III) showed a similar behaviour, whereas MEF 75 (Table IV) increased significantly both at rest and after exercise owing to dipyridamole.

Furthermore, exercise determined a slight decrease of actual plasmatic pH (Table V) both in basal conditions ($p<0.025$) and after dipyridamole infusion ($p<0.0025$) and after ASA pretreatment and dipyridamole infusion ($p<0.025$).

Plasmatic carbon dioxide tension showed a significant decrease at rest both after dipyridamole infusion ($p<0.01$) and after ASA pretreatment and dipyridamole infusion ($p<0.025$) (Table VI).

Table I. Behaviour of FEV_1 in patients with chronic obstructive lung disease before and after exercise.

	BASE	AFTER DIPYRIDAMOLE INFUSION	AFTER ASA PRETREATMENT AND DIPYRIDAMOLE INFUSION
A. Rest	1550±353.8	1600±357.7	1650±382.8
B. Exercise	1900±348.5	1733.3±365.8	1700±324.4
Significance (p<)			
A vs B	N.S.	N.S.	N.S.

Table II. Behaviour of MEF 25 in patients with chronic obstructive lung disease before and after exercise.

	BASE	AFTER DIPYRIDAMOLE INFUSION	AFTER ASA PRETREATMENT AND DIPYRIDAMOLE INFUSION
A. Rest	500±159	450±117.9	600±146.8
B. Exercise	600±176	583±148	583±161
Significance (p<)			
A vs B	N.S.	N.S.	N.S.

Table III. Behaviour of MEF 50 in patients with chronic obstructive lung disease before and after exercise.

	BASE	AFTER DIPYRIDAMOLE INFUSION	AFTER ASA PRETREATMENT AND DIPYRIDAMOLE INFUSION
A. Rest	1316±440.8	1166±396.8	1300±404.8
B. Exercise	1416.8±302.8	1333.8±452.7	1150.4±427.9
Significance (p<)			
A vs B	N.S.	N.S.	N.S.

Table IV. Behaviour of MEF 75 in patients with chronic obstructive lung disease before and after exercise.

	1	2	3	SIGNIFICANCE (p<)		
	BASE	AFTER DIPYRIDAMOLE INFUSION	AFTER ASA PRETREATMENT AND DIPYRIDAMOLE INFUSION	1 vs. 2	1 vs. 3	2 vs. 3
A. Rest	2566.6±656.4	3800±1180	3100±910	0.05	N.S.	N.S.
B. Exercise	3033±621.0	4066±1005	3533±865.0	0.05	N.S.	N.S.
Significance (p<)						
A vs. B	N.S.	N.S.	N.S.			

Table V. Behaviour of actual plasmatic pH in patients with chronic obstructive lung disease before and after exercise.

	BASE	AFTER DIPYRIDAMOLE INFUSION	AFTER ASA PRETREATMENT AND DIPYRIDAMOLE INFUSION
A. Rest	7.37±0.02	7.41±0.02	7.37±0.01
B. Exercise	7.32±0.03	7.33±0.02	7.34±0.02
C. 30 min. after	7.37±0.04	7.36±0.02	7.38±0.04
Significance	(p<)		
A vs. B	0.025	0.0025	0.025
A vs. C	N.S.	0.01	N.S.
B vs. C	0.05	0.05	0.05

Table VI. Behaviour of carbon dioxide tension (PCO_2=mm Hg) in patients with chronic obstructice lung disease before and after exercise.

	BASE	AFTER DIPYRIDAMOLE INFUSION	AFTER ASA PRETREATMENT AND DIPYRIDAMOLE INFUSION
A. Rest	44.0±1.32	34.0±5.22	39.5±3.12
B. Exercise	41.3±5.13	37.8±6.50	36.5±2.12
C. 30 min. after	42.8±2.46	40.1±2.07	39.5±1.40
Significance	(p<)		
A vs. B	N.S.	N.S.	N.S.
A vs. C	N.S.	N.S.	N.S.
B vs. C	N.S.	N.S.	0.05

Exercise induced no significant modifications of CO_2 in all conditions studied (Table VI).

Actual plasmatic bicarbonate at rest did not show significant changes either after dipyridamole infusion or after ASA pretreatment plus dipyridamole infusion (Table VII).

Exercise, moreover, induced a significant decrease of this parameter in all conditions investigated (Table VII).

Betathromboglobulin plasmatic levels (Table VIII) did not show significant changes after dipyridamole infusion and decreased slightly after ASA pretreatment both at rest and after exercise ($p<0.05$).

Furthermore, the difference between BTG levels during exercise and 30 minutes after in the recovery period was significant after dipyridamole infusion ($p<0.05$).

Circulating plasmatic TxB_2 (Table IX) was undetectable at rest (less than 0.5 pMol/ml); during exercise TxB_2 increased to 0.95 ± 0.32 pMol/ml in basal conditions and to 0.625 ± 0.15 pMol/ml after dipyridamole infusion. This difference was significant ($p<0.05$).

After ASA pretreatment TxB_2 levels during exercise were lower than 0.5 pMol/ml ($p<0.025$).

6-keto-$PGF_{1\alpha}$ at rest increased but not significantly after dipyridamole infusion and was undetectable after ASA pretreatment ($p<0.0005$) (Table X). A similar pattern was observed after exercise and 30 minutes after in the recovery period.

The difference between 6-keto-$PGF_{1\alpha}$ levels at rest and after exercise after dipyridamole infusion was significant ($p<0.05$).

2. Patients of group B (smoking)

In patients of group B, smoking, in basal conditions, induced a significant decrease of actual pH with a tendency to return at control values after 15 minutes (Table XI).

After dipyridamole infusion, smoking did not influence plasmatic pH like after ASA pretreatment. On this treatment actual pH decreased slightly but significantly ($p<0.005$) 15 minutes after smoking (Table XI).

Plasmatic carbon dioxide tension increased not significantly in basal conditions after smoking and and returned to control values after 15 minutes (Table XII).

Conversely, after dipyridamole infusion and after ASA pretreatment plus dipyridamole, PCO_2 did not change after smoking and increased only 15 minutes after smoking (N.S. after dipyridamole, $p<0.0025$ after ASA pretreatment and dipyridamole infusion) (Table XII).

Actual plasmatic bicarbonate in basal conditions decreased significantly after smoking ($p<0.05$), whereas it did not show any changes after dipyridamole infusion and ASA pretreatment plus dipyridamole (Table XIII).

Cigarette smoking increased betathromboglobulin plasmatic levels (Table XIV) , whereas after dipyridamole infusion BTG decreased significantly also after smoking. A similar pattern of BTG was observed after ASA pretreatment plus dipyridamole.

Table VII. Behaviour of actual plasmatic bicarbonate (mEq/1) in patients with chronic obstructive lung disease before and after exercise.

	BASE	AFTER DIPYRI-DAMOLE INFUSION	AFTER ASA PRETREAT-MENT AND DIPYRIDA-MOLE INFUSION
A. Rest	24.0±1.73	22.8±2.02	23.16±2.08
B. Exercise	20.5±2.17	20.0±1.00	19.5 ±1.03
C. 30 min. after	19.6±2.35	21.6±3.05	23.16±2.89
Significance (p<)			
A vs. B	0.025	0.025	0.0125
A vs. C	0.025	N.S.	N.S.
B vs. C	N.S.	N.S.	0.05

Table VIII. Behaviour of circulating betathromboglobulin (ng/ml) in patients with chronic obstuctive lung disease before and after exercise.

	BASE	AFTER DIPYRI-DAMOLE INFUSION	AFTER ASA PRETREAT-MENT AND DIPYRIDA-MOLE INFUSION
A. Rest	64.06±15.12	63.5 ±20.46	58.2±16.04
B. Exercise	82.23±22.18	86.26±32.52	54.1±18.08
C. 30 min. after	66.16±26.6	47.16±36.66	52.7±15.48
Significance (p<)			
A vs. B	N.S.	N.S.	N.S.
A vs. C	N.S.	N.S.	N.S.
B vs. C	N.S.	0.05	N.S.

Table IX. Behaviour of circulating TxB_2 (pMol/ml) in patients with chronic obstructive lung disease before and after exercise.

	1	2	3	SIGNIFICANCE (p<)		
	BASE	AFTER DIPYRIDAMOLE INFUSION	AFTER ASA PRETREATMENT AND DIPYRIDAMOLE INFUSION	1 vs. 2	1 vs. 3	2 vs. 3
A. Rest	Undetectable	Undetectable	Undetectable	N.S.	N.S.	N.S.
B. Exercise	0.95±0.32	0.625±0.15	Undetectable	0.05	0.025	N.S.
C. 30 Min. after	Undetectable	Undetectable	Undetectable	N.S.	N.S.	N.S.

UNDETECTABLE = plasmatic concentrations of TxB_2 less than 0.5 pMol/ml.

Significance (p<)			
A vs. B	0.0125	0.025	N.S.
A vs. C	N.S.	N.S.	N.S.
B vs. C	0.0125	0.025	N.S.

Table X. Behaviour of 6-keto-$PGF_{1\alpha}$ in patients with chronic obstructive lung disease before and after exercise.

	1	2	3	SIGNIFICANCE (p<)		
	BASE	AFTER DIPYRIDAMOLE INFUSION	AFTER ASA PRETREATMENT AND DIPYRIDAMOLE INFUSION	1 vs. 2	1 vs. 3	2 vs. 3
A. Rest	102.4±57.2	142.7±68.1	Undetectable	N.S.	0.0005	0.0005
B. Exercise	145.7±72.3	200.6±67.5	Undetectable	N.S.	0.0005	0.0005
C. 30 Min. after	112.5±58.5	125.2±59.7	Undetectable	N.S.	0.0005	0.0005
Significance (p<)						
A vs. B	N.S.	N.S.	N.S.			
A vs. C	N.S.	0.05	N.S.			
B vs. C	N.S.	N.S.	N.S.			

Table XI. Behaviour of actual pH in patients with chronic obstructive lung disease before and after smoking.

	BASE	AFTER DIPYRIDAMOLE INFUSION	AFTER ASA PRETREATMENT AND DIPYRIDAMOLE INFUSION
A. Before smoking	7.4 ±0.002	7.38±0.03	7.43±0.02
B. Just after smoking	7.34±0.03	7.38±0.07	7.42±0.18
C. 15 min. after	7.36±0.02	7.37±0.014	7.37±0.02
Significance (p<)			
A vs. B	0.01	N.S.	N.S.
A vs. C	0.025	N.S.	0.005
B vs. C	N.S.	N.S.	0.01

6-keto-$PGF_{1\alpha}$ in basal conditions increased significantly after dipyridamole infusion ($p<0.05$) and was undetectable after ASA pretreatment plus dipyridamole (Table XV).

After cigarette smoking 6-keto-$PGF_{1\alpha}$ decreased but not significantly in basal conditions. After dipyridamole infusion 6-keto-$PGF_{1\alpha}$ levels diminished but remained significantly higher than in basal conditions ($p<0.05$). After ASA pretreatment 6-keto-$PGF_{1\alpha}$ levels were undetectable both before and after smoking (Table XV).

DISCUSSION

Physical exercise induces an increase of forced expiratory volume (FEV) and of maximum expiratory flow (MEF) at 25%, 50%, 75% of vital capacity, but only MEF 75 increases significantly after dipyridamole infusion both at rest and after bicycle ergometer test ($p<0.05$).

At the same time, after dipyridamole infusion and after ASA pretreatment plus dipyridamole infusion there is an increase of pulmonary ventilation demonstrated by the plasmatic levels of PCO_2 lower than in basal conditions.

These changes of respiratory function could depend from a major synthesis and/or pulmonary prostacyclin release determined by

Table XII. Behaviour of carbon dioxide tension (PCO_2=mm Hg) in patients with chronic obstructive lung disease before and after smoking.

	BASE	AFTER DIPYRIDAMOLE INFUSION	AFTER ASA PRETREATMENT AND DIPYRIDAMOLE INFUSION
A. Before smoking	43.0±4.24	43.5±4.94	38.5±2.5
B. Just after smoking	46.5±3.5	43.0±1.41	39.0±3.7
C. 15 min. after	43.5±4.94	46.5±5.19	49.0±2.82
Significance (p<)			
A vs. B	N.S.	N.S.	N.S.
A vs. C	N.S.	N.S.	0.0025
B vs. C	N.S.	N.S.	0.005

Table XIII. Behaviour of actual plasmatic bicarbonate (mEq/l) in patients with chronic obstructive lung disease before and after smoking.

	BASE	AFTER DIPYRIDAMOLE INFUSION	AFTER ASA PRETREATMENT AND DIPYRIDAMOLE INFUSION
A. Before smoking	25.5±1.4	24.0±0.7	25.0±0.8
B. Just after smoking	24.5±0.9	24.2±1.7	25 ±1.2
C. 15 min. after	23.8±0.4	24.2±1.7	25.7±1.9
Significance (p<)			
A vs. B	N.S.	N.S.	N.S.
A vs. C	0.05	N.S.	N.S.
B vs. C	N.S.	N.S.	N.S.

Table XIV. Behaviour of betathromboglobulin in patients with chronic obstructive lung disease before and after smoking.

	1	2	3	SIGNIFICANCE	(p<)	
	BASE	AFTER DIPYRIDAMOLE INFUSION	AFTER ASA PRETREATMENT AND DIPYRIDAMOLE INFUSION	1 vs. 2	1 vs. 3	2 vs. 3
A. Before smoking	80.4±15.65	35.4±7.85	32.75±9.4	0.0025	0.0025	N.S.
B. Just after smoking	92.45±18.36	46.05±10.43	39.0±13.54	0.005	0.005	N.S.
C. 15 min. after	75.4±16.10	43.6±8.37	44.7±14.8	0.01	0.025	N.S.
Significance	(p<)					
A vs. B	N.S.	N.S.	N.S.			
A vs. C	N.S.	N.S.	N.S.			
B vs. C	N.S.	N.S.	N.S.			

Table XV. Behaviour of 6-keto-$PGF_{1\alpha}$ in patients with chronic obstructive lung disease before and after smoking.

	1	2	3	SIGNIFICANCE (p<)		
	BASE	AFTER DIPYRIDAMOLE INFUSION	AFTER ASA PRETREATMENT AND DIPYRIDAMOLE INFUSION	1 vs. 2	1 vs. 3	2 vs. 3
A. Before smoking	122.7±47.4	185.5±59.7	Undetectable	0.05	0.0005	0.0005
B. Just after smoking	77.4±30.2	137.4±57.1	Undetectable	0.05	0.0005	0.0005
C. 15 min. after	99.1±43.2	142.3±59.4	Undetectable	N.S.	0.0005	0.0005
Significance	(p<)					
A vs. B	N.S.	N.S.	N.S.			
A vs. C	N.S.	N.S.	N.S.			
B vs. C	N.S.	N.S.	N.S.			

dipyridamole infusion, expression of which are the higher plasmatic 6-keto-$PGF_{1\alpha}$ levels both at rest and after exercise (30).

This agrees with the releasing action of smooth musculature of the respiratory tract demonstrated for PGI_2 in man (2).

All the same, a direct action of dipyridamole releasing smooth bronchial musculature independently from the prostaglandin mediation is more likely from the moment that such effect is present even after pretreatment with elevated doses of aspirin such as to inhibit completely PGI_2 synthesis (25, 26, 27).

On the other hand, concerning the behaviour of platelet function, physical exercise in patients with COLD induces a platelet activation demonstrated by the increase of the plasmatic levels of betathromboglobulin and TxB_2.

Dipyridamole infusion, as has been demonstrated by other authors, (21, 22, 23, 24) prevents platelet activation decreasing BTG and TxB_2 levels ($p<0.05$) during exercise and increasing at the same time 6-keto $PGF_{1\alpha}$ circulating levels a stable metabolite of PGI_2 (30).

Vice versa aspirin at the dosage employed by us (2400 mg in 36 hours) depresses contemporaneously platelet function and prostacyclin production (25, 26, 27) (undosable 6-keto-$PGF_{1\alpha}$ levels) without being this action influenced in any way by the further infusion of dipyridamole.

As for the action of cigarette smoke,it is known to cause a constriction of the smooth muscles of the respiratory system mediated by nervous reflexes triggered by the contact of smoke with the nasal epithelium of the high respiratory ways through stimulation of the sensitive receptors present in the respiratory tract (31).

The spasm of the small airways thus caused, determines a double or treble increase of resistances to the expiratory flow lasting from 10 to 80 minutes (31, 32, 33).

On the other hand cigarette smoking is known to exalt platelet function and to decrease prostacyclin release from the lungs (7).

In our study the smoke of two cigarettes, in patients with COLD, determined a reduction of pH and an increase of PCO_2, expression of the spasm of the small arways.

This action of smoke is antagonized both by dipyridamole infusion and by aspirin pretreatment.

It is probable that dipyridamole prevents the spasm of the bronchial smooth musculature both because of a direct action and indirectly promoting a major release of PGI_2 expressed by the higher levels of 6-keto-$PGF_{1\alpha}$ (30).

The fact that such action persists also after aspirin pretreatment with doses inhibiting PGI_2 production (25, 26, 27) brings to the conclusion that aspirin can prevent the contracting action of smoke on the smooth musculature of the vessels inhibiting the synthesis of some intermediate endoperoxides whose production by platelets could be stimulated by smoke and that can increase the airways resistances (3).

Platelet function is exalted by cigarette smoke and this is demonstrated in our study by the higher circulating BTG levels that though tend to return to normal 15 minutes after cigarette smoking. After dipyridamole infusion instead, BTG levels lowered before smoking remain substantially unchanged and the same can be said after aspirin pretreatment.

Furthermore, smoking is in agreement with what is sustained by Gryglewski (7), inhibits PGI_2 release by the lung (lower circulating levels of 6-keto-$PGF_{1\alpha}$ metabolite) (30) even in patients with COLD but such action is validly antagonized by dipyridamole infusion, while aspirin at high dosage seems to inhibit completely the release or synthesis of PGI_2 (undosable 6-keto-$PGF_{1\alpha}$ levels) as has been demonstrated by other authors (25, 26, 27).

In conclusion our study demonstrates that:
1) Both physical exercise and cigarette smoking activate platelet function in patients with COLD. This is demonstrated by a greater BTG release and by higher TxB_2 levels (reached after exercise); and that such activation is antagonized both by dipyridamole infusion and by aspirin pretreatment with following dipyridamole infusion;
2) Muscular exercise increases PGI_2 release by the lung and cigarette smoke inhibits it; in the first case dipyridamole increases PGI_2 release, in the second case antagonizes partially the action of smoke that inhibits PGI_2 release. Vice versa, aspirin at high doses inhibits completely PGI_2 synthesis and dipyridamole does not exert any further action on this effect;
3) Exercise tends to increase pulmonary ventilation while smoke tends to diminish it; this is demonstrated in the first case by the slight FEV and MEF 25-50-75 increase and by the reduction of plasmatic CO_2 and in the second case by the increase of plasmatic CO_2 and by the pH reduction; dipyridamole strengthens the action of exercise and inhibits the action of smoke. These effects occur also after aspirin pretreatment and therefore, rather than being a consequence of the increased PGI_2 release, could depend from a direct spasmolitic action of dipyridamole independently from prostaglandins or from the removal operated by aspirin of the action of some intermediate endoperoxides that can stimulate the contraction of the smooth musculature of the respiratory tract and increase thus the airways resistances.

REFERENCES

1. Y. Bakhle, J.R. Vane, Metabolic function of the lungs. In: Marcel Dekker, Inc, New York and Basel, 1977.
2. S.M.M. Karim, P.G. Adaikan, S.R. Cottegoda, Prostaglandins and human respiratory smooth muscle: structure-activity relationship. In: Advances in prostaglandins and thromboxane research, Vol. 7, edited by Samuelsson B., Romvell P.W. and Paoletti R., Raven Press, New York, p. 969, 1980.
3. P.I. Kadowitz, E.W. Spannhake, J.L. Levin, A.L. Hyman, Differential actions of prostaglandins and the pulmonary vascular

bed. In: Advances in prostaglandins and thromboxane research, Vol. 7, edited by Samuelsson B., Romvell P.W. and Paoletti R., Raven Press, New York, p. 731, 1980.

4. A.P. Smith, Advances in prostaglandin research. Practical applications of prostaglandins and their synthesis inhibitors, edited by S.M.M. Karim, M.T.P. Press Ltd, Lancaster, 83, 1976.
5. P.J. Kadowitz, A.L. Hyman, Vasoconstrictor effects of thromboxane B_2 on the canine and feline pulmonary bed. In press.
6. R. J. Gryglewski, R. Korbutt, A. Ocėtkiewicz, Generation of prostacyclin by the lungs in vivo and its release into the arterial circulation. Nature 273:765 (1978).
7. R.J.Gryglewski, Is the lung an endocrine organ that secretes prostacyclin. In: Prostacyclin, edited by J.R. Vane and S. Bergstrom, Raven Press, New York, p.275, 1979.
8. A. Musca, C. Cordova, F. Violi, A. Perrone, C. Alessandri, F. Pavone, F. Balsano, Fibrin polymerization behaviour in patients with chronic respiratory failure. In: (Abstract),VIII European Congress of Cardiology, Paris, June 22-26, 1980.
9. A. Paunesco-Podeanu, C. Bratu, T. Tarachiu, M. Cotsecu, V. Bratu, A. Bucur, Les thromboses pulmonaires qui compliquent l'insuffisance respiratoire et le coeur pulmonaire chronique. Med. Int. (Buc.) 25:473 (1973).
10. F. Balsano, C. Cordova, A. Musca, A. Perrone, F. Violi, Metabolismo polmonare ed emocoagulazione in fisiologia, patologia e clinica. Clin. Ter. 80:513 (1977).
11. P. Steel, H.R. Ellis, S. Weily, E. Genton, Platelet survival time in patients with hypoxemia and pulmonary hypertension. Circulation 55:660 (1977).
12. R. Breda, B. Bizzi, R. Landolfi, Ruolo del polmone nell'emocoagulazione. Clin. Ter. 94 (Suppl. 1), 1, 41 (1980).
13. E. Tremoli, L. Bertoli, P. Maderna, F. Conti, R. Marlini, O. Mantero, Platelet antiaggregating therapy in chronic obstructive lung disease. Clin. Resp. Physiol. 16:84 (1980).
14. C. Cordova, A. Musca, F. Violi, G.C. De Mattia, A. Perrone, C. Alessandri, F. Balsano, Plasma beta-thromboglobulin levels in patients with chronic respiratory failure. In: Abstracts. VIII European Congress of Cardiology, Paris, June 22-26, 1980.
15. D.A. Rickaby, C.A. Dawson, M.B. Maron, Pulmonary inactivation of serotonin and site of serotonin pulmonary vasoconstriction. J. Appl. Physiol. 48:606 (1980).
16. J. Svensson, T. Strandberg, T. Tuveno, M. Hamberg, Thromboxane A_2: effects on airway and vascular smooth muscle. Prostaglandins 14:426 (1977).
17. J.D. Dusting, S. Moncada, J. Vane, Prostaglandins, their intermediates and precursors: cardiovascular actions and regulatory role in normal and abnormal circulatory system. Progr. Cardiovasc. Dis. 21:405 (1979).
18. J.C. Frölich M. Ogletree, B.A. Peskar, K.L. Brigham, Pulmonary

hypertension correlated to pulmonary thromboxane synthesis. In: Advances in prostaglandin and thromboxane research, Vol. 7, edited by Samuelsson P. Romwell P.W. and Paoletti R., Raven Press, New York, p. 745, 1980.

19. K. Radegran, S.E. Bergentz, D.H. Lewis, U. Ljungquist, P. Olsson, Pulmonary effects of induced platelet aggregation. Intravascular obstruction or vasoconstriction? Scand. J. Clin. Lab. Invest. 28:423 (1971).
20. G. Bo, J. Hognestad, Effects on the pulmonary circulation of suddenly induced intravascular aggregation of blood platelets. Acta Physiol. Scand. 85:523 (1972).
21. S. Moncada, R. Corbutt, Dipyridamole and other phosphodiesterase inhibitors act as antithrombotic agents by potentiating endogenous prostacyclin. Lancet 1:1268 (1978).
22. K.A. Jorgensen, J. Dyeberg, E. Stoffersen, Prostacyclin (PGI_2) and the effect of phosphodiesterase inhibitors on platelet aggregation. Pharm. Res. Commun. 11:605 (1979).
23. K.E. Blass, H.U. Block, W. Förster, K. Ponicke, Dipyridamole, a potent stimulator of prostacyclin (PGI_2) biosynthesis. Br. J. Pharmacol. 68:71 (1980).
24. G.G. Neri Serneri, G. Masotti, L. Poggesi, G. Galanti, S. Castellani, Dipyridamole stimulates prostacyclin biosynthesis in man and in vitro. In: 6th International Congress on Thrombosis, Montecarlo, October 23-25, 1980,
25. G.G. Neri Serneri, G. Masotti, R. Abbate, S. Fabilla, L. Poggesi, G.F. Gensini, G. Galanti, R. Laureano, Enhanced prostacyclin production and decreased thromboxane formation by dipyridamole. In: Florence International Meeting on Myocardial Infarction, Experta Medica, Vol. I, p.489, 1979.
26. G. Masotti, G. Galanti, L. Poggesi, R. Abbate, G.G. Neri Serneri, Differential inhibition of PGI_2 production and platelet aggregation by aspirin in humans. In: 5th International Congress on Thromboembolism, Bologna May 29-June 2 (Abstract) p.46, 1978.
27. G. MAsotti, R. Abbate, G. Galanti, L. Poggesi, G.G. Neri Serneri, Are conventional doses of acetylsalicyclic acid advisable in prevention of thrombosis? In: Florence International Meetings on Myocardial Infarction, Experta Medica, Vol. I, p.489, 1979.
28. C.A. Ludlam, B. Moores, A. Boctona, D.S. Pepper, J.D. Cash, The release of a human platelet specific protein measured by radioimmunoassay. Thromb. Res. 6:543 (1975).
29. R.J. Lewy, J.B. Smith, M.J. Silver, J. Saia, P. Walinsky, L. Weiner, Detection of thromboxane B_2 in peripheral blood of patients with Prinzmetal angina. Prostaglandins Med. 42:425 (1979).
30. J.A. Salmon, A radioimmunoassay for 6-keto $PGF_{1\alpha}$. Prostaglandins 3:383 (1978).
31. J.A. Nadel, J.H. Comore, Acute effect of inhalation of cigarette smoke on airway conductance. J. Appl. Physiol. 16:713 (1961).
32. G.M. Starling, Mechanism of bronchoconstriction caused by

cigarette smoking. Br. Med. J. 3:275 (1967). 1:

33. J.M. Miller, B.J. Sproule, Acute effects of inhalation of cigarette smoke on mechanical properties of the lungs. Am. Rev. Resp. Dis. 94:721 (1966).

VASODILATOR TREATMENT OF PRIMARY PULMONARY HYPERTENSION

L. Cotter

Brompton Hospital
Fulham Road
London SW3 6HP
England

Primary pulmonary hypertension has been defined as pulmonary artery hypertension and normal pulmonary capillary wedge pressure with right ventricular hypertrophy for which no aetiology is apparent (1). The clinical diagnosis is made by excluding other causes of pulmonary hypertension, although differentiation from chronic pulmonary thromboembolic disease may be impossible ante-mortem. It predominantly affects young women causing their death after median period of 2 - 3 years (2) although long term follow up (3) and even spontaneous remission (4) have been reported in exceptional cases. Although its cause is unknown the pathological changes include medical hypertrophy and laminar intimal arteriolar fibrosis suggesting a vasoconstrictive element in the genesis of the disease (5). Some cases are familial (6) and as autoimmune disease is present in about the third of cases (7), immunological mechanisms have been suggested in the genesis of the disease. A disease indistinguishable from primary pulmonary hypertension occurred in patients in central Europe who took the weight reducing agent aminorex fumarate (8), and 4 others taking the anti-diabetic agent phenformin (9,10).

The effects of various agents on the pulmonary vasculature of such patients have been observed but until recently no treatment had been shown to be of therapeutic benefit. Our own study was of the effects of diazoxide on 9 such patients (11).

Diazoxide

Diazoxide is a benzothiadiazine derivative related to the thiazide diuretics but with no diuretic activity (12). It is a potent dilator of resistance vessels and has been widely used intravenously in the treatment of hypertensive emergencies (13). Although it is effective orally, its use in the treatment of systemic hypertension has been limited by its side effects, particularly the causation of diabetes mellitus by direct effects on the cells of the islets of Langerhans.

Parenteral Diazoxide

All the patients in our study were females aged from 25 - 62 years. All nine had diagnostic cardiac catheterization performed with pulmonary arteriography in 7, and none showed any evidence of any congenital heart lesion, pulmonary thromboembolism or pulmonary veno-occlusive disease. During cardiac catheterization, catheters placed in the main pulmonary trunk and a systemic artery allowed continuous monitoring of pulmonary and systemic artery pressure and blood sampling for oxygen tension measurement. Oxygen uptake was measured continuously using respiratory mass speedometry (14) so that changes in cardiac output could be measured by direct Fick analyses. The maximum cumulative effects of up to 600 mg of diazoxide injected into the pulmonary artery of the patients on mean pulmonary artery pressure and pulmonary blood flow are shown in figures 1 and 2. The effects on pulmonary vascular resistance calculated from these measurements and left atrial (or pulmonary artery wedge) mean pressure are shown in figure 3.

There was no effect on mean pulmonary artery pressure but pulmonary blood flow increased from an average of 3.1 l/min to an average of 5.4 l/min ($p<0.001$), so that the calculated pulmonary vascular resistance fell in every case by 3.9 to 17.0 units, from an average of 20.6 units to an average of i7.0 units.

Oral Diazoxide

Of 7 patients who were given oral diazoxide, 5 had side-effects (table 1), which were severe enough to stop the administration of the drug, particularly as it had caused no improvement in symptoms. Two patients improved, one dramatically. This latter patient, initially crippled by syncope, chest pain and dyspnoea was releieved of syncope and chest pain and showed a marked improvement in her exercise tolerance. This patient, along with 4 others was catheterized while on oral therapy (400 mg/day), and at catheterization had increased her pulmonary blood flow from 2.2 l/min to 4.3 l/min with a fall in her pulmonary vascular resistence from 27.1 to 14.2 units (figures 4 and 5) but with no change in her pulmonary artery pressure (figure 6).

Discussion

In the thirty years since Dresdale et al. (15) clearly described the haemodynamic features of primary pulmonary hypertension, the search for an effective treatment for the disease has continued. This quest has been hampered by the rarity of the disease so that reports are usually about very few patients, and by the absence of a non-inva-

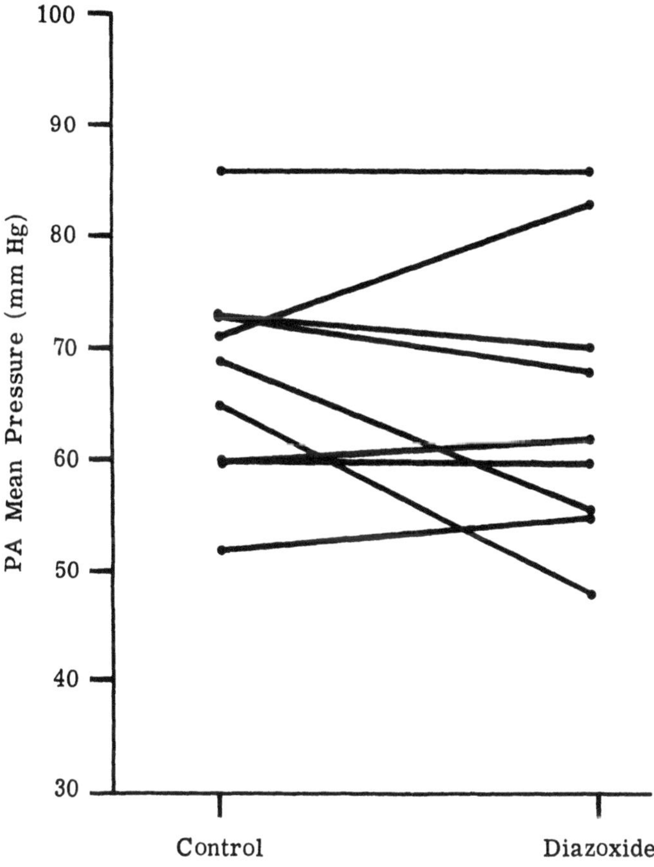

Fig. 1

sive method of assessing pulmonary artery pressure on pulmonary vascular resistance. Most attention has focused on vasodilator drugs, but acetylcholine, alpha-adrenergic blockers (16), beta-adrenergic stimulaters (17), anticoagulants (18), antihistamines (19), anti prostaglandins (20) and of course corticosteroids (21) have all been assessed with dissapointing results. Of these acetylcholine and the alpha-adrenergic blocker tolazoline hydrochloride reduce the pulmonary artery pressure in primary pulmonary hypertension given parenterally (16), but both are ineffective by mouth. Phentolamine, another alpha-adrenergic blocker has haemodynamic effects on the pulmonary vasculature, whether given parenterally or orally (22), and caused subjective improvement in the patient so treated by Ruskin et al. The beta-adrenergic stimulator isoproterenol may be effective when given sublingually but the need for 2 hourly doses is limiting and its effect

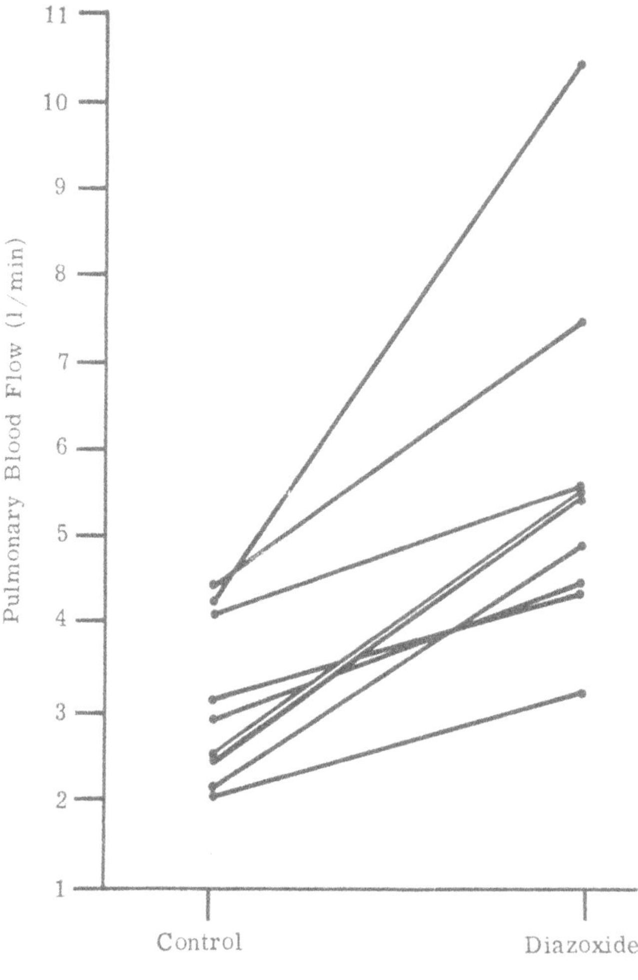

Fig. 2

on symptoms and the disease process may not be favourable (23).

More recently systemic vasodilators have been assessed and Rubin and Peter reported impressive improvements in 4 patients whom they treated with oral hydrallazine (24). They found diminution in the pulmonary vascular resistance from an average of 17.5 units to 7.7 units with an increase in pulmonary blood flow from 3.8 l/min to 7.1 l/min. The pulmonary artery pressures were unchanged. These haemodynamic improvements were present at rest and following exercise, and persisted at repeat studies 3 to 6 months later.

Similar effects were noted in a single patient given nifedipine, a calcium antagonist with vasodilatory properties, described by

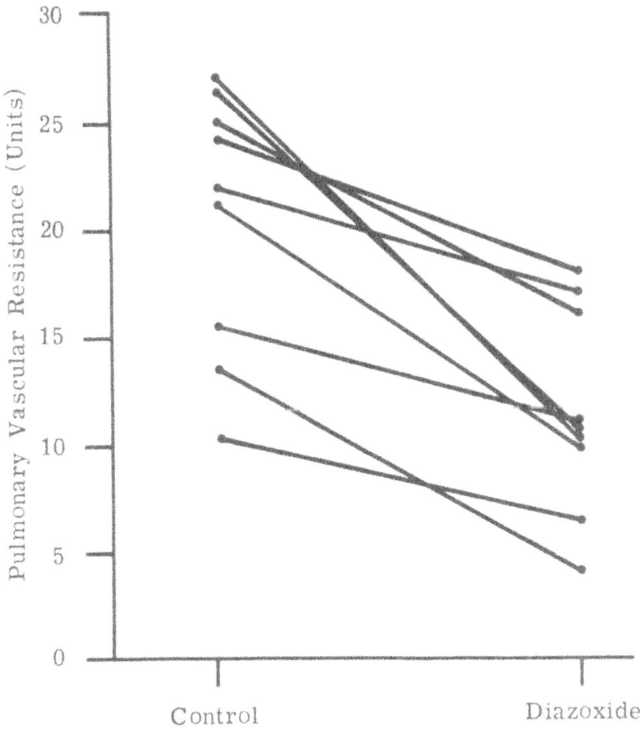

Fig. 3

Camerini et al. (25). They documented a fall in pulmonary vascular resistance by 50% with a rise in pulmonary blood flow of 90%. These findings also persisted at a 3 month follow and were accompanied by clinical improvement.

Oral diazoxide was first used by Wang and his colleagues in Manchester (26). They observed the haemodynamic effects of parenteral and oral diazoxide in 3 patients with primary pulmonary hypertension and 1 with pulmonary thromboembolic disease. Two of the 3 patients with primary pulmonary hypertension improved subjectively and objectively on the oral drug. This report was followed by a case report from Klinke and Gilbert (27), whose patient also improved haemodynamically and became entirely asymptomatic. In the combined experience of Wang et al., Klinke and Gilbert and ourselves, of 9 patients given oral diazoxide, 3 have improved markedly, 1 of our patients also improved appreciably while 1 other of Wang et el.'s group improved temporarily.

The use of diazoxide in our hands was severely limited by side-effects which did not occur in Klinke and Gilbert's case and which were not problematic in Wang et al.'s series. The Manchester group

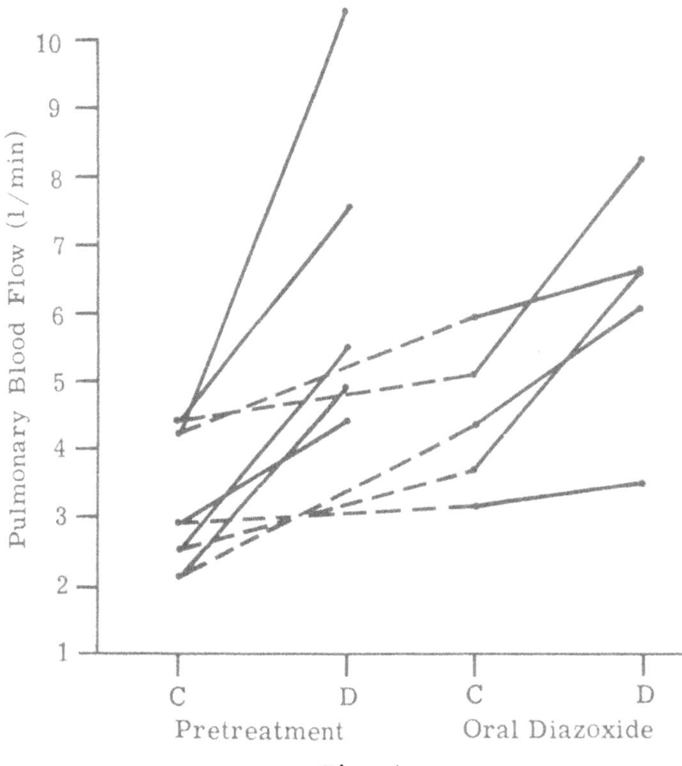

Fig. 4

are, however, very experienced in the use of diazoxide in severe systemic hypertension (28) and it may be that our management of the diazoxide side-effects was imperfect. Lack of control of the side-effects led to the withdrawal of the drug in 5 cases, even though haemodynamic improvements, though not symptomatic improvements, were present.

Thus, diazoxide and hydrallazine are now available as possible therapy for primary pulmonary hypertension, while phentolamine and nifedipine may also prove useful. Although Rich has pointed out the dangers of empirical treatment of primary pulmonary hypertension with vasodilators (29), it now seems justifiable to measure the parenteral effects of diazoxide or hydrallazine in such patients and if the response is favourable to embark on carefully supervised oral therapy, accompanied by periodic repeat assesments.

It may be that the long period of therapeutic nihilism in this disabling and distressing condition is drawing to a close (30).

Table 1. Side Effects of Oral Diazoxide

Peripheral oedema	4
Diabetes mellitus	3
Nausea and vomiting	2
Postural hypotension	1
Hirsutes	2

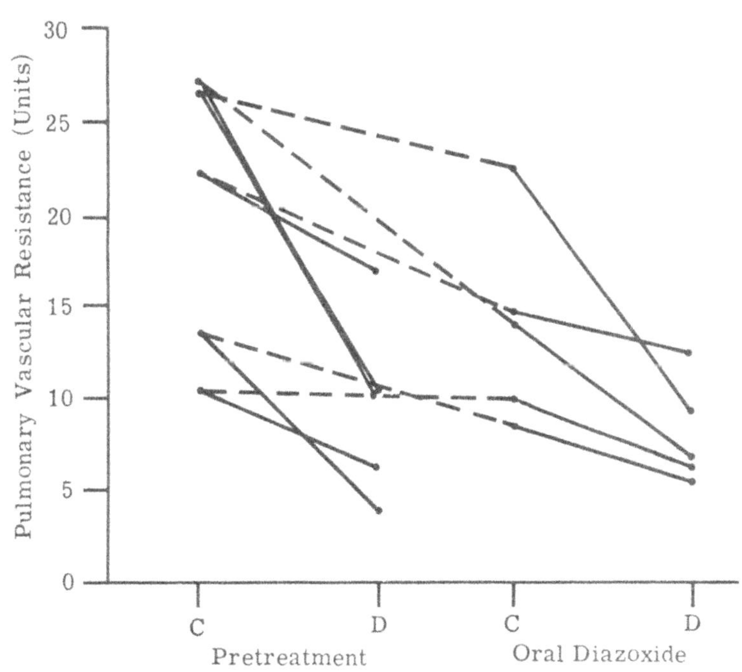

Fig. 5

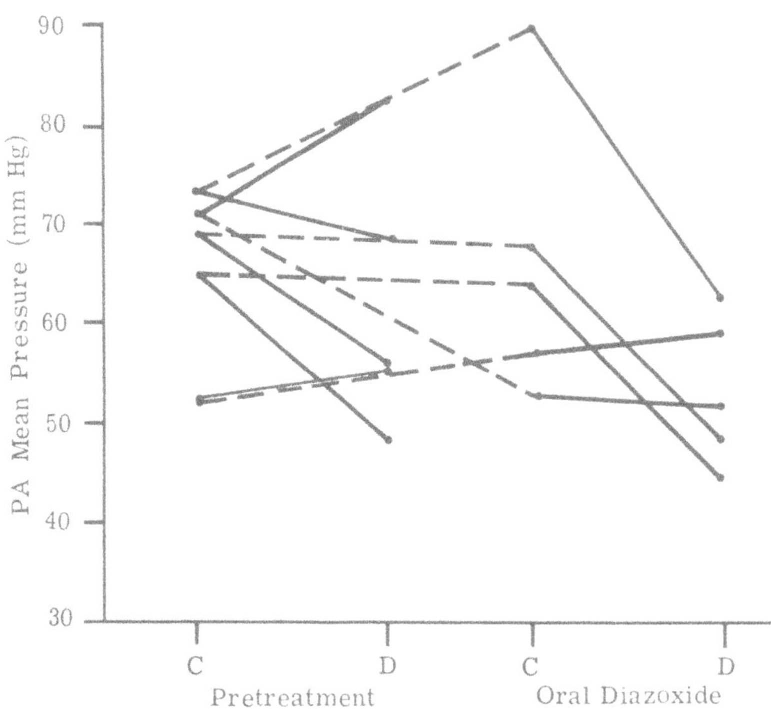

Fig. 6

Acknowledegement

All figures are by kind permission of the editor of Thorax.

REFERENCES

1. S. Hatano, T. Strasser, Primary pulmonary hypertension report on a WHO meeting. World Health Organization. (1975).
2. R.P. Gatewood, P.N. Yu, Primary pulmonary hypertension. Prog. Card. (1979).
3. L. Suarez, Long-term follow-up in primary pulmonary hypertension. Br. Heart J. 41: 702 (1979).
4. P.D.V. Bourdillon, C.M. Oakley, Regression of primary pulmonary hypertension. Br. Heart J. 38: 264 (1976).
5. P. Wood, Pulmonary hypertension with special reference to the vasoconstrictive factor. Br. Heart J. 21: 557 (1959).
6. R.C. Clarke, C.F. Coombs, G. Hadfield, A.T. Todd, On certain abnormalities congenital and aquired of the pulmonary arteries. Q. J. Med. 21: 51 (1927).

7. C.A. Wangevoort, N. Wangevoort, Pathology of pulmonary hypertension. New York, John Willey and Sons. (1977).
8. J.M. Kay, P. Smith, D. Heath, Aminorex and the pulmonary circulation. Thorax 26: 262 (1971).
9. M. Fahlen, H. Bergman, Phenformin and pulmonary hypertension. Br. Heart J. 35: 82 (1973).
10. B.J. Sproule, E.A. Phillipson, C.M. Couves, R.T. Brownlee, Acute pulmonary hypertension in idiopathic lactic acidosis. Canadian Medical Association Journal 94: 141 (1966).
11. M. Honey, L. Cotter, N. Davies, D. Denison, Clinical and haemodynamic effects of diazoxide in primary pulmonary hypertension. Thorax 35: 269 (1980).
12. J. Koch-Weser, Drug therapy: diazoxide. N. Engl. J. Med. 294: 1271 (1976).
13. M. Moser, Diazoxide: an effective vasodilator in accelerated hypertension. Am. Heart J. 87: 791 (1974).
14. N.J.H. Davies, D.M. Denison, The measurement of metabolic gas exchange by mass spectrometry alone. Respir. Physiol. 36: 261 (1979).
15. D.T. Dresdale, M. Schultz, R.J. Michton, Primary pulmonary hypertension. Am. J. Med. 11: 686 (1951).
16. R.F. Grover, J. Reeves, S.G. Blount, Tolazoline hydrochloride: an effective pulmonary vasodilator. Am. Heart J. 61:5 (1961).
17. U. Shettigar, H.N. Hultgren, M. Speatr, R. Martin, H.D. Davies, Primary pulmonary hypertension: favorable effect of isoproterenol. N. Engl. J. Med. 295: 1414 (1976).
18. D.E.L. Wilckin, K.M. Mac Kenzie, J.F. Goodwin, Anticoagulation therapy of obliterative pulmonary hypertension. Lancet 1: 781 (1960).
19. F. Rengo, B. Trimarco, M. Chiarello, Histamine and hypoxic pulmonary hypertension: a quantitative study. Cardiovasc. Res. 12: 752 (1978).
20. J. Szczeklik, Effects of prostaglandin E1 on the pulmonary circulation in patients with pulmonary hypertension. Br. Heart J. 40: 1397 (1978).
21. F.S. Daoud, J.T. Reeves, D.B. Kelly, Isoproterenol as a potential pulmonary vasodilator in primary pulmonary hypertension. Am. J. Cardiol.42: 817 (1978).
22. J.N. Ruskin, A.M. Hutter, Primary pulmonary hypertension treated with phentolamine. Ann. Intern. Med. 90: 772 (1979).
23. U. Elkayam, W. Frishman, C. Yoran, J. Strom, M. Cohen, Unfavourable haemodynamic and clinical effects of isoproterenol therapy in primary pulmonary hypertension. Card. Med. 3: 1177 (1978).
24. R.J. Rubin, H.R. Peter, Oral Hydrallazine therapy for primary pulmonary hypertension. N. Engl. J. Med. 302: 69 (1980).
25. F. Camerini, E. Alberti, S. Klugman, A. Salvi, Primary pulmonary hypertension: effects of Nifedipine. Br. Heart J. 44: 352 (1980).

26. S.W.S. Wang, J.E.F. Pohl, D.J. Rowlands, E.G. Wade, Diazoxide in treatment of primary pulmonary hypertension. Br. Heart J. 40: 572 (1978).
27. W.P. Klinke, J.A.L. Gilbert, Diazoxide in primary pulmonary hypertension. N. Engl. J. Med. 302: 91 (1980).
28. J.E.F. Pohl, B. Thurstan, Use of diazoxide in hypertension with renal failure. Br. Med. J. 1: 142 (1971).
29. S. Rich, Vasodilator therapy for pulmonary hypertension (letter N. Engl. J. Med. 302: 1260 (1980).
30. J.T. Reeves, Hope in primary pulmonary hypertension. N. Engl. J. Med. 302: 81 (1980).

THE THROMBOGENIC RISK IN CHRONIC RESPIRATORY FAILURE

A. Musca, C. Cordova, and F. Violi

IV Clinica Medica
Università degli Studi di Roma
Roma - Italy

The problem of a thrombogenic risk in chronic respiratory failure (CRF) can easily be collected within t-epulmonary hypertension picture. The relationships between these two factors are reciprocal and ambivalent: hypertension and pulmonary vascular damage are a thrombogenic risk where the eventual thrombosis favours pulmonary localization, while the complex thrombophilic dyscoagulation in patients with CRF, which is the other condition for thrombogenic risk, could cause the aggravation of pulmonary hypertension and of the linked anatomico-cunctional lesion by means of a more or less generalized microthrombosis.

The more recent acquisitions in the clinical and experimental field make of this pathogenic bipolarity a condition more than just hypothetical. This mechanism, which is the subjects of this symposium, is already largely accepted for other analogous conditions like peripheral arteriopathy, arteriosclerotic and not, myocardial ischemia, transient amaurosis or cerebral ischemia. In other words, it is a meeting point between two pathogenic poles: vascular damage and thrombophilic dyscoagulation.

However, while for the above forms the relationship of cause and effect between vascular occlusion and ischemic symptoms is obvious and sufficiently specific, this is not so as far as the pulmonary field is concerned. In fact, the entity of the role played by the eventual, more or less generalized microthrombosis (11) in determining a recurrence, in bronchial forms refractory to traditional therapy (12), and in the rapid evolution of the basic disease, is practically an arduous if not impossible evaluation. From this there is a sense of scepticism and disinterest for the pathophysiologic, diagnostic and therapeutic turnovers that this problem presents; certainly not by part of researchers closely tied with this problem but by part of a not insignificant number of Internists and Pneumologists.

For several years our research group has been studying this problem at both its pathologic and clinical -diagnostic points of view.

Besides confirming the data already existing in literature like hyperfibrinogenemia, increased prothrombin time and an increase of the "am" tract of the thromboelastogram (11, 12), in our patients we showed the presence of significant reductions of the plasma AT III levels, which is noted condition of risk for the onset of disseminated intravascular coagulation (DIC) (10). Also in more than 80% of the cases a significant increase of plasma antiplasmin activity was found (10). Regarding platelets, a significant hyperaggregation was found in approximately 70% of the cases (1). The platelet aggregation (PA) undergoes a further significant increase two hours after therapeutic bleeding (300-400 ml) (4). This is not the place to refer how much we have done to explain the pathogenesis of this hyperaggregation. We believe that sufficient documentation has been made on the presence in platelet poor plasma of these patients with CRF of a "hyperaggregating factor" (5), that platelets show an increased activability of the thromboxane metabolic pathway (7) and that acute increases of plasma 5-HT could be at least partly responsible for the hyperaggregation from therapeutic bleeding (6).

If everything seen up to now affirms that a complex and often a multifactorial prothrombotic condition, in other words a thrombotic risk, frequently exists in CRF, then one becomes aware that none of these knowledges proves that the thrombotic risk in these patients could pass or have passed to the actual thrombotic condition. That is, it does not inform us if, when and how much the thrombotic risk becomes a thrombotic reality affecting the pathogenesis of the basic disease.

We would like to show you results of our more recent studies that could contribute to prove this goal. Figure 1 shows the behaviour of the fibrin(ogen) polymerization curve. The method used for this study was that of Ferry and Morrison, modified by Dettori et al. (8). A Beckman Trace III photometer was used which gives reliable readings. We studied 20 patients with CRF and 20 normal volunteers for control. Only subjects with normal fibrinogen plasma levels were included in our study; while plasma AT III levels were low in five patients with CRF. The kinetics of the fibrin(ogen) polymerization curve were significantly faster in the sharp raising phase of the curve with final optical density readings clearly and significantly higher in the patients with CRF with respect to controls (Fig. 2). This behaviour was present indifferently in patients with either low or normal AT III plasma levels. This finding suggests that the fibrinogen in these patients is polymerized more rapidly and in a greater amount. Because the fibrinogenic system is physiologically always in function, the normal subject is perfectly balanced by an efficient fibrinolysis. It could be suggested therefore that from the same thrombogenic stimulus the chronic respiratory patient forms a greater amount of fibrin.

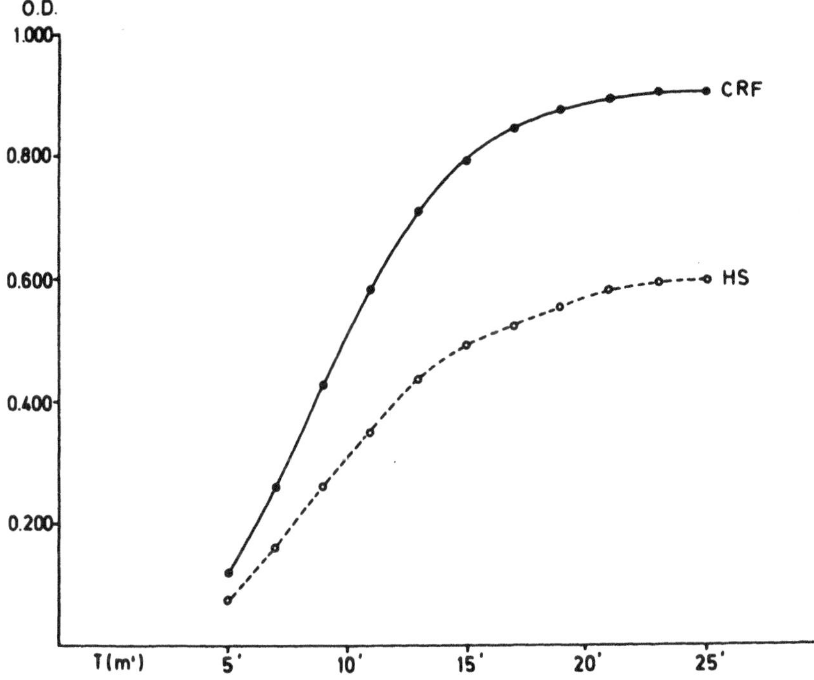

Fig. 1. General feature of the fibrinogen-fibrin polymerization curve (mean values) in healthy subjects (HS) and in patients with chronic respiratory failure (CRF).

We get a more direct evidence of the thrombotic event from studying the beta-Thromboglobulin (beta-TG) plasma levels. As it is well known, this globulin is released from the platelet mostly during the phase of release reaction II. A study of the beta-TG levels could give some ideas about the entity of the actual platelet activation. The data in table I show the beta-TG plasma values of 24 patients with CRF. The blood samples were collected using the method of Ludlan et al. (9). The beta-TG assay was determined in RIA (AHERSHAM) and Born's method was used for evaluating the platelet aggregation induced by ADP (2). A comparative control study was carried out on 10 normal volunteers. Significantly higher values of beta-TG plasma levels were found in the patients with CRF. The statistical correlation between platelet aggregation and beta-TG was fairly good ($r = 0.745$) (Fig. 3). A clear and acute increase of beta-TG levels can be observed after therapeutic bleeding (Fig. 4); however, this increase is less significant regarding PA. In fact the statistical correlation (Fig. 5) between the two increases is clearly inferior to the one observed for the base values ($r = 0.559$).

We suggest that the high beta-TG values found in the patients

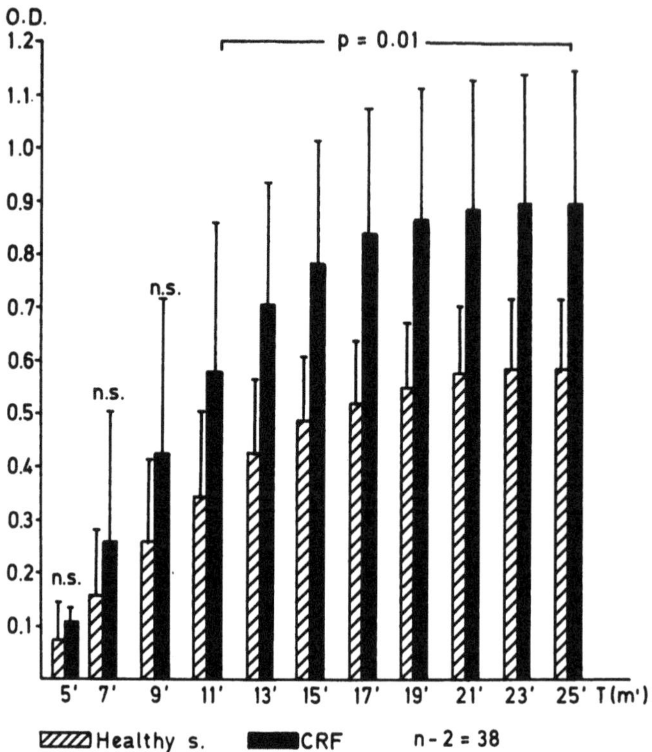

Fig. 2. Statistical evaluation of fibrinigen-fibrin polymerization curves.

Table 1. PA and plasma beta-TG in patients with CRF (24) and in healthy volunteers (20).

	Healthy volunteers	Patients with CRF
PA (% Trasmittance)	55.6±9.5	75.3±9.8 (p=0.01)
Beta-TG (ng/ml)	25.6±2.7	76.5±29.9 (p=0.01)

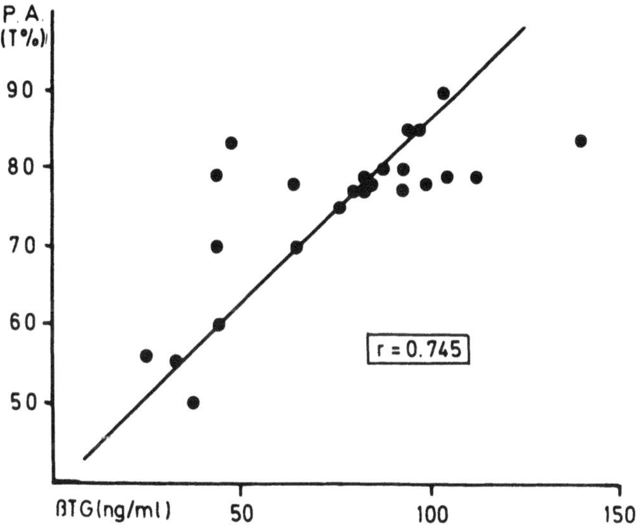

Fig. 3. Statistical correlation between PA and plasma beta-TG in 24 patients with CRF (n = 23).

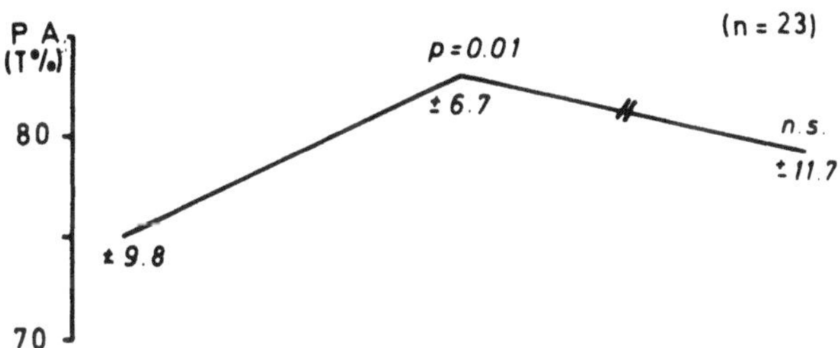

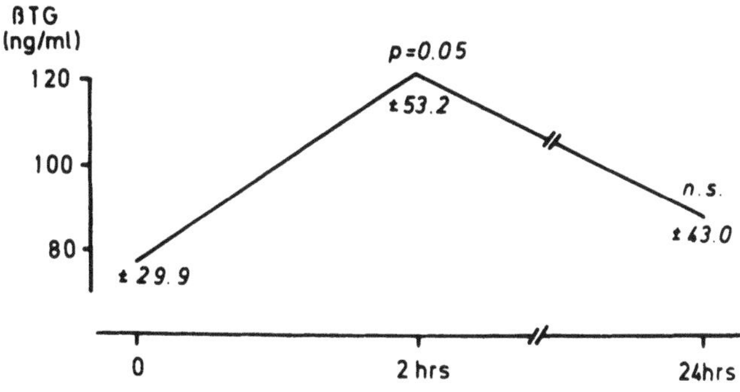

Fig. 4. PA and plasma beta-TG behaviour before and after a blood-letting in patients with CRF.

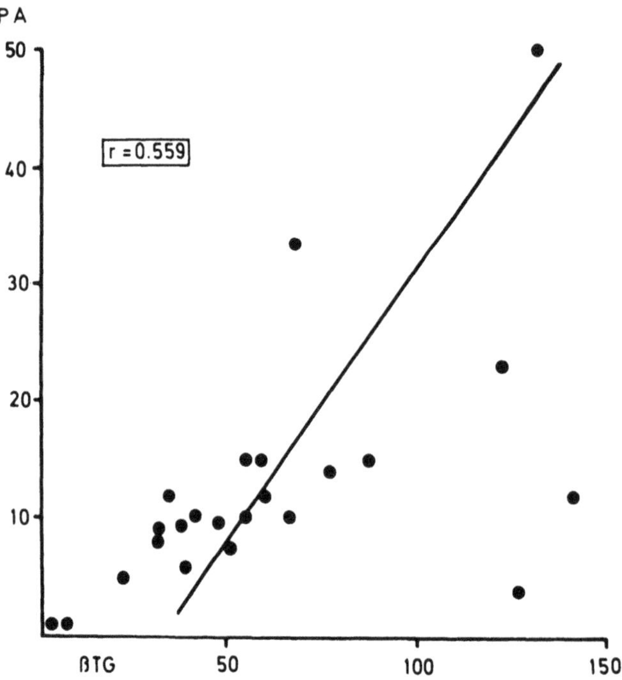

Fig. 5. Statistical correlation between PA and plasma beta-TG increases 2 hrs. after a bloodletting (n = 23).

with CRF, which are more or less similar to those found by Smith et al., for example, in patients with clinical peripheral deep vein thrombosis (13), can be considered as being reliable evidence in favour of a more or less generalized state of platelet activation actually present in these patients, which is often increased after therapeutic bleeding.

However, it should be clear that, in accordance with other authors, we do not intend to give a strictly quantitative meaning to this method, but rather a qualitative value to a possible indication that a greater amount of platelets are activated in these patients.

REFERENCES

1. F. Balsano, C. Cordova, A. Musca, A. Perrone, F. Violi, Metabolismo polmonare ed emocoagulazione in fisiologia, in patologia ed in clinica. Clin. Ter. 80:513 (1977).
2. G.V.R. Born, Aggregation of blood platelet by adenosine diphosphate and its reversal. Nature 19:927 (1962).

3. C. Cordova, A. Musca, A. Perrone, F. Violi, V. Marigliano, Turbe emocoagulative in corso di broncopatia cronica. Progr. Med. 32:925 (1976).
4. C. Cordova, A. Musca, A. Perrone, F. Violi, V. Marigliano, Aggregazione piastrinica e salassoterapia nei soggetti affetti da insufficienza respiratoria cronica. Clin. Ter. 82: 415 (1977).
5. C. Cordova, A. Musca, A. Perrone, F. Violi, C. Alessandri, V. Marigliano, La iperaggregazione piastrinica del soggetto con insufficienza respiratoria cronica é legata ad un fattore plasmatico? Progr. Med. 34:1007 (1978).
6. C. Cordova, A. Musca, A. Perrone, F. Violi, V. Marigliano, C. Alessandri, Platelet hyperaggregation after bleeding in patients with chronic respiratory failure: role of serotonin. In: XIV Int. Intern. Med. Rome 16-19 October 1978.
7. C. Cordova, A. Musca, F. Violi, A. Perrone, C. Alessandri, V. Marigliano, F. Balsano, Pathophisiological and clinical research on the platelet hyperaggregation in patients with chronic respiratory failure. In: International Symposium on "Pulmonary Circulation III". Prague 2-4 July 1979.
8. A.S. Dettori, O. Ponari, E. Civardi, A. Megha, M. Pini, R. Poti, Impaired fibrin formation in advanced cirrhosis. Haemostasis 6:137 (1977)
9. C.A. Ludlam; A.E. Bolton, S. Moore, J.D. Cash, New rapid method for diagnosis of deep vein thrombosis. Lancet 2:259 (1975)
10. A. Musca, C. Cordova, F. Violi, A. Perrone, C. Alessandri, M.S. Bonavita, Alterazioni del versante fibrinico dell'emocoagulazione nella patologia polmonare cronica. In: Convegno su "Turbe emocoagulative nelle broncopneumopatie croniche". Roma 11 Aprile 1979.
11. A. Paunescu-Podeanu, M. Costescu, G. Dobrin, Modificari ale coagulabilitatii sanguine in corul pulmonar cronic. Stud. Cerc. Med. Int. 13:243 (1972).
12. A. Paunescu-Podeanu, C. Bratu, T. Tarachiu, M. Costescu, V. Bratu, A. Bucur, Les thromboses pulmonaires qui compliquent l'insuffisance respiratoire et le coeur pulmonaire chronique. Med. Int. 25:437 (1973).
13. R.C. Smith, R.C. Ducanson, C.V. Rukley, R.G. Webber, N.C. Allan, J. Dawes, A.E. Bolton, W.M. Hunter, D.S. Pepper, J.D. Cash, Beta-thromboglobulin and deep vein thrombosis. Thromb. Haemostas. (Stuttg.) 39:338 (1978).

ROUND TABLE ON "PULMONARY VASCULAR DISEASES": FINAL REMARKS

F. Balsano

IV Clinica Medica
Università degli Studi di Roma
Roma - Italy

This session examined Pulmonary Vascular Diseases. We listened to reports regarding pulmonary hypertension and its relationship with hypoxemia and platelet function; we heard about the therapeutic correction of these diseases using therapy tending to modify the noted thrombophilic condition of both the platelet and fibrinogenic systems present in a high percentage of these patients, who, therefore, are also affected with secondary pulmonary hypertension.

Up to a few years ago, not more than five or six, the pathogenic relationship between dyscoagulation and pulmonary hypertension was an unknown problem or it was approached in a superficial and fragmentary manner.

Essentially the French research works reported (Bignon et al.) called attention to the presence of a more or less generalized microthrombosis of the pulmonary vascular tree in 85% of patients deceased from chronic respiratory failure. Other works indicated the efficiency of heparin therapy in some recurring cases of chronic respiratory failure refractory to traditional treatment.

In the light of what was done during these past years, and to what we heard today, I think that the concept of pulmonary hypertension cannot be divided from the concept of a thrombophilic condition in chronic pulmonary diseases. The pathogenic problem is related to the lesion of the vascular and pulmonary structures brought by the pulmonary disease which carry an important part in both the general and local blood coagulation systems.

Since 1975 in occasion of the Symposium of Pulmonary Hypertension, I sustained this pathogenic bipolarity: on the one hand, hypertension and pulmonary vascular damage are a thrombogenic risk that conditions a prevalent pulmonary localization of enentual thrombosis; on the other hand, the complex thrombophilic dyscoagultion in patients with chronic respiratory failure, which is the other condition for thrombogenic risk, could cause the aggravation of hypertension in the pulmonary circulatory system and of the pulmonary anatomico-functional lesion by means of a more or less generalized microthrombosis.

As you can see, these two conditions pursue each other creating a classical situation of auto-maintainance and aggravation.

I think we are the first to report personal data indicating that elevated platelet aggregation was frequently present in these patients. At that time our study referred to about 20 cases; today our experience depends on over 150 cases in whom we systematically studied both the platelet and the fibrinogenic systems of blood coagulation.

Much of this interesting symposium was dedicated to hypoxemia. I was very pleased by this because it substantially confirmed that the relationship between hypoxemia and pulmonary hypertension has been amplified to include platelet aggregation also. In 1978 Steele reported a significant increase of platelet half-life after many days of oxygen administration to hypoxemic patients suffering from chronic respiratory failure. This demonstrated a tangible reduction of platelet consumption in these patients, that, as you know, have a greatly decreased basal platelet half-life.

During the Italian Congress of Internal Medicine in Rome, we reported the results of our research concerning the relationship between platelet aggregation and oxygen saturation of blood. In patients with chronic respiratory failure the platelet aggregation of the venous blood was significantly higher than that of arterial blood samples which were collected simultaneously. The oxygen saturation of 100% in the blood of these patients, who were basically hypoxemic, determined a significant decrease of the basal hyperaggregation.

The problem is fascinating for everyone and particularly for us. However, it is far from being solved and more effort is still needed from those who in future intend to dedicate their attention to this aspect, certainly not neglectable, of pulmonary vascular pathology.

PART 8

HAEMORHEOLOGY AND VASCULAR DISEASE

BASIC RHEOLOGY OF MAMMALIAN BLOOD: FACTORS PROMOTING AND FACTORS INTERFERING WITH FLUIDITY OF BLOOD

Th. Wetter and H. Schmid-Schönbein

Department of Physiology of RWTH-Aachen
Schneebergweg 211
D-5100 Aachen F.R.G.

Introduction

Blood flow in the microvasculature is determined by rheological phenomena related to the behaviour of single red blood cells. This behaviour can be characterized in terms of deformability, aggregation tendency, tank tread motion, and haematocrit adaptation to the flow situation. The last mechanism induces a separation of the paths, that plasma and blood cells take through a micronetwork.

All effects have been documented by microphotographs or motion picture scenes, part of which is given below. They have been taken from in vitro geometries of a few microns of inner dimension and from in vivo preparation.

Methods

Preparation and microscopic technique

Several thin tissues allow transillumination and in vivo microscopic observation of microvessel blood flow. Descriptions of preparations of mammalian micronetworks can be found e.g. in the publications of Chambers and Zweifach 1944 (mesentery), Strock and Majno 1969 (m. cremaster), Burton 1973 (m. sartorius) or Webb and Nicoll 1954 (bat wing). Several other preparations and improvements of details are available by now, which will, however, be omitted in this text. Two in vitro techniques have been developed that allow the seemingly paradox combination of blood cells moving fast relative to their immediate neighbourhood though being stationary with respect to the microscopic view. This has to be achieved by two absolute movements of equal speed but opposite direction, being added to zero absolute speed at the very point of the blood cell under view.

In the first case this is achieved by a modified cone-plate-viscosimeter, where cone and plate both rotate in different directions. The instrument developed by Th. Fischer* is called a Rheoscope for being manufactured of plexiglass, transillumination and microscopic observation is possible and shows stationary erthrocytes flowing with respect to the surrounding medium, in the center of the gap (Fig. 1).

The second technique involves a moving glass capillary (Gaehtgens 1981 i.p.). Its principle can be understood by means of the following model:

Imagine a trian moving forward in front of you at a low speed. A passenger in the train walks backwards at that same speed. He will then remain stationary in front of you. In the case of the moving capillary the passenger is the blood cell, driven to flow at constant speed by a constant pressure difference between two ends of a glass tube of a few microns in diameter, which is the "train", driven in a different direction by a slow electro-motor. If pressure difference and voltage are adjusted to each other, we see the cells flowing but stationary and can again try to detect details of flow behaviour.

Blood samples

In the case of in vivo preparations the blood of the experimental animal was used without modification. For in vitro deformability studies washed human erythrocytes were suspended in dextran solutions either without modification or after spectrin cross linking using a membrane permeant SH-group oxidant (Fischer et al. 1978).

For aggregation studies human whole blood of normal subjects was compaired with that of diabetics.

Results

Deformability

It is well known from in vivo and in vitro experiments that the deformability of mammalian red blood cells, in contrast to avian erythrocytes (Gaehtgens et al. 1979) has a great positive effect on whole blood fluidity in large and small vessels. The red blood cell has been shown in vitro to pass through glass tubes of inner diameter near 3μm (Jay and Canham 1977). Microvessel photographs and films support the importance of the fact, that the mammalian RBC with its undisturbed diameter of approximately 7μm enters and easily passes capillaries with a diameter much less than this.

After the membrane was artificially stiffened, the cells as a whole could no longer be elongated - or made to change their outer form in shear (Fig. 2). Nevertheless, whenever the cytoplasm was fluid and when subjected to high shear stress RBC's do not interfere with blood fluidity in vitro. In vivo measurements of capillary flow velocities (Driessen et al. 1980) show little effects under normal pressure. The effect of membrane stiffening become very evident at low pressure when permanent capillary blockage effects are seen especially

---

* A description of its functional principles can be found in Schmid-Schönbein et al. 1973.

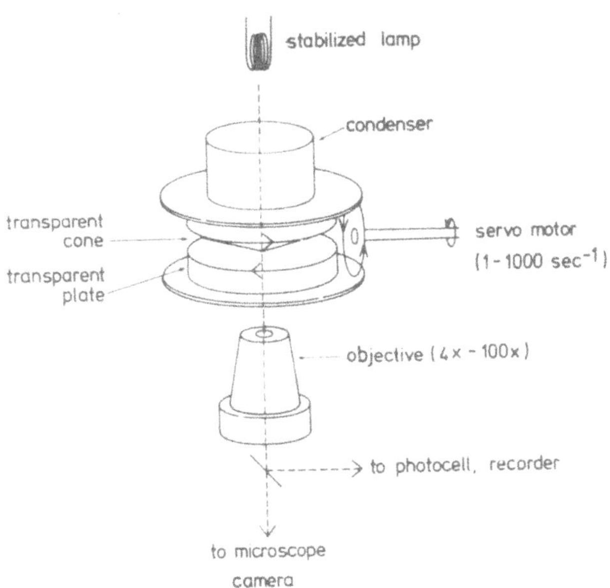

Fig. 1. Schematical drawing of the Rheoscope (Schmid-Schönbein et al., 1973). Blood cells are observed in the gap between the counterrotating plexi-glass cone and plate.

in hemorrhagic shock. The reasons for this differential behaviour will be given in the paragraph about membrane rotation ("tank treading"), which is still possible after membrane stiffening.

Aggregability

Red cell aggregation is well known as a factor having a capability of interfering with blood fluidity, whenever there is a lack of forces to disperse aggregates. Complications are known to arise from raised protein concentrations of plasma; fibrinogen and globulins play the most important role, thus focusing interest e.g. in diabetes mellitus and pregnancy.

What should be mentioned, however, from the viewpoint of basic rheology, is the fact that raised aggregability seems to have practically no effect at times or in domains of high shear forces, which is demonstrated by the lowest row of fig. 3 taken in the rheoscope with shear rates near 1000 s^{-1}. This marks the range of well perfused arterioles and capillaries. Venules, however, are perfused at shear rates of about 100 s^{-1} or below and so have flow conditions offering the chance of aggregate formation, which is enhanced by any reduction of shear rate, also demonstrated in fig. 3. An even more pronounced effect arises from augmented aggregability of e.g. blood samples from diabetics; this is shown by comparing the two scenes in one row of fig. 3 at shear rates of 80 s^{-1} or less.

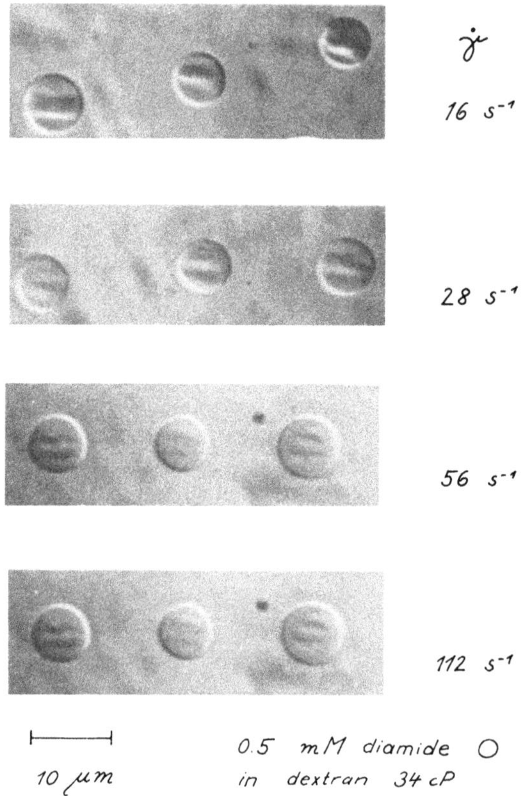

Fig. 2. Diamide RBC's (Fischer et al., 1978). Instead of increasing elongation with increasing shear rate buckling takes place.

Rotation of membrane and cytoplasm

In large vessels whole blood can be shown to be a fluid of viscosity of about 5 cP (5mPa/s) at high shear rates. As plasma viscosity is about 1.2 cP (1.2mPa/s), blood as a 40% suspension shows a fourfold fluidity decrease, which is much less than with 40% suspensions of solid, ordinary particles (Wilkinson 1960). This relatively small decrease of fluidity in spite of considerable volume concentration of cellular components is even much lower when blood moves through capillaries of 4.4 μm inner diameter (Albrecht et al. 1979). The mechanism which so effectively reduces the flow hinderance produced by the red cell membrane and cytoplasm has now been elucidated. It is only present in non-nucleated mammalian red blood cells.

New experimental demonstrations in the rheoscope and the moving capillary show that there is a highly effective transmission of shear

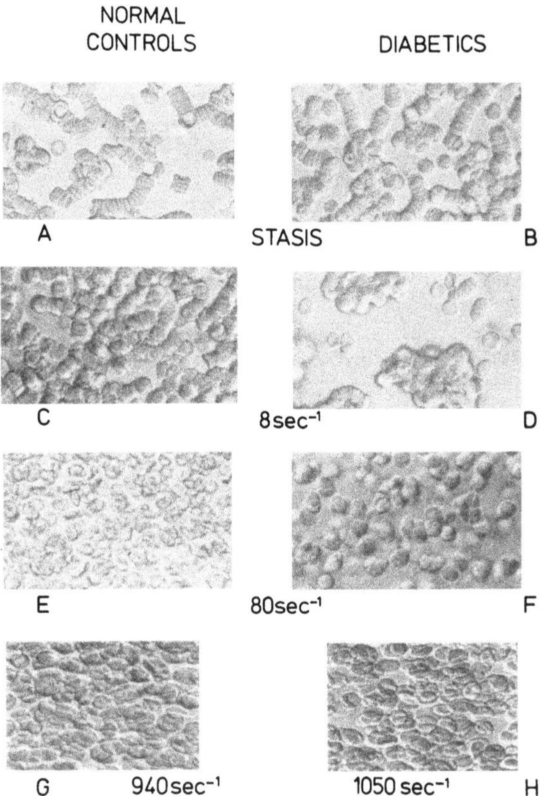

Fig. 3. Human RBC's of normal (left panel) and diabetic subjects. Decreasing shear rate in the Rheoscope (Schmid-Schönbein et al., 1973) demonstrates normal and enhanced aggregation tendency.

forces from the plasma to the cell membrane and from the cell membrane into the cytoplasm. The experimental approach starts with latex particles attached to the cell membranes of cells, which are then observed in the rheoscope and moving capillary geometries. Fig. 4 and 5 schematically draw the action of shear forces.

In the rheoscope there are idealized forces from left to right above and from right to left below the particle (e.g. a sphere), which, if solid, rotates as a whole and tumbles, as nucleated bird erythrocytes do. This involves higher energy dissipation in suspension flow. Mammalian RBC, which do not tumble, but remain elongated and orientated in shear as indicated in the lower part of fig. 4, show membrane rotation around the cytoplasm. This type of motion is associated with minimal energy dissipation and is a phenomenon also

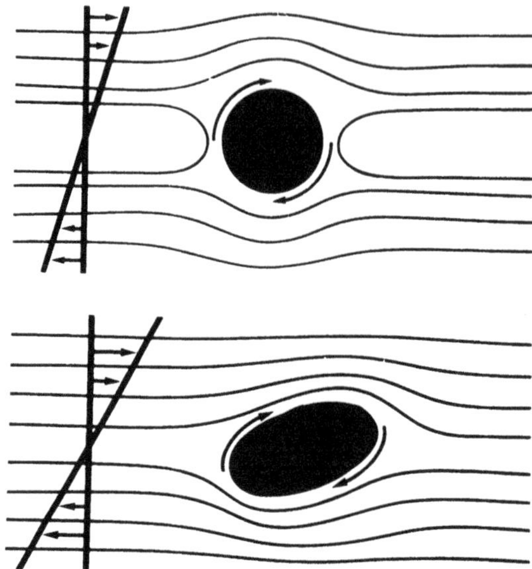

Fig. 4. Schematic drawing of flow adaption of non deformable sphere and deformable ellipsoid.

occurring, when ordinary fluid droplets are subjected to shear. In RBC's this rotation can be traced by the latex particles, whose migration along the cell shape can indeed be followed in the frames of the motion picture scene. To demonstrate vortex-like rotation of the cytoplasm when sheared by the rotation or tank-treading membrane, Heinz-bodies were artificially induced and rheoscope experiments were carried out in the way described above. Fig. 6 reveals rotation of intracellular laminae at decreasing speeds from outer to inner regions of the cell*.

At any time and in any place, where this rotation takes palce,

---

* Interpretation of details visible from the film projected at the conference, go beyond the physical scope of this text and should be taken from the publications of Th. Fischer, some of which are cited at the end of the text.

MEMBRANE ROTATION IN CAPILLARY FLOW
RED CELLS SUBJECTED TO ASYMMETRICIALLY
VISCOUS DRAG $D = \tau \cdot a$

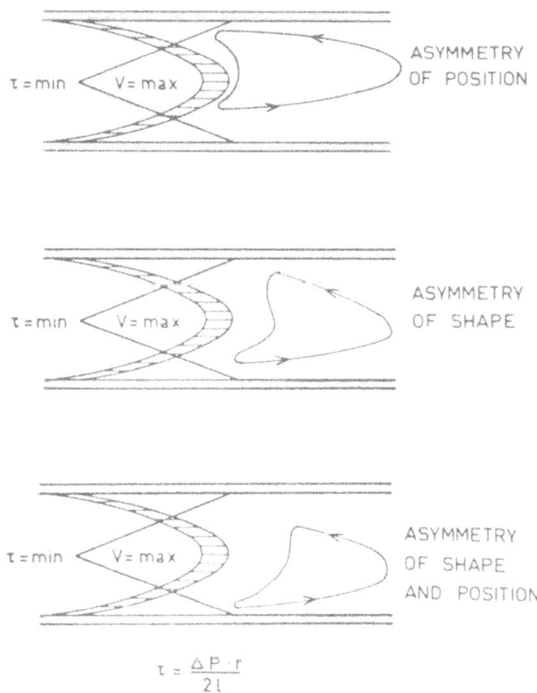

Fig. 5. Any slight asymmetry of suspended particles in tube flow induces some kind of rotational motion.

it considerably promotes fluidity, for the particle behaviour does not primarily disturb the flow field but participates in the externally induced flow pattern.

Fig. 5 and 7 prove that the membrane rotation is also possible in capillaries. The schematical drawing shows that any occurrence of asymmetry of cell position, vessel or forces will result in unequal shear forces acting on two parts of the membrane and producing rotation . The scenes from a motion picture with schematic drawings of one cell with its latex particle in the right of the corresponding film scenes indicate the existence of that membrane rotation.

So membrane rotation, and probably also cytoplasm rotation is not limited to rheoscope geometries and should be memorized as a factor that highly enhances fluidity in mammalian blood vessels.

It should be pointed to the fact that spectrin cross-linking as mentioned in the paragraph about deformability, is in a very

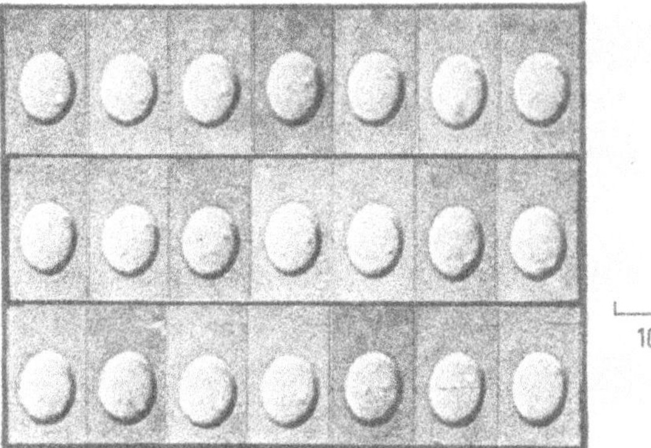

Movement of a membrane-bound and a freely floating cytoplasmic Heinzbody (frequency = 3.1/sec and 1.7/sec). Time interval 21 msec. Shear rate = 71/sec. Viscosity of continuous phase = 22 cP.

Fig. 6. Cytoplasm rotation can also be demonstrated in the Rheoscope (Fischer et al., 1978, (2)).

indirect way related to the ability of membrane rotation : Diamide RBC's could be shown to exhibit the same membrane rotation in the rheoscope but could not be elongated. This explains the in vivo observation of unaffected flow velocities as long as a high pressure gradient and high shear forces rotate the cell membranes. Once stoppage occurs, the cells cannot be elongated and practically irreversibly clog the capillaries. The stiff cells resist static pressure gradients, which do not induce rotation but bulk motion.

Haematocrit regulation

It is well known that the haematocrit value in the peripheral small blood vessels is significantly different from that found in a large vessel (from where the blood is usually taken for rheological measurements (Fahraeus 1929), Albrecht et al., 1979). It is now known that the haematocrit in the microvessel can fall to zero: this is the consequence of "plasma skimming" or its equivalent, the "screening" of cells away from a capillary entrance.

On the other hand, the haematocrit under conditions of high flow has been found to be as high as 40% (Klitzman and Duling 1979). We now understand that the haematocrit can be actively controlled by the vasomotor activity of the precapillary resistance vessels (Schmid-Schönbein et al., Wetter et al. 1981 i.p.).

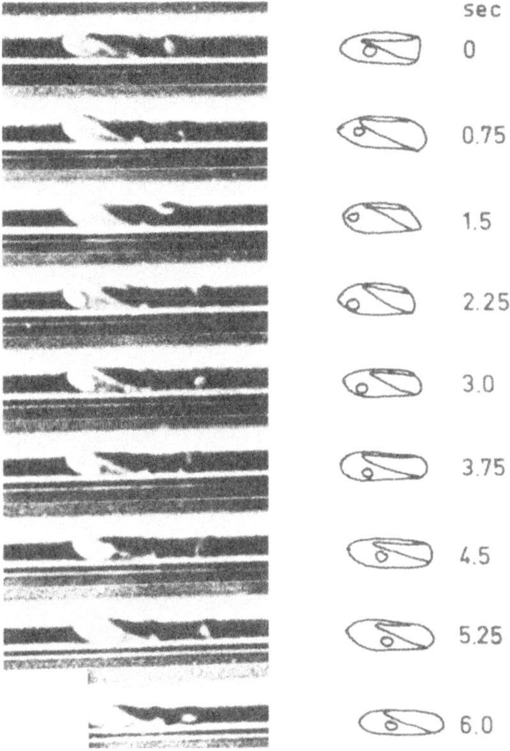

Fig. 7. Motion picture scenes from the travelling capillary (Gaehtgens, 1981, i.p.) demonstrate membrane rotation in tube flow by latex particles attached to the membrane.

The basic principle of the haematocrit control is related to the well known fact that at a branch point the red blood cells have the tendency to enter the faster of two channels. The principle held not only in a large sample of stochastically selected blood vessels, where momentary haematocrit and flow were compared (Klitzman and Duling 1979), but also when at individual branch points the temporal variation of haematocrit and flow rate were correlated. In the latter experiments flow rate was either regulated by spontaneous vasomotion or modified by suddenly induced changes of pressure (Wetter et al., 1981, i.p.).

Therefore, in the intact microvasculature the fluidity of the blood is regulated in the sense that the mass of the red cells are funnelled into those vessel with high flow (and therefore high shear stresses). Similarly, red cells are screened away from capillaries with low flow (and low shear stresses), which therefore are only perfused with plasma, a "thin" Newtonian fluid.

The slow onset of both vasoconstriction and vasodilation provides a safety mechanism that protects against the failure as the reduction of haematocrit in the constrictor phase clearly precedes the drop of flow to values associated with very low shear stresses. Conversely, when the vasodilation begins, the capillaries are first perfused only with plasma - haematocrit rising gradually and strictly simultaneously with increases in shear stress.

The control mechanism fails, whenever the rhythmic vasomotion breaks down, simply because in the dilated state of the vasculature the velocity differences at the branch point tend to be minimal. When other factors are kept equal the flow is therefor most homolgeniously distributed - but at the same time, the cells no longer have a choice to go into one of the two channels. Under these conditions (which were first induced by pharmacological or pH-dependent dilation by Klitzman and Duling 1979) the haematocrit in all microvessels (including the capillaries) is elevated. It is well known that many disease states, most notably diabetes mellitus in association with chemical dilatation, i.e. a loss of vascular tone in all tissues where this has been tested (for a review see H. Schmid-Schönbein 1976). As long as the shear forces are high, the resulting high haematocrit in the microvessels is of no great significance. When however, the flow velocities in the diabetic vascular bed are reduced (for whatever reason) the situation is highlighted by the simultaneous presence of a high haematocrit, elevated plasma viscosity, enhanced tendency to aggregation; in other words: a combination of factors capable of interfering with the fluidity of blood co-exist and are capable of potentiating the flow retardation to full stagnation.

Conclusions

Normal blood flow in the microvessels is characterized by very high fluidity of the blood - which is a consequence of red cell properties as well as of the physiological haematocrit regulation.

Obviously, it is possible to assign distinct pathogenetic roles to the different rheological abnormalities: it is very likely that sick-ling red blood cells should occlude capillaries - whereas a flow disturbance by either enhanced aggregability or elevated haematocrit is most likely to cause venular flow disturbances as often described - e.g. by Knisely 1965.

There have been a number of attempts at haemorheological therapy, one of the more successful appears to be simple isovolemic haemodilution. Its most likely effect is a reduction of the microvascular haematocrit - but also an interference with the actual formation of venular aggregates - simply because venular flow is then again too fast. The preferential effect of haemodilution on the venular and venous side of the vasculature is related to an augmentation of venous return and a subsequent increase in stroke volume and thence cardiac output.

REFERENCES

Albrecht, K.H., Gaehtgens, P., Pries, A. and Heuser, M., 1979, The Fahraeus effect in narrow capillaries. Microvasc. Res. 18:33.

Burton, K.S., 1973, Cat sartorius muscle: An isolated perfused skeletal muscle preparation for microvascular research. Microvasc. Res. 5:401-409.

Chambers, R. and Zweifach, B.W., 1944, Topography and function of the mesenteric circulation. Am. J. Anat. 75:173-205.

Driessen, G.K., Haest, C.W.M., Heidtmann, H., Kamp, D. and Schmid-Schönbein, H., 1980, Effect of reduced red cell "deformability" on flow velocity in capillaries of rat mesentery. Pflüger's Arch. 388:75-78.

Fahraeus, R., 1929, The suspension stability of blood. Physiol. Rev. 9:241.

Fischer, T.M., Haest, C.W.M., Stöhr, M., Kamp, D. and Deuticke, B;, 1978, Selective alteration of erythrocyte deformability by SH-reagents. Evidence for an involvement of spectrin in membrane shear elasticity. In: Biochimica et Biophysica Acta, 510:270-282 (1).

Fischer, T.M., Stöhr-Liesen, M., Schmid-Schönbein, H., 1978, Red cells as a fluid droplet; tank tread like motion of human erythrocyte membrane in shear flow. Science 202:894-896(2).

Gaehtgens, P., 1981, In press (Biorheology).

Gaehtgens, P., Schmidt, F. and Will, G., 1979, Microrheology of nucleated erythrocytes (NRBC) during flow through narrow capillaries. Microvasc. Res. 17:23, 7.

Jay, A.W.L. and Canham, P.B., 1977, Viscoelastic properties of the human red blood cell membrane. II. Area and volume of individual red cells entering a micropipette. Biophys. J. 17:169.

Klitzman, B. and Duling, B.R., 1979, Microvascular hematocrit and red cell flow in resting and contracting striated muscle. Am. J. Physiol. 237:H 481 - H 490.

Knisely, M.H., 1965, Intravascular erythrocyte aggregation (blood sludge). In: Handbook of physiol., W.F. Hamilton and P. Dow (eds.), Sect. 2, Vol. III, Washington D.C.

Schmid-Schönbein, H. and Volger, E., 1977, Abnormes Fliessverhalten des Blutes beim Diabetes mellitus: Über die Rolle gestörter Fliesseigenschaften und veränderter Fliessbedingungen bei der Pathogenese der diabetischen Retinopathie. In: Diabetische Angiopathien, Hrsg.: K. Alexander - M. Cachovan, Verlag Gerhard Witzstock, Baden-Baden-Brüssel-Köln-New York, S. 38-48.

Schmid-Schönbein, H., Klitzman, B., and Johnson, P.J., 1981, Vasomotion and blood hemorheology fluidity: maintenance of blood fluidity in the microvessel by rhythmic vasomotion. In press (Bibl. Anat.).

Schmid-Schönbein, H., Gosen, J., Heinrich, L., Klose, H.J. and Volger, E., 1973, A counter rotating "rheoscope-chamber" for the study of the microrheology of blood cell aggregation by microscopic observation and microphotometry. Microvasc. Res. 6:366-376.

Strock, P.E. and Majno, G., 1969, Microvascular changes in acutely ischemic rat muscle. Surgery Gyn. Obstetrics 129: 1213-1224.

Webb, R.L. and Nicoll, P.A., 1954, The bat wing as a subject for studies in homeostasis of capillary beds. Anat. Rec. 120: 253.

Wetter, Th., Schmid-Schönbein, H., Johnson, P.C. and Klitzman, B., Simultaneous variation in flow velocity and hematocrit in skeletal muscle. Wetter el al. in press (Bibl. Anat.).

Wilkinson, W.L., 1960, Non-Newtonian fluids: fluid mechanism, mixing and heat transfer. New York-London-Oxford-Paris: Pergamon Press.

THE RED CELL AS A RISK FACTOR IN CIRCULATORY DISEASES

John A. Dormandy

St. James' and St. George's Hospitals
Sarsfeld Road
London SW12, England

The vitally essential function of the red cell distributing oxygen through the body has perhaps stopped us from appreciating that the red cells may also represent a risk factor predisposing to circulatory insufficiency. Our recent interest and increasing knowledge of the rheological or flow properties of blood has shown that this risk to the circulation may be manifested in two different ways: by an increase in the whole blood viscosity associated with a raised concentration of red cells , and by a maldistribution of flow in the microcirculation due to increased rigidity of the red cells. The second of these mechanisms is much more speculative.

The red cell as a danger and potential risk was perhaps already hinted at in the Hippocratic literature of the 5th and 4th centuries before Christ, which first advocated blood letting; a practice in favour with our predecessors for over two millenia. But there has been increasing evidence in the last few years that, even in the normal range, a high haemoglobin level or haematocrit is an important cardiovascular risk factor (whilst it had previously been assumed that this was only true of polycythaemia). In the province of the cerebral circulation Kannel (1972) showed as part of the Framingham study that the risk of cerebral infarction over a 16 year period was proportional to the initial haemoglobin value within the normal range. Men with haemoglobin values over 15g and women over 14g had twice as many cerebral infarctions as comparable groups with lower haemoglobin values. In a beautiful series of clinical experiments, Thomas et al., (1977) demonstrated the probable link between haemoglobin level and cerebral infarction by showing that there was a very close correlation between haemoglobin, blood viscosity and total cerebral blood flow.

In the same Framingham study it was also found that at least part of the effect of haemoglobin on the incidence of cerebral infarction is due to a significant correlation between haemoglobin level and blood pressure, particularly the diastolic ($p<0.01$). But it is in the territory of the coronaries that the circulatory implications of the risk of high normal haematocrit are most serious. It is now 15 years since Burch and De Pasquale first pointed out that patients with myocardial ischaemia have an abnormally raised haematocrit, and in their later paper (1965) they summarised the evidence linking high haematocrit to diminished coronary blood flow and the therapeutic implications of these findings. They did not however look for a direct correlation between the haematocrit and the development of subsequent 'myocardial events'. This has only been demonstrated in the excellent Stockholm Prospective Study where over 6,000 apparently healthy individuals were examined originally in 1961 and then observed for the development of new events of coronary heart disease. At the end of 9 years' follow-up there was a significant correlation between the original haemoglobin level and the development of new ischaemic events (Bottiger, 1972). Preliminary results after 15 years, presented by Carlson in 1977, showed an increased significance of the initial haemoglobin, which now became a better predictor for myocardial ischaemia than abnormalities in the plasma lipids.

An overabundance of red cells can also be a risk to our attempts at improving the circulation by surgery. Bouhoustos (1974) followed up 445 patients after arterial reconstructive surgery and showed that the immediate pre-operative haemoglobin was an important determinant of post operative complications. Patients with a pre-operative haemoglobin level between 16.0 and 16.4g had six times higher incidence of complications than patients with a pre-operative haemoglobin below 16.0g. This dramatic and unexpected result has received insufficient attention ; many vascular surgeons still believe that the more haemoglobin, the better. We have carried out a rather similar survey in patients undergoing local amputations of the foot for diabetic ischaemic disease. There was a clear separation between the preoperative haemoglobin of the amputations which healed and those that failed requiring a further higher resection (Bailey, 1979). Again, the presence of a low haemoglobin seemed to be a better predictor of success than any other laboratory or clinical measurement.

There is no doubt that the principal and possibly the only explanation for the cardiovascualr complications associated with a high haematocrit is the well-established relationship to whole blood viscosity. It is generally agreed that this is approximately a semilogarithmic relationship so that the effect of blood viscosity of altering a high haematocrit is greater than the effect of the same change at a lower haematocrit. The subsequent effect of blood viscosity on blood flow is also generally accepted.

The increasing number of reports of the clinically beneficial effects of haemodilution lends further support to the proposition that red cells can be an important risk factor in certain circumstances. In the study from Queen Square already quotated (Thomas, 1977), patients with clinical and objective evidence of cerebral ischaemia were venesected in small stages reducing their mean haematocrit from 52% to 46%. This was accompanied by a clinical improvement and an increase in actual blood flow from 36.2 to 62.7ml/100g/min. Haemodilution therefore resulted in an overall improvement in oxygen delivery. In myocardial ischaemia, venesection and haemodilution have been reported to be beneficial by Burch and De Pasquale (1965) and Langsjoen (1973). Whilst in the treatment of ischaemia of the legs we (Yates et al., 1979) as well as others have reported good objective results. In our experience the calf blood flow increased by 51% at rest and by 170% after reactive hyperaemia. The haemoglobin delivery increased by less as the blood was more dilute, but on average it still rose by 13% at rest and, most importantly from the clinical point of view, it increased by 100% at peak flow.

All this lends support to the proposition that a high normal red cell concentration may be a risk factor and to what may at first seem the unlikely hypothesis that the normal range of haematocrit is not necessarily the optimal range. But is this indeed so implausible? Not if we look at it from the evolutionary point of view. We have evolved our normal range of haematocrit over a very long period during which the principal danger to the cardiovascualr system was from trauma and haemorrhage. A relatively high natural or initial haematocrit would have favoured the survival of repeated blood loss. It is only very recently during modern civilisation that the risk of accidental trauma has been diminished and the principal cardiovascular risk has come to be arterial narrowing and ischaemia. Under these very new conditions the optimal haematocrit may well be less than the normal range we have inherited.

Equally exciting, but for the moment much more debatable, is the second possible mechanism whereby the red cell may be an important circulatory risk factor. That is the proposition that a decrease of the normal flexibility of the red cell may impair its ability to negotiate the narrow channels of the microcirculation. Theoretically this is perfectly plausible, but its practical proof depends on our assessment of the validity of the techniques available for measuring red cell deformability. The very multiplicity of techniques advocated suggests that this is an area where the clinical significance of haemorheology is, for the moment, more open to doubt. The most commonly used techniques are based on the filtration of red cells in various suspensions through pores smaller in diameter than the undeformed red cell; and it is only the validity of this group of techniques which will be considered.

There is no direct experimental evidence, even in animals, that the filterability of red cells is directly related to tissue perfusion. By contrast there is much accumulated evidence that a significant decrease in red cell filterability can be demonstrated in many circulatory diseases and often the degree of abnormality has a prognostic significance in terms of progression of the disease; for instance we have shown that red cell filterability has decreased in patients with ischaemia of the legs and that those who subsequently come to amputation have even more rigid red cells than those who do not (Dormandy et al., 1977). More recently, a decrease in red cell deformability has been shown in all patients with myocardial infarction (Dormandy et al., 1981). The abnormality seems to take approximately ten hours to reach maximum effect and this lowest value for red cell filterability can be very closely correlated with the subsequent clinical progress of the infarction. Patients who develop pulmonary oedema, cardiogenic shock, or died had progressively more rigid red cells within hours of the infarction. An abnormality in red cell filterability has also been demonstrated in a number of other circulatory diseases such as angina pectoris (Nicolaides et al.,1977) and diabetes (Barnes et al., 1977).

As regards the last criteria, there are very few drugs which definitely improve red cell deformability in vivo, although there are a number of other possible approaches to this problem such as prevention of ATP depletion in red cells, altering the red cell membrane-plasma surface tension, altering the surface zeta potential or altering the ratio of polymerised and unpolymerised spectrine which is the principal skeletal protein of the red cell. Although a number of drugs acting through one or more of these mechanisms are already available and do seem to alter the filterability of red cells, they have not yet been conclusively proven to be of clinical value. It is interesting that the parallel improvement in filterability and clinical condition has been shown using plasmapheresis in Raynaud's disease (Dodds et al., 1979).

In conclusion, there would now seem to be overwhelming evidence that the red cell is a very real circulatory risk factor, in terms of its contribution to whole blood viscosity. It may be equally important in terms of an abnormality in its deformability, although this relatively new concept is yet to be fully explored.

REFERENCES

Bailey, M.J., Johnston, C.L.W., Yates, C.J., Somerville, P.G. and Dormandy, J.A., 1979, Pre-operative haemoglobin as a predictor of outcome of diabetic amputations. Lancet 2: 168.

Barnes, A.J., Locke, P., Scudder, P.R., Dormandy, T.L., Dormandy, J.A. and Slack, J., 1977, Hyperviscosity: a treatable component of diabetic microcirculatory disease. Lancet 2: 789-791.

Bottiger, L.E. and Carlson, L.A., 1972, Stockholm prospective study 2. In: Skandia International Symposium, 1-362. Nordiska Bokhandelns Förlag, Stockholm.

Bouhoustos, J., Morris, T., Chavatz, D. and Martin, P., 1974, The influence of haemoglobin and paltelet levels on the results of arterial surgery. Brit. J. Surg. 61:984.

Burch, G.E. and De Pasquale, N.P., 1965, Haematocrit viscosity and coronary blood flow. Diseases of the Chest 48:225.

Carlson, L.A., 1977, Presentation at International Conference on Atherosclerosis in Milan.

Dodds, A.J., O'Rielly, M.J.G., Yates, C.J., Cotton, L.T., Flute, P.T. and Dormandy, J.A., 1979, Haemorheological response to plasma excange in Raynaud's syndrome. Brit. Med. J. 2:1186-1187.

Dormandy, J.A., Boyd, M. and Ernst, E., 1981, Red cell filterability after myocardial infarction. To be published in Scand. J. of Lab. and Clin. Invest. Jan.

Kannel, W.B., Gordon, T., Wolf, P.A. and McNamara, P., 1972, Haemoglobin and the risk of cerebral infarction: The Framingham Study. Stroke 3:490.

Langsjoen, P.H., 1973, The value of reducing blood viscosity in acute myocardial infarction. Bibl. Anat. 2:180.

Nicolaides, A.N., Bowers, R., Horbourne, J., Kinder, P.H., Besterman, E.M., 1977, Blood viscosity, red cell flexibility, haematocrit, and plasma fibrinogen in patients with angina. Lancet 2:943.

Reid, H.L., Dormandy, J.A., Barnes, A.J., Lock, P.J. and Dormandy, T.L., 1977, Impaired red cell deformability in peripheral vascular disease. Lancet 2:666

Thomas, D.J., Marshall, J., Ross-Russel, R.W., Wetherley-Main, G., Duboulay, G.H., Pearson, R., Symon, L., and Zilkha, E, 1977, Effect of haematocrit on cerebral blood flow in man. Lancet 2:941.

Yates, C.J., Berent, A., Andrews, V. and Dormandy, J.A., 1979, Increase in leg blood flow by normovolaemic haemodilution in intermittent claudication. Lancet 2:166.

HEMORHEOLOGICAL PARAMETERS IN SOME VASCULAR DISEASES

J.F. Stoltz

Hemorheology Department
Regional Blood Transfusion Centre
Barbois
54500 Vandoeuvre-lès-Nancy, France

The origin of arterial diseases (acrosyndromes or peripheral vascular diseases is undoubtedly more generally attributed to parietal and vasomotor anomalies than to hemorheological disorders. However, in the light of recent investigations it would seem that increased erythrocyte aggregation is generally observed during arterial disease and is sometimes accompanied by reduced red cell deformability resulting in the appearance of a hyperviscosity syndrome. These rheological disturbances may have very significant bearing on the complications observed via three primary mechanisms: hemolysis (resulting in ADP release and promoting platelet aggregation), erythrocyte aggregation (resulting in a decreased blood flow (sludge)), and reduced erythrocyte deformability accompanied by reduced oxygen availability in the small blood vessels.

In this paper we have attempted to investigate the main hemorheological disturbances described during peripheral arteriopathy and acrosyndromes by trying to define the implications of these changes from the therapeutic point of view.

1) HEMORHEOLOGICAL PARAMETERS AND PERIPHERAL ARTERIAL DISEASES

Few rheological studies have been undertaken on peripheral arterial diseases and where the studies do exist, they are often incomplete. Three main types of changes have, however, been regularly observed by various authors:

This work was supported by DRET (Biological department)

a) Appearance of a hyperviscosity syndrome revealed by Dormandy et al., (1973) in a study on 126 patients. It was noted the viscosity, measured at two deformation rates (23 and 230 sec^{-1}), was higher in patients with associated ischaemic heart disease (Figure 1).
The authors also compared blood viscosity with claudication distance and noted that the higher the patient's blood viscosity, the lower his walking periphery (Figure 2). The authors put forward the notion of 'rheological claudication'. These results are in full agreement with those obtained by Störmar et al. (1974) who also noted the appearance of plasma and blood hyperviscosity (Figure 3), as well as with our own results (Figure 4) obtained during a pharmacological study on 8 patients. It is noted that plasma hyperviscosity and an increased tendency for red blood cell aggregation have also been found by Dintenfass and Ibels (1975).
It is necessary to mention the recent work carried out by Anadere et al (1979). They applied the theory of linear viscoelasticity to blood ($\eta^* = \eta' - i\eta^*$) and showed that the elastic and viscous modulus of blood are increased in patients with peripheral arterial disease (Figure 5).

b) Modifications associated with erythrocyte filterability. In fact, according to the work carried out by Ehrly et al. (1976) it seems that erythrocyte filterability, tested by two different techniques, is reduced. It must be noted that this decrease is all the more marked in patients suffering from decubitus or gangrene. In fact erythrocyte deformability could be an important factor in determining the symptoms of an inadequate peripheral blood flow. However, before concluding, it would be better to carry out more detailed studies.

c) Biochemical plasma modifications. Most of the authors (Stormer et al., 1974) agree on the rheological modifications and also on important modifications in the level of plasma proteins (increase in fibrinogen and a reduction in the albumin/globulin and albumin/fibrinogen ratios) (Figures 6 and 7). Considering the importance of these proteins on blood and plasma viscosity, these variations can partly explain the hyperviscosity at low shear rates and the increase in red blood cell aggregation.

2) HEMORHEOLOGICAL PARAMETERS AND RAYNAUD'S DISEASE OR SYNDROMES

Acrosyndromes are above all, functional, permanent or paroxystic 'dystonic' syndromes which affect one of the sectors of the terminal vascular bed (the arteriole sector in the case of Raynauds disease or the veinlet sector in the case of acrocyanosis) leading to repercussions in the capillary network. Whether the phenomenon is clearly

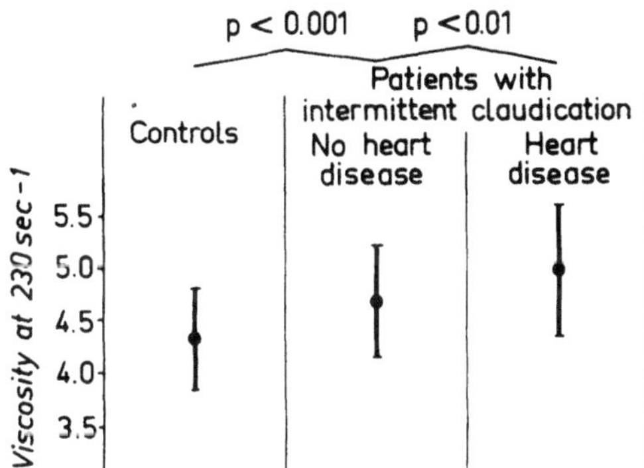

Fig. 1. Correlation between blood viscosity ($\dot{\gamma}$ = 230 sec^{-1}), intermittent claudication with evidence of ischaemic heart disease. (Viscosity in centipoises) (from Dormandy)

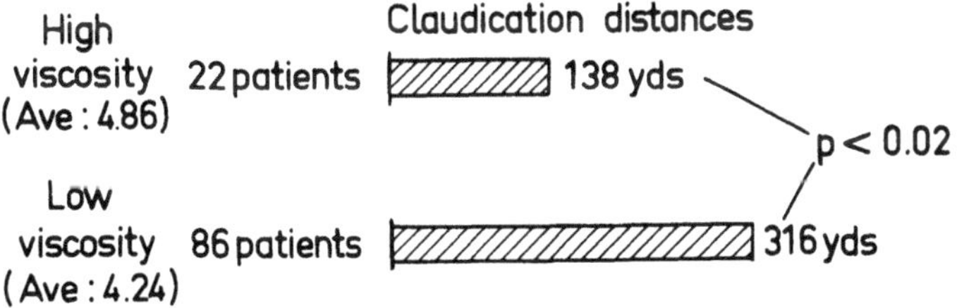

Fig. 2. Claudification distances and blood viscosity (from Dormandy et al.)

a secondary incident, or whether it has a more essential action, it is always conventionally attributed to vasomotor pathogenesis, in other words to mechanisms which involve the vascular wall, its tonicity, its innervation, etc. In other cases the acrosyndromes cor-

	Plasma		Blood				K
	η or η_0 cP	$\frac{\eta}{\eta_0}$	η or η_0 $\dot{\gamma}=4.6\ sec^{-1}$ cP	η or η_0 $\dot{\gamma}=0.01\ sec^{-1}$ cP	$\frac{\eta}{\eta_0}$ $\dot{\gamma}=4.6\ sec^{-1}$	$\frac{\eta}{\eta_0}$ $\dot{\gamma}=0.01\ sec^{-1}$	$\frac{\eta}{\eta_0}$ Blood / $\frac{\eta}{\eta_0}$ Plasma
Normal	1.32 ± 0.08 (n=46)	1	10.45 ± 2.3 (n=54)	109 ± 28.5 (n=55)	1	1	1
Peripheral arterial disease	1.54 ± 0.18 (n=49)	1.16	12.5 ± 1.6 (n=45)	139 ± 24.4 (n=40)	1.14	1.3	1.12
	$p < 0.0005$		$p < 0.0005$	$p < 0.0005$			

Fig. 3. Mean apparent viscosity ± SD of plasma and blood in peripheral arterial diseases (from Störmer et al. - 1974)

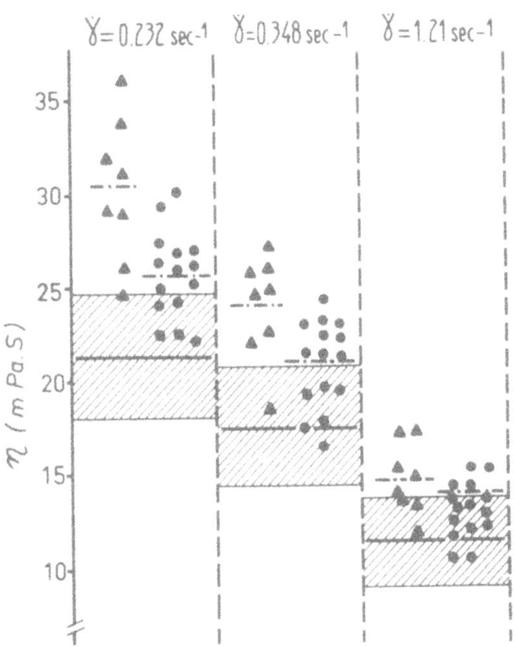

Fig. 4. Mean apparent viscosity of blood in patients with peripheral arterial diseases (▲ n = 8) and with Raynaud's disease (● n = 15) H = 40% _._. mean value for patients, ____ control (Personal results)

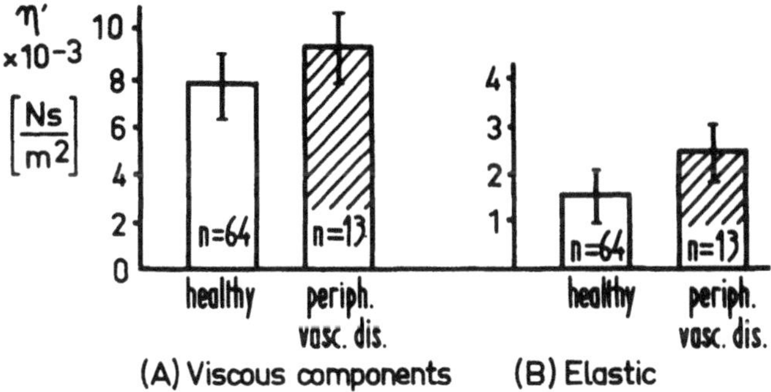

Fig. 5. Viscous (A) and elastic components (B) for healthy donors and patients with peripheral vascular disease (γ = 10 sec^{-1}) (from Anadere et al.)

	Total protein (g%)	Albumin (%)	Globulins			
			α_1 %	α_2 %	β %	γ %
Normal	7.35 ± 11.5 (n=60)	65.9 ± 4.6 (n=60)	2.3 ± 1.2 (n=60)	5.7 ± 1.9 (n=60)	9.6 ± 1.8 (n=60)	16.0 ± 3.5 (n=60)
Peripheral arterial disease	8.16 ± 1.0 (n=20)	53.7 ± 7.9 (n=20)	4.1 ± 1.4 (n=20)	11.3 ± 2.6 (n=20)	11.3 ± 2.9 (n=20)	19.5 ± 6.1 (n=20)
	0.005 > p > 0.0025	p < 0.0005	p < 0.0005	p < 0.0005	0.0025 > p > 0.0005	0.0025 > p > 0.0005

Fig. 6. Mean plasma proteins ± SD in peripheral arterial diseases and controls (from Störmer)

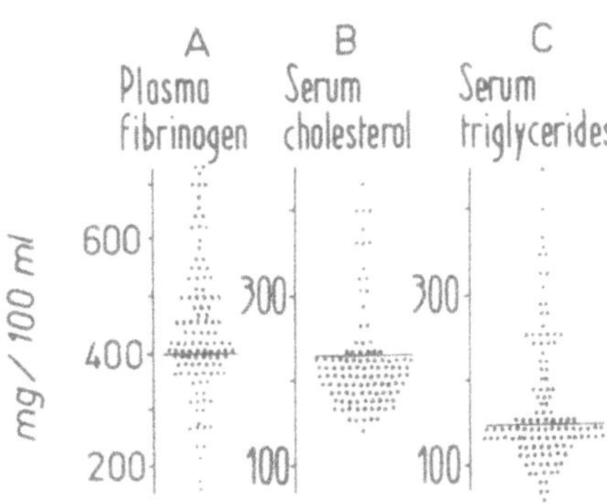

Fig. 7. Distribution of (A) plasma fibrinogen, (B) serum cholesterol, and (C) serum triglyceride concentrations. Upper limits of normal ranges (normal mean ± S.D.) in a non-aged-matched population are indicated. (from Dormandy et al)

Factor *	Shear rate (sec-1)	Raynaud (20 patients) (Mean ± SE)	Control (12 patients) (Mean ± SE)	P Value
Hematocrit, %	...	39.0 ± 1.12	42.6 ± 1.20	<.05
Whole blood viscosity	52	5.26 ± 0.94	4.88 ± 0.17	>.05
Whole blood viscosity	0.52	33.0 ± 2.33	30.9 ± 1.14	>.05
RBC viscosity +	52	6.0 ± 0.11	5.0 ± 0.09	<.01
RBC viscosity +	5.2	12.1 ± 0.58	9.49 ± 0.24	<.01
RBC viscosity +	0.52	44.8 ± 1.90	28.4 ± 1.14	<.01
Plasma viscosity	...	1.50 ± 0.045	1.188 ± 0.03	<.01
Relative viscosity ×	0.52	31.0 + 0.78	25.0 ± 1.0	<.01

* Viscosity is expressed in centipoises

+ Represents RBC viscosity in autologous plasma at a hematocrit value of 45 %

× Obtained by dividing RBC viscosity by plasma viscosity; relative viscosity is an index of RBC aggregation

Fig. 8. Rheologic changes in Raynaud syndrome (from Tietjen et al. 1975)

Plasma Protein gm/100 ml Blood	Raynaud *	Control ×	P Value
Gamma globulin	1.48 ± 0.173	0.77 ± 0.04	< .01
Fibrinogen	0.400 ± 0.0025	0.259 ± 0.003	< .01
Fibrinogen and globulins	4.32 ± 0.178	2.80 ± 0.11	< .01

* Group of 20 patients; values expressed as mean ± SE.
× Group of 12 patients; values expressed as mean ± SE.

Fig. 9. Plasma protein changes in Raynaud syndrome (from Tietjen et al.)

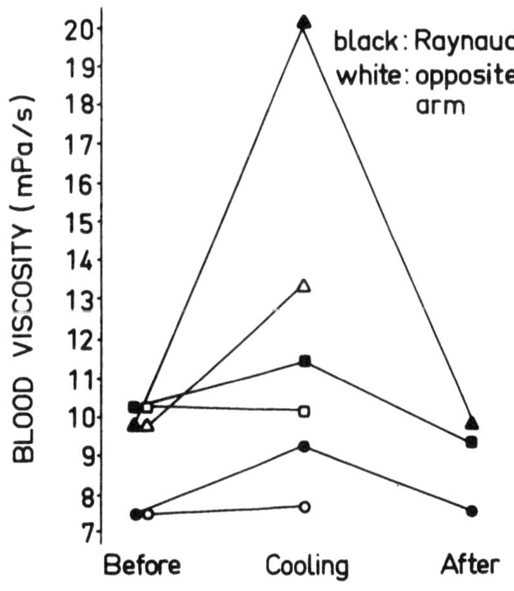

Fig. 10. Blood viscosity (shear - rate 3.75 s^{-1}) in three patients with Raynaud's disease before, during and after the cooling-induced phenomenon (from Forgoni et al. 1976)

respond to organic micro-angiopathies and are dystrophic. In general, the part played by circulating blood and the actual hemorheological changes are more rarely put forward than are vasomotor or parietal phenomena.

From a rheological point of view, the secondary hemorheological changes which are related to the vasomotor phenomenon must be differentiated from the primary changes.

Thus, arteriole vasoconstriction or veinlet stasis results in a hemodynamic related slackening in blood circulation causing more severe intravascular erythrocyte aggregation than the aggregation which can be physiologically observed in the veinlet sector (sludge phenomenon). These secondary hemorheological changes are extremely difficult to investigate and would have to be studied by taking blood in situ. Even then the results would be open to criticism. We might assume, however, that the red cells have a tendency to aggregate and perhaps also become fragile resulting in reduced red cell deformability. Because of the changes often associated with vascular permeability we might also assume that changes occur in local hematocrit and protein values as well as in the distribution of these factors.

Apart from these secondary changes, it is also possible to identify primary hemorheological anomalies which are likely to give rise to acrosyndromes. Goyle and Dormandy have even voiced the assumption that increased viscosity might be at the origin of Raynaud's syndrome.

The eventual responsibility of the rheological factors such as erythrocyte aggregation and deformability as the cause of Raynaud's disease or syndromes has been investigated, but the results obtained are not always convergent. In a study on 22 patients, Pringle et al. (1965) revealed an increase in viscosity during certain Raynaud syndromes. Their results showed that during the syndrome, blood viscosity increased 2.5 cp on average to reach a value of 5.2 cp. A conjunctival sludge phenomenon was also some times observed. Moreover, in a large number of cases, the authors observed high plasma fibrinogen levels.

In a very extensive investigation Tietjen et al. (1975) revealed an increase in plasma and blood viscosity which was particularly noticeable at low shear rates ($\gamma = 0.52\ sec^{-1}$) (Figure 8). Concurrently, the authors observed an increase in IgG and plasma fibrinogen levels (Figure 9). From their results, the authors concluded that the constant increase in viscosity was partly due to the "inflammatory" syndrome. In a recent investigation (Figure 4) we ourselves have confirmed these results and have shown that the increase in blood viscosity was more significant at low shear rate values.

We should also mention the work carried out by Goyle and Dormandy who observed high blood and plasma viscosity during Raynaud's syndrome at temperatures of 27° and $37^{\circ}C$ and at low shear rate values ($0.77\ 22.62\ sec^{-1}$). Also worthy of note is the study carried out by Forconi et al. (1976) on three patients which revealed an increase in blood viscosity after immersing the patients' hands in ice cold water (Figure 10). Since no rheological changes were observed in the two reference subjects studied, the authors attributed these changes to the disease.

In a general study on 17 patients, Dintenfa-s (1977) attempted an analysis of the disturbed rheological factors. He observed that the most frequently recurring anomalies were the tendency towards erythrocyte aggregation and greater red blood cell rigidity. Moreover, the albumin/fibrinogen and albumin/globulin ratios were frequently lower than normal.

Finally, we should mention the work carried out by Johnson et al. (1977) as well as the study undertaken by McGrath et al. (1978) who observed no change in blood and plasma viscosity in patients suffering from a primary Raynaud phenomenon (Raynaud's disease).

To summarize, it could be said that although increased total protein and hematocrit levels are factors that have been rarely observed, several authors have reported the tendency towards increased red blood cell aggregation, probably plasma related (primarily the albumin/globulin ratio and fibrinogen). This would explain the frequency with which changes in viscosity are observed in Raynaud's syndromes related to general inflammatory disease and why these changes have not been found in nerve related vasomotor syndromes for example. It is obvious that an order to define whether the general hemorheological anomalies cause or aggravate certain acrosyndromes, extensive rheological studies must be carried out on a specific clinically defined series of patients.

3) DISCUSSION - CONCLUSION

A change in the rheological properties of blood during vascular diseases may be either a significant factor revealing inevitable signs of change in blood flow, or a simple indication, with no particular significance of a more general disturbance associated with the vascular disease. There is no doubt that in the first case, if it were possible to correct the disturbed hemorheological factors, this would represent a new pharmacological approach to this type of disease.

In this way, we should mention the benefits of difibrinogenation suggested by studies on peripheral arterial disease (Ehrly et al., 1976; Vinazzer, 1977). The drugs which act on the fibrinogen level (Arvin De-fibrase) produce a decrease in blood and plasma viscosity (7 to 15% at high shear rates and 20-30% at low shear rates). Platelet aggregates, which might contribute to microvascular occlusion, also appear to be reduced after defibrinogenation (Lowe et al., 1979ab). As concerns the effects on blood flow, increases in resting ankle systolic pressure, calf muscle blood flow and foot skin blood flow have been described.

We should also mention the work undertaken by Dodds et al. (1979) who showed that the weekly use of the plasma exchange technique on 8 patients with Raynaud's syndrome resulted in an approximately 20% decrease in blood viscosity with an increase in a blood deformability index.

Broadly speaking, it would undoubtedly be most worthwhile to study the various possibilities of substitute techniques i.e. hemodilution and plasma exchange, on patients with peripheral arteriopathy or Raynaud's syndrome. Both techniques produce a temporary decrease in blood viscosity. At this point it would be interesting to compare the hemorheological and hemodynamic changes with the clinical improvements observed.

Moreover, if the results confirmed, beyond doubt, that the changes were more microrheological, the use of specific action drugs on this parameter should also be considered.

However, the present state of research would seem to suggest that the blood hyperviscosity syndrome observed during vascular disease and Raynaud's syndrome is perhaps an indication of an increased tendency towards rouleaux formation. The biochemical changes observed seem to confirm this assumption. It is, however, conceivable that these anomalies may also lead to changes in the red blood cell membrane resulting in a decrease in its deformability.

REFERENCES

1. I. Anadere, H. Chmiel, H. Hess, G.B. Thurston, Clinical blood rheology. Biorheology 16:171-178 (1979).
2. L. Dintenfass, Hemorheological factors in Raynaud's phenomenon. Angiology 28:472-481 (1977).
3. L. Dintenfass, L.S. Ibels, Blood viscosity factors and occlusive arterial disease in renal transplant recipients. Nephron 15: 456-465 (1975).
4. A.J. Dodds, M.J.G. O'Reilly, C.J.P. Yates, L.T. Catton, P.T. Flute, J.A. Dormandy, Haemorheological response to plasma exchange in Raynaud's syndrome. Br. Med. J. 1186-1187 (1979).
5. J.A. Dormandy, E. Hoare, J. Colley, D.E. Arrowsmith, T.L. Dormandy, Clinical, haemodynamic, rheological and biochemical findings in 126 patients with intermittent claudication. Br. Med. J. 4:576-581 (1973).
6. J.A. Dormandy, J.M.C. Gutteridge, E. Hoare, T.L. Dormandy, Effect of clofibrate on blood viscosity in intermittent claudication. Br. Med. J. 4:259-262 (1974).
7. J. A. Dormandy, E. Hoare, J. Postlethwaite, Blood viscosity of patients with intermittent claudication - concept of "rheological claudication". Biorheology 13:161-164 (1976).
8. H. Ehringer, R. Dudczek, K. Lechner, A new approach in the treatment of peripheral arterial occlusions: Defibrination with Arvin. Angiology 25:279 (1974).
9. A.M. Ehrly, Influence of arvin on the flow properties of blood. Biorheology 10:453 (1973).
10. A.M. Ehrly, H.J. Köhler, Impaired erythrocyte deformability in patients with chronic occlusive arterial disease. In: Abstract book, Xe International Congress of Angiology - Tokio 1976.

11. S. Forconi, M. Guerrini, D. Agnusdei, F. Laghi Pasini, T. Di Perri, Abnormal blood viscosity in Raynaud's phenomenon. The Lancet 7985:586 (1976).
12. T. Jahnsen, S.L. Nielsen, F. Skovborg, Blood viscosity and local response to cold in primary Raynaud's phenomenon. The Lancet 1001-1002 (1977).
13. G.D.O. Lowe, J.J. Morrice, C.D. Forbes, C.R.M. Prentice, A.J. Fulton, J.C. Barbenel, Subcutaneous ancrod therapy in peripheral arterial disease: Improvement in blood viscosity and nutritional blood flow. Angiology 30:594 (1979a).
14. G.D.O. Lowe, M.M. Reavey, R.V. Johnston, C.I.D. Forbes and C.R.M. Prentice, Increased platelet aggregates in vascular and non-vascular illness: Correlation with plasma fibrinogen and effect of ancrod. Thromb. Res. 14:377 (1979b).
15. M.A. McGrath, R. Peek, R. Penny, Raynaud's disease: Reduced hand blood flows with normal blood viscosity. Aust. N.Z.J. Med. 8: n°2, 126-131 (1978).
16. Th. von Neuhann, Untersuchungen über Plättchenfunktion und Blutviskosität bei M. Raynaud und Sklerodermie. Fortschr. Med. 89:376-379 (1971).
17. R. Pringle, D.N. Walder, J.P.A. Weaver, Blood viscosity and Raynaud's disease. The Lancet 1:1086-1089 (1965).
18. H. Schmid-Schönbein, J. Weiss, E. Volger, H.J. Klose and H. Malotta, Microhaemorheology and defibrination. Zeitschrift fur Allegemeine Medizin 54:1635 (1978).
19. J.F. Stoltz, S. Gaillard, C. Schmidt, M. Verry, A. Larcan, F. Streiff, Viscosité sanguine et syndromes de Raynaud. Ann. Med. Nancy 19:209-212 (1980).
20. B. Stormer, R. Horsch, F. Kleinschmidt, D. Loose, H. Bruster, K. Kremer, Blood viscosity in patients with peripheral vascular disease in the area of low shear rates. J. Cardiovasc. Surg. 15:577-584 (1974).
21. G.W. Tiejen, S. Chien, E.C. Leroy, I. Gavras, H. Gavras, F.E. Gump, Blood viscosity, plasma proteins, and Raynaud syndrome. Arch. Surg. 110:1343-1346 (1975).
22. H. Vinazzer, Zur Wirkung von Arvin auf die Blutgerinung. Wiener Zeitschrift für Inner Medizin 52:378 (1971).

EVALUATION OF THE HAEMORHEOLOGICAL DETERMINANTS IN CORONARY HEART DISEASE

A. Sarno, A. Raineri*, P. Assennato*, and G. Caimi

Chair of Clinical Medicine and Medical Therapy III
* Chair of Cardiovascular Physiopathology
University of Palermo - Italy

Increased blood viscosity has been described in patients with coronary artery disease (1, 2, 3, 4, 5, 6, 7, 8).

The behaviour of blood viscosity determinants in different clinical situations and the relation of viscosity to ischaemia are, however, not well known.

We studied blood and plasma viscosity (Wells-Brookfield cone-on-plate microviscosimeter), haematocrit, plasma fibrinogen and Tk (9) in a population of patients with acute myocardial infarction (n=83), previous myocardial infarction (n=26), angina (n=25). The patients were subdivided according to the presence or absence of diabetes.

Haemorheological determinants were studied also in 69 normal controls matched for age and sex.

The difference in averages was evaluated with the variance analysis at one way.

Subsequently a group of patients with previous myocardial infarction and a group with angina underwent a submaximal exercise test.

Difference in mean values was analysed with Student's t-test for paired data.

ACUTE MYOCARDIAL INFARCTION

At the early stage, all the haemorheological determinants are altered in comparison with normal controls. The deceased patients have much higher averages than survivors in all parameters, including Tk (Tab. I).

In the patients subdivided according to diabetes, all the determinants, except Tk, have significant differences of averages in controls and in patients with acute myocardial infarction, diabetics and non diabetics (Fig. 1). Student's t-test, used to verify the role of diabetes on the single determinant, shows that only the haematocrit is dependent on it. Two weeks after myocardial infarction averages of all haemorheological determinants, except for blood and plasma viscosity, are different (Fig. 2). Here again diabetes is not responsible for the trend of blood rheology.

Table 1. A.M.I. early stage

	Controls (n = 69)	MI patients survived (n = 75)	MI patients deceased (n = 8)
Blood viscosity cP at 230 sec^{-1}	3.93 ± 0.53	4.66 ± 0.86	5.25 ± 0.94
Blood viscosity cP at 46 sec^{-1}	5.60 ± 1.16	6.31 ± 1.71	8.21 ± 3.36
Plasma viscosity cP at 230 sec^{-1}	1.47 ± 0.16	1.74 ± 0.42	1.67 ± 0.30
Haematocrit %	43.37 ± 3.97	44.73 ± 5.03	41.75 ± 6.45
Fibrinogen mg/100ml	279.69 ± 109.65	490.84 ± 184.81	590.60 ± 327.70
Tk	0.74 ± 0.09	0.73 ± 0.14	0.89 ± 0.23

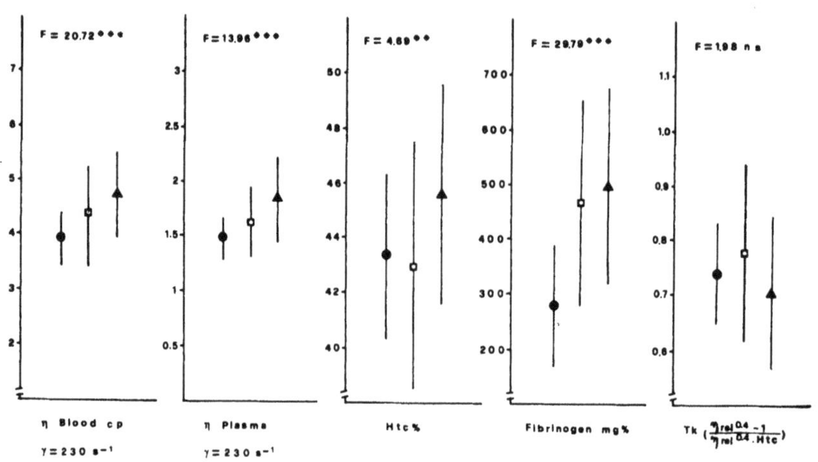

Fig. 1. A.M.I. early stage

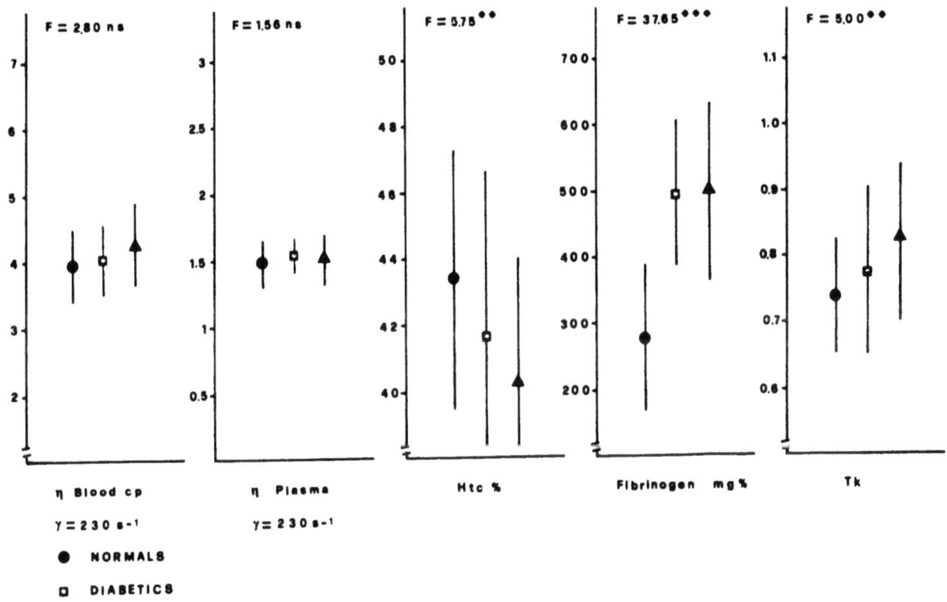

Fig. 2. A.M.I. after two weeks

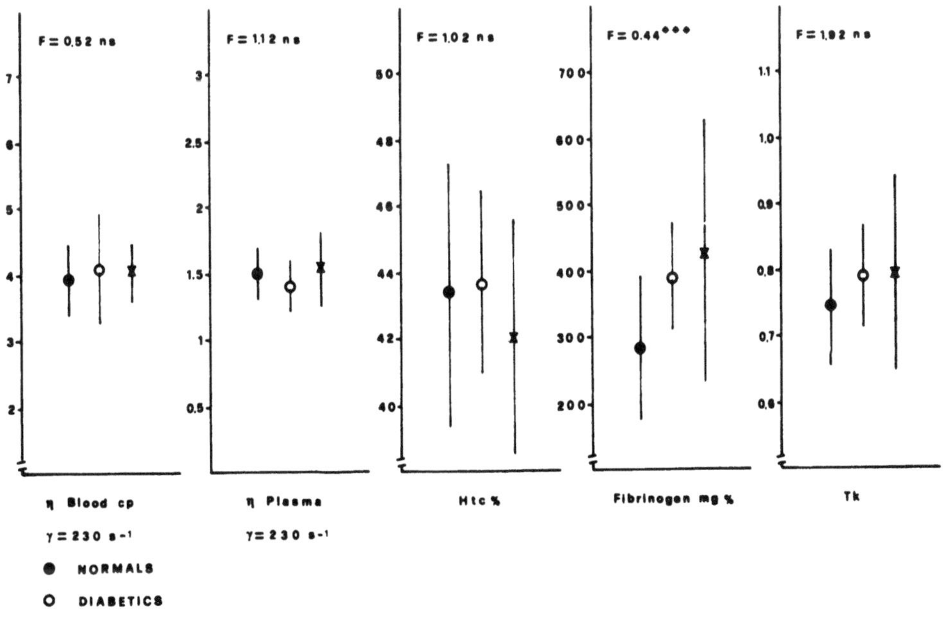

Fig. 3. Patients with previous myocardial infarction

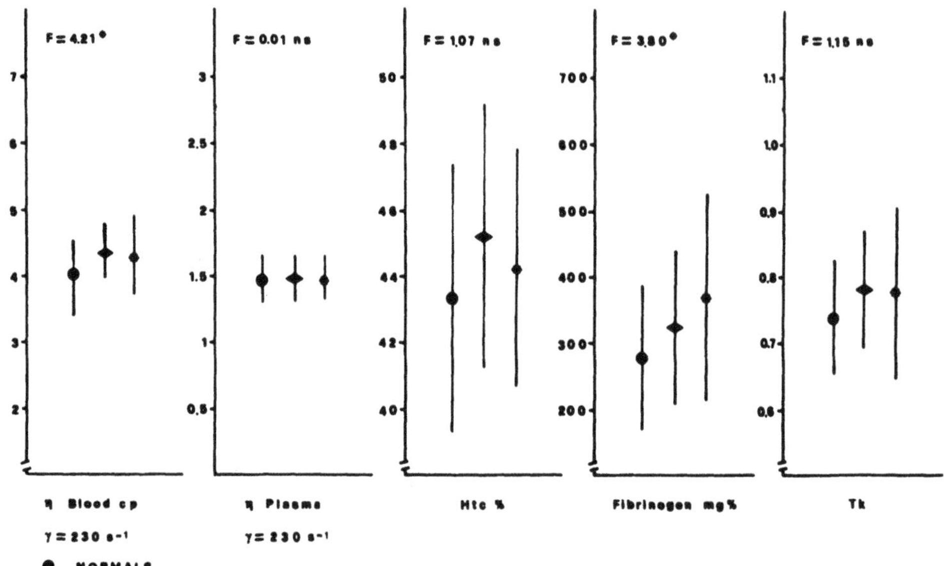

Fig. 4. Angina

CHRONIC CORONARY DISEASE

In the patients with previous myocardial infarction, diabetics and non diabetics, the only significant different averages are those of fibrinogen (Fig. 3). Diabetes does not affect the behaviour of any determinant .

An analogous trend can be observed in the group of angina patients (Fig. 4) even if the difference of the fibrinogen averages is less significant. Blood viscosity averages are also different in this group. Diabetes has no influence at all.

EXERCISE

Normal subjects at the end of an exercise exhibit a significant increase in plasma viscosity, haematocrit and fibrinogen. Previous infarct patients after exercise show, in addition, a highly significant increase in blood viscosity (Fig. 5). Thirty minutes after exercise neither group shows any significant modifications as compared to initial levels.

A similar behaviour, although the modifications are less significant, is found in the patients with angina (Fig. 6).

Exercise therefore induces distinctive haemorheological alterations in subjects with coronary heart disease and this enables us to differentiate them from normal subjects, who are otherwise indistinguishable from patients.

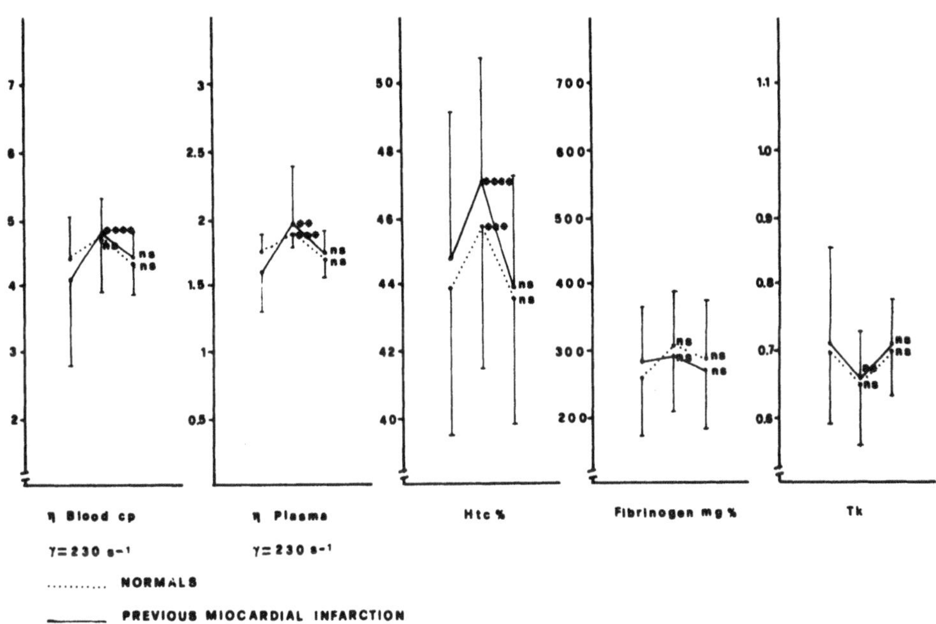

Fig. 5. Exercise test

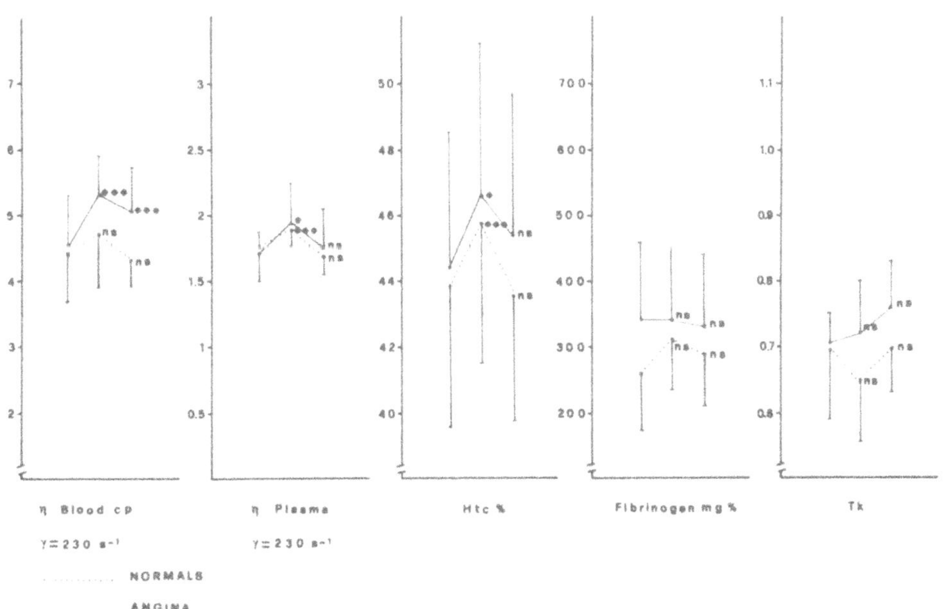

Fig. 6. Exercise test

CONCLUSION

In the initial stage of myocardial infarction there are impressive alterations of all haemorheological determinants, which seem to be correlated to the severeness of the clinical situation.

In the other stages of coronary disease it is generally impossible to detect any particular rheological behaviour suitable for chronic coronary patients from normal subjects.

An exercise test, however, enables us, confirming the observation of other authors (10), to differentiate between normal subjects and those with coronary disease.

REFERENCES

1. F. Kellog, J.R. Goodman, Viscosity of blood in myocardial infarction. Circ. Res. 8:972 (1960).
2. G.A. Mayer, Blood viscosity in healthy subjects and patients with coronary heart disease. Canad. Med. Ass. J. 91:951 (1964).
3. V. Kallio, M. Salimivalli, P. Brummer, Blood viscosity changes in patients hospitalized because of acute chest pain. Cardiologia 50:323 (1967).
4. J. Ditzel, H.O. Bang, N. Thorsen, Myocardial infarction and Whole-blood viscosity. Acta Med. Scand. 183:577 (1968).
5. J. Ditzel, J. Dyerberg, P. Grinsted, Increased whole-blood viscosity at low rates of shear and haematocrit levels in patients with previous myocardial infarction. 6th Europ. Conf. Microcirculation, Aalborg 1970, p. 56 (Karger, Basel 1971).
6. K.M. Jan, S. Chien, J.T. Bigger, Observations on blood viscosity changes after acute myocardial infarction. Circulation 51:1079 (1975).
7. A.N. Nicolaides, R. Bowers, T. Hourbourne, P.H. Kindner, E.M. Besterman, Blood viscosity, red-cells flexibility, haematocrit and plasma fibrinogen in patients with angina. Lancet 2:943 (1977).
8. J.A. Dormandy, A. Dodds, A. Boyd, D. Bennet, Haemorheological changes associated with myocardial infarction and their clinical significance. Symposium Europeen de Hemorheologie et Pathologie, Nancy, Octobre 1979.
9. L. Dintenfass, Theoretical aspects and clinical applications of the blood viscosity equation containing a term for the internal viscosity of the red cell. Blood Cells 3:367 (1977).
10. T. Di Perri, Rheological factors in circulatory disorders. Angiology 30:480 (1979).

SUBJECT INDEX

GPSR Compliance
The European Union's (EU) General Product Safety Regulation (GPSR) is a set of rules that requires consumer products to be safe and our obligations to ensure this.

If you have any concerns about our products, you can contact us on

ProductSafety@springernature.com

In case Publisher is established outside the EU, the EU authorized representative is:

Springer Nature Customer Service Center GmbH
Europaplatz 3
69115 Heidelberg, Germany

www.ingramcontent.com/pod-product-compliance
Ingram Content Group UK Ltd.
Pitfield, Milton Keynes, MK11 3LW, UK
UKHW051131260726
13967UKWH00010B/2978
* 9 7 8 1 4 6 8 4 8 6 1 7 9 *